THE
Evidence-Based Practice Manual
FOR Nurses

SECOND EDITION

Edited by

Jean V Craig MSc RSCN RGN
Research Associate, Evidence-Based Child Health Unit,
University of Liverpool Institute of Child Health, Alder Hey
Children's Hospital, Liverpool, UK

Rosalind L Smyth MA MBBS MD MRCP DCH FRCPCH
Brough Professor of Paediatric Medicine, University of
Liverpool Institute of Child Health, Alder Hey Children's
Hospital, Liverpool, UK

Forewords by
Christine Beasley
Chief Nursing Officer, Department of Health, London, UK

Sarah Mullally
Former Chief Nursing Officer, Department of Health, London, UK

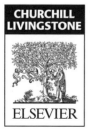

CHURCHILL
LIVINGSTONE

ELSEVIER

Edinburgh London New York Oxford Philadelphia St Louis Sydney Toronto 2007

CHURCHILL
LIVINGSTONE
ELSEVIER

© Elsevier Science Limited 2002
© 2007, Elsevier Limited. All rights reserved.

The right of Jean V Craig and Rosalind L Smyth to be identified as the editors of this work has been asserted by them in accordance with the Copyright, Designs and Patents Act 1988.

First edition 2002
Second edition 2007
  Reprinted 2007

ISBN-13 978 0 443 10230 1

British Library Cataloguing in Publication Data
A catalogue record for this book is available from the British Library

Library of Congress Cataloging in Publication Data
A catalog record for this book is available from the Library of Congress

Note

Knowledge and best practice in this field are constantly changing. As new research and experience broaden our knowledge, changes in practice, treatment and drug therapy may become necessary or appropriate. Readers are advised to check the most current information provided (i) on procedures featured or (ii) by the manufacturer of each product to be administered, to verify the recommended dose or formula, the method and duration of administration, and contraindications. It is the responsibility of the practitioner, relying on their own experience and knowledge of the patient, to make diagnoses, to determine dosages and the best treatment for each individual patient, and to take all appropriate safety precautions. To the fullest extent of the law, neither the Publisher nor the Editors or Authors assume any liability for any injury and/or damage to persons or property arising out of or related to any use of the material contained in this book.

The Publisher

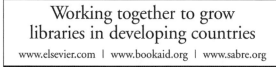

Working together to grow libraries in developing countries

www.elsevier.com | www.bookaid.org | www.sabre.org

ELSEVIER   BOOK AID International   Sabre Foundation

The Publisher's policy is to use paper manufactured from sustainable forests

Printed in China

Contents

SECTION 1 THE CONTEXT FOR EVIDENCE-BASED PRACTICE

SECTION 2 SKILLS FOR EVIDENCE-BASED PRACTICE

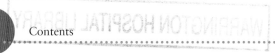

10. Implementing best evidence in
clinical practice 267
Lin Perry

11. How can we develop an
evidence-based culture? 305
Carl Thompson

Contributors

Jean V Craig MSc RSCN RGN (Chapters 1, 2 and 3) Research Associate, Evidence-Based Child Health Unit, University of Liverpool Institute of Child Health, Alder Hey Children's Hospital, Liverpool, UK

Rosalind L Smyth MA MBBS MD MRCP DCH FRCPCH (Chapter 7) Brough Professor of Paediatric Medicine, University of Liverpool Institute of Child Health, Alder Hey Children's Hospital, Liverpool, UK

Olwen Beaven BSc(Hons) MSc (Chapter 3) Information Specialist, BMJ Knowledge, BMJ Publishing Group, BMA House, London, UK

Faith Gibson PhD MSc RGN RSCN RNT Onc Cert Cert Ed (Chapters 4 and 5) Senior Lecturer in Children's Nursing Research, Centre for Nursing and Allied Health Professions Research, Institute of Child Health and Great Ormond Street Hospital for Children NHS Trust, London, UK

Anne-Marie Glenny BSc MMedSci PhD (Chapters 4 and 5) Lecturer in Evidence-Based Oral Healthcare, University of Manchester, Manchester, UK

Michelle Howarth MSc RGN PGCE (Chapter 8) Lecturer in Nursing, University of Salford, Manchester, UK

Ann Jacoby BA(Hons) PhD (Chapter 6) Professor of Medical Sociology, Division of Public Health, University of Liverpool, Liverpool, UK

Andrea Litva BA(Hons) MA PhD (Chapter 6) Lecturer in Medical Sociology, Department of Primary Care, University of Liverpool, Liverpool, UK

Joan Livesley BSc MA RN RSCN (Chapter 8) Senior Lecturer, Faculty of Health and Social Care, School of Nursing, University of Salford, Manchester, UK

Maggie Pearson MA PhD HonMFPHM (Chapter 1) Professor of Health and Social Care and Deputy Vice-Chancellor, Keele University, Keele, UK

Lin Perry MSc RN PhD (Chapter 10) Senior Research Fellow, St Bartholomew School of Nursing and Midwifery, London, UK

Lois Thomas PhD BA(Hons) RN (Chapter 9) Senior Research Fellow, Department of Nursing, University of Central Lancashire, Preston, UK

Carl Thompson PhD BSc(Hons) RN (Chapter 11) Senior Research Fellow, Department of Health Sciences, University of York, York, UK

Foreword to second edition

I am delighted to have the opportunity to introduce this, the second edition, of The Evidence-Based Practice Manual for Nurses. I know it will prove a valuable resource for individual nurses and nursing teams everywhere.

Like many commentators I have been amazed at how quickly evidence-based nursing has become accepted as a core professional value and foundation for everything we do in nursing. We owe much of this to the pioneers of nursing research who, over the years, have shifted nursing from a profession based on ritual and routine to one that today generates and uses a wide range of evidence across the spectrum of professional activity. With evidence firmly located at the core of educational curricula, nurses have changed the way they think and lead clinical practice locally and nationally.

Whilst this is an achievement, it is not the end. We live in a fast-moving world where advances in science and technology constantly reframe our understanding of what can be achieved for patients. Patient expectations have increased commensurately – and continue to do so as healthcare moves from a professional and provider led system to one that is patient-centric. As well as good clinical outcomes, patients rightly expect a good service, a positive experience of healthcare with greater choice about what happens to them.

The context for nursing practice is changing as well. Increasing emphasis on public health and prevention will mean that hospitals are reserved for the very ill with more routine care and long term conditions managed closer to home. At the same time there will be a continued drive throughout the system for quality, productivity and best use of resources.

The imperative for evidence-based nursing is therefore stronger than ever. It will ensure greater accountability to stakeholders and best value for investment. It will help nurses lead quality and caring, and will drive up standards at every level. Crucially it will place nurses and nursing at the forefront of enterprise and innovation in healthcare.

If they are to do this, individual nurses and nursing teams must continuously develop and extend their knowledge and skills in evidence-based nursing. This book helps by offering a wide ranging and comprehensive approach to evidence-based nursing, set within the context of contemporary policy, regulation and professional standards before focusing down on the knowledge and skills required to generate evidence, examine issues, and make decisions regarding current and future practice. It provides a patient focused approach to using best evidence incorporating multiple methods and strategies, and helps to develop the critical skills required for working collaboratively with patients and other professionals on issues of care.

I would like to end this piece by reminding readers of a point made by Florence Nightingale well over a century ago. An early pioneer of evidence-based nursing herself, she said that if nursing is not moving forwards, it is moving backwards. A point that is surely as true today as it was then.

Chris Beasley
Chief Nursing Officer
For England

Foreword to first edition

Nurses are committed to delivering high-quality care that meets the needs of their patients, but it is in identifying and indeed recognising what constitutes high quality that the challenge lies.

Nurses are rising to this challenge. They are increasingly listening to, and working with, their patients to identify what it is they want from the health service. They accept that it is not sufficient to purely base practice on tradition. Practice must be continuously reviewed, continuously questioned and, where appropriate, decisions made based upon available evidence.

This evidence is not purely focused upon clinical interventions and therapies but, as nursing research continues to flourish, relates to all aspects of health, health care and the patient experience. Therefore, many types of evidence from many sources will need to be considered. This will require nurses to develop or utilise an array of skills, to not only review the evidence but also to then apply it to their practice. This is where this manual provides that practical support.

Through the use of real-life examples it will help individual nurses in their efforts to achieve an evidence-based approach to clinical practice, supporting them in asking the right questions, developing the skills they need to explore and evaluate evidence, all to the eventual benefit of the patients. Developed by leading researchers and clinicians, the manual provides a very valuable tool for your personal professional development. I commend it to you.

Sarah Mullally
Former Chief Nursing Officer

Preface

'Evidence-based' is one of the most used adjectives in health care today. It was previously applied almost exclusively in the term 'evidence-based medicine' but happily, terms such as 'evidence-based practice' are becoming more widespread and emphasise that this is a concept that should apply to all of health care. Nurses, the largest group of professionals who provide health care, have been at the forefront in recognising the need to identify, evaluate and apply best evidence to their clinical practice. Since this manual was first published, awareness of evidence-based practice has become widespread throughout clinical practice, but professional groups can find it difficult to keep pace with the requisite knowledge and skills. This manual presents these techniques in a straightforward and relevant style which will enable nurses to understand and apply evidence-based practice in their own individual settings.

As with the first edition, the manual is divided into three sections. Section 1 provides the background and context for evidence-based practice in nursing and gives details of some of the challenges (and solutions) which nurses meet in ensuring that patient care is informed by scientific evidence.

Section 2 focuses on the practical skills required for identifying best evidence to support health-care decisions. It provides detailed, step-by-step guidance in formulating focused clinical questions, conducting successful searches of electronic databases, critically appraising research studies that use qualitative or quantitative methods, and integrating research findings into clinical decisions. There is also a chapter on systematic reviews and meta-analyses, which highlights the importance of this form of research in informing best patient care.

Section 3 focuses on how to make evidence-based practice a reality. Firstly, clinical guidelines, as a method for implementing best evidence, are considered together with tools for assessing their rigour. The practical strategies that clinical teams and organisations need to consider if they are to promote and sustain an evaluative, evidence-based approach to their work are discussed.

For this new edition, all chapters have been revised. A new chapter entitled 'Integrating research evidence into clinical decisions' has been added (Chapter 8). It focuses on understanding the impact that clinical expertise and patient preferences have on the interpretation or implementation of research evidence. One of the strengths of this manual has been the number of worked examples and case studies. To keep this volume relevant and contemporary, many have been replaced with new examples, which illustrate how recent evidence has changed practice.

Finally, we wish our readers well as they develop and use their skills to ensure that their clinical decisions are informed by the best available research evidence. Nurses, as a profession, are uniquely placed to understand patients' needs, priorities and beliefs and to integrate these considerations with their own expertise and with clinical evidence in making decisions. The result of these endeavours is that better clinical decisions will be made and patient care will improve.

Jean V Craig
Rosalind L Smyth

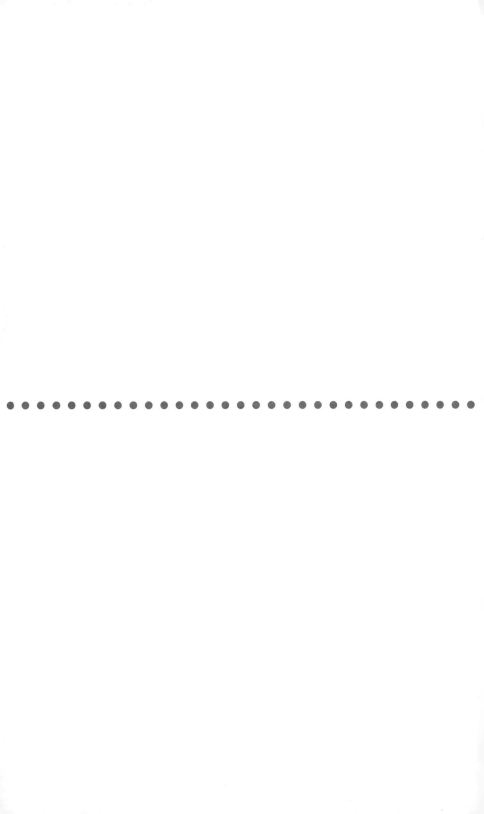

SECTION 1

The context for evidence-based practice

CHAPTER 1

Evidence-based practice in nursing

Jean V Craig and Maggie Pearson

KEY POINTS

- An evidence-based approach to clinical practice aims to deliver appropriate care in an efficient manner to individual patients.

- The process entails the integration of research evidence, clinical expertise and the interpretation of patients' needs and perspectives in making decisions.

- Nursing care involves a wide range of interventions and therefore draws on a diverse evidence base, including, for example, evidence from psychology, sociology and public health.

- Individual nurses need to develop key skills in order to access and use evidence appropriately in clinical practice.

- Sources of synthesised evidence are evolving and are being made accessible to nurses.

- In terms of developing nurse researchers, issues such as organisational culture, management support, and career paths that accommodate both clinical and research work need to be addressed.

Introduction

At the heart of government's drive to modernise health care is a commitment to the development of quality health services based on evidence (Australian Government Department of Health and Ageing 2006, Department of Health 1997 and 2006, National Institutes of Health 2005). In the UK, the strategy for nursing, *Making a Difference*, reflects this commitment and emphasises the need for a robust evidence base for nursing, midwifery and health visiting (Department of Health 1999). The vision for nursing in the 21st century is for all nurses to seek out evidence and apply it in their everyday practice, with an increasing proportion actively participating in research and development, and some developing into research leaders (Department of Health 2000, 2006).

Evidence-based health care: what is it and why do we need it?

Within the campaign to improve the quality of health care, there is a great deal of talk about 'evidence-based practice'. This phrase trips lightly off the tongue and can engender a reassuring warm glow that all is well: we know what needs to be done and all that is required is for practitioners to implement the evidence. If only it were that simple!

Evidence-based practice has been described as 'doing the right things right' (Muir Gray 1997, p.18). This means not only doing things more efficiently and to the best standard possible, but also ensuring that that which *is* done, is done 'right' – so that more good than harm results.

Intuitively, few practitioners would disagree with this approach, but there are several hurdles on the way to this goal: we need the evidence base to know what it is 'right' to do; we have to be clear to whom the evidence really applies; and we also have to be clear at what stage in a person's trajectory of health or illness the evidence-based intervention is indicated. All this, at a time when the pressures are increasing to deliver challenging service targets, to reduce waiting at all stages of the patient experience and to give patients more personal choice as to how, when and where they are treated (Department of Health 2004). The key point here is that, if we can get it right, evidence-based practice *will* help to improve people's experiences of illness and health care, and good established nursing practice already does.

It is important to remember that the concept of evidence-based practice is not a new one. We would be doing our predecessors a great disservice to pretend otherwise. Let us take two basic examples: infection control and prevention of deep vein thrombosis are long-established aspects of nursing care, undertaken daily in hospitals and in people's homes, which can prevent complications arising from immobility or vulnerability to infection. These long-established practices avoid 'unnecessary' distress, treatments, days immobilised at home or in hospital. Indeed, it is salutary to reflect that the number of hospital inpatient days attributed to hospital-acquired infection (HAI) is rising dramatically and is reported to be between 4% and 10% in the United States, Australasia and most European countries (Department of Health 2003a). The associated economic burden is high. In the UK alone it is estimated to amount to at least £1 billion a year (Plowman et al 1999, 2001). Reasons for the increase in HAI are multiple: patient factors (such as increased numbers of people with weakened immunity); therapeutic factors (increased availability of devices that breach normal defence mechanisms, inappropriate use of antibiotics); organisational factors (such as increased movement of patients) and behavioural factors (inadequate hygiene practices by staff) are all implicated (Department of Health 2003a). This increase in HAI is especially worrying in view of the risk of antibiotic-resistant infections such as methicillin-resistant *Staphylococcus aureus*.

There is a particularly cruel irony in the rise of hospital-acquired infections in an era in which evidence-based practice is generally accepted as a key component of modern health care: evidence-based approaches to preventing cross-infection were already clearly evident in the 19th century. For example, in the 1840s, Semmelweis's insistence that doctors performing autopsies should wash their hands before going on to deliver babies was associated with a dramatic reduction in mortality due to sepsis, from over a fifth to 3% (Rotter 1997). Similarly, it was careful observation that led John Snow (Figure 1.1) in the 1840s to pinpoint a water tap in Broad Street as the cause of the outbreak of cholera in London. These two examples from the 19th century encapsulate the variety of domains of professional health practice which can and should be evidence based but they also demonstrate powerfully how reflective questioning and acutely observant practitioners can uncover evidence within their own everyday practice which, when acted upon, can improve health, although not all examples will be quite so dramatic!

John Snow's observation in respect of cholera serves to remind us that evidence-based practice is as relevant and important in public health interventions and community developments as it is in the care of individual

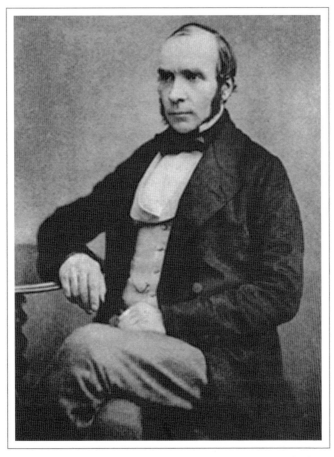

Figure 1.1 John Snow, English anaesthetist and epidemiologist. Photograph of oil painting by Thomas Jones Barker (1847). From the Wellcome Library, London, with permission. Videodisc no. 51428

patients in, say, intensive care units. Indeed, the UK Economic and Social Research Council has invested in a network of research centres that pull together the evidence base for public policy and its implementation.

It is clear that no aspects of nursing practice for health, whether in the community, home or hospital, should be 'safe' from the concept of evidence-based practice. In some areas, acceptance of the concept is not the problem, but the reality is! In those (largely hospital clinical) areas where there has been a great deal of research, it is almost impossible to keep on top of the burgeoning body of knowledge that emerges daily, and the challenge is to manage that knowledge so that busy practitioners can find it accessible and be alert to its quality. Amidst the mass of publications, it is important to be able to discern how robust the evidence is: how the study was designed, and the extent to which the results can be generalised to a wider population. It is important to remember that different kinds of 'evidence' and knowledge are generated by different kinds of research methodologies: all have their place, but we need to be mindful of the strengths and weaknesses of each.

Furthermore, where we do have robust evidence, we need to be clear and careful about to whom it applies. It is crucial that evidence from clinical trials undertaken with a specific population subsample is not inappropriately extrapolated to other population subgroups. For example, the majority of clinical trials are undertaken in samples of people under the age of 65. Clinical trials in the very elderly (people over 80 years of age) are extremely scarce (Le Quintrec et al 2005). Care should therefore be taken in extrapolating that evidence, which will of necessity have been generated in people with few co-morbidities that could 'confuse' the results, to older people who could have several co-existing conditions. Randomised controlled trials have shown, for example, that thrombolytic therapy significantly reduces the risk of death in patients with acute myocardial infarction (MI) (Fibrinolytic Therapy Trialists 1994), but only 10% of the sample populations in the trials were >74 years of age, and when the results for these participants were examined, the efficacy of the therapy was found to be ambiguous. The potential risks of applying extrapolated evidence from studies conducted in adults to children has prompted the establishment of the Medicines for Children Research Network (mcrn.org.uk) which facilitates the conduct of studies of medicines for children.

In other spheres of health-related interventions and health care, however, we simply do not have enough robust evidence to really know what it is 'right' to do. The priority is to generate the evidence required, but that takes time if it is to be done properly. So what should be done in the meantime? Where there is no robust evidence base, the ethos of evidence-based practice should, at the very least, stop us in our tracks to reflect on the impact of what we are doing in the name of health, and why. Reflective practice is a key component of evidence-based health care; the very ethos of good professional practice is to reflect on the taken-for-granted assumptions that underpin everyday practice, and to routinely assess the impact and outcomes of interactions and interventions with patients, clients and the public. And we need to do all this without becoming 'frozen' and disempowered by the lack of robust evidence for much of what we do.

The evidence-based movement across health care

In the early years of the evidence-based 'movement', the discourse was limited to 'medicine', rather than health care (Sackett et al 1997), but the principles of evidence-based medicine have subsequently been applied to other spheres of professional practice in health and social care such as pharmacy (Tully & Cantrill 1999), the therapies (Bury & Mead 1998), orthodontics (Harrison 2000) and nursing (DiCenso et al 1998). Whereas the Cochrane Collaboration reviews and syntheses evidence on the impact of healthcare interventions, the Campbell Collaboration reviews and syntheses evidence of the impact of educational and social interventions.

Development of the evidence-based concept

The first textbook on evidence-based medicine (EBM) defined it as: 'the conscientious, explicit and judicious use of current best evidence in making decisions about the health care of patients' (Sackett et al 1997, p.2). The authors elaborated that the practice of EBM entailed the integration of individual clinical expertise with the best available external clinical evidence from systematic research, and involved taking account of the patient's perspective in making clinical decisions.

Contrary to the assertions of its critics, therefore, that EBM was narrowly concerned with the conduct of randomised controlled trials and the implementation of their results in routine practice (Grahame Smith 1998), the 'product champions' of EBM never argued that it was 'simply' a matter of slavishly following rigid guidelines based solely on the findings of clinical trials: the need to tailor care on the basis of research evidence and clinical experience to the needs of patients was always acknowledged.

In 2000, Sackett and colleagues included the value of clinical expertise and patient perspectives more explicitly in their definition of EBM as 'the integration of best research evidence with clinical expertise and patient values' (Sackett et al 2000, p.1).

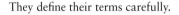

They define their terms carefully.

• Best research evidence is defined as:

> *clinically relevant research, often from the basic sciences of medicine (sic), but especially from patient-centred clinical research . . . (Sackett et al 2000, p.1)*

They go on to assert that:

> *New evidence from clinical research both invalidates previously accepted diagnostic tests and treatments and replaces them with new ones that are more powerful, more accurate, more efficacious and safer. (Sackett et al 2000, p.1)*

Note that the discourse is about 'diagnostic tests' and 'treatments', whereas the broader concept of 'care' which embodies nursing practice in all settings involves much more: communication, comfort, observation, for example. This means that, in applying these principles to the variety of nursing practice, we need to draw on a range of evidence bases in psychology, sociology and possibly, for improving comfort, ergonomics!

• Clinical expertise is defined as:

> *the ability to use our clinical skills and past experience to rapidly identify each patient's unique health state and diagnosis, their individual risks and benefits of potential interventions, and their personal values and expectations. (Sackett et al 2000, p.1)*

Personal professional experience, clinical judgement and even intuition have a role to play.

• By 'patient values', the authors mean:

> *the unique preferences, concerns and expectations each patient brings to a clinical encounter and which must be integrated into clinical decisions if they are to serve the patient. (Sackett et al 2000, p.1)*

In reality, then, EBM is manifest not 'simply' by the implementation of 'patient-centred clinical research', but by the integration of systematically derived research-based knowledge with the practitioner's tacit knowledge drawn from experience and their interpretation of the needs and perspectives of each person with whom they interact in individual clinical encounters. What is implied is that truly evidence-based practice must involve the patient in the clinical decisions.

The principles enunciated by Sackett and colleagues are clearly of direct relevance to all professional practice, but for any practitioner this is a daunting agenda. It means having access to an up-to-date synthesis of research findings in a form that can be assimilated, having confidence in one's own professional judgement and having the communication skills, insight and empathy to 'read' and respond to the patient's circumstances and needs. Narrowing the concept down to 'investigations and treatments' perhaps makes the concept and requisite evidence base more manageable, but the majority of nursing practice cannot retreat into such a focused definition. Nursing care involves a wider range of interventions and needs to draw on a wide range of research-based evidence. For example, whilst there is an emerging body of research-based evidence about how best to manage and prevent leg ulcers (Cullum et al 2001, 2004), nurses do not 'simply' treat leg ulcers: they care for the person with the leg ulcer.

Challenges

The challenge, then, for nursing practice (as for all professional practice) is to develop and draw on the well-focused evidence base relating to specific clinical treatments to improve the quality of clinical procedures, whilst also drawing on a more diverse evidence base for the wider concept of care which nurses provide (Pursey et al 1997). This challenge is not straightforward: if it is to become a reality rather than a vain but noble hope, there are several imperatives to be addressed. These will take both time and resources.

First, the relevant research-based evidence bases are not comprehensive: there are yawning gaps in the robust evidence for much of what nurses do in the course of their daily work. Rigorous research to address these gaps takes time, and established research expertise in nursing, although increasing, is in relatively short supply (Department of Health 1998b, Pearson 2000). It is important that the recognition of the need for evidence-based practice does not result in a misguided and undiscerning dash to seek out *any* 'knowledge' available, irrespective of the quality of research on which it is based. Critical appraisal skills will be crucial to enable practitioners thirsty for knowledge to discriminate between high- and poor-quality evidence.

Second, the relevant evidence bases are not static: there has been an explosion in the volume of research publications over the last few decades and it is impossible for any busy practitioner to keep abreast of the literature. More than 74,000 health service research publications were produced in the UK alone in 1997 with an average annual growth rate of almost 4% (Wellcome Trust 2001). In a single year (2005), more than 660,000 new articles were included in the Pubmed database. Over 12,000 of these are randomised controlled trials. We urgently need effective means of synthesising the emerging evidence and making this updated knowledge base accessible. In England, the National Library for Health is intended to fulfil that function.

Third, life-long learning is generally accepted as an important principle in the 21st century, not just for busy professionals who need to keep abreast of the knowledge in their field and adapt to role changes (Department of Health 2001), but for citizens generally, whose roles and opportunities in work and socially are constantly changing as the technological and social revolutions leave no holds barred. For professions such as those involved in health care, steeped in tradition and an ethos of established expertise, the notion that established procedures may not be based on robust evidence, or that new knowledge may challenge some established shibboleths is not comfortable. Furthermore, if busy practitioners are to have the time to access the evidence base and update their knowledge, there are clear human and financial resource implications: all at a time when recruitment and retention of staff are acknowledged to be key constraints which the service faces in meeting public expectations and increasingly challenging targets set by government.

Finally, the fact that a piece of research has been conducted does not automatically mean that the findings should be transferred directly into the clinical setting. Individual research studies need to be examined in the context of other evidence before a practice change is initiated. Consider, for example, the management of gastro-oesophageal reflux, a condition in which recurrent vomiting, failure to thrive, feeding difficulties and abdominal pain may be present. Infants who are placed in the prone or left lateral position have been shown to experience significantly improved outcomes (measured using the 'reflux index') compared with infants nursed on their backs (Kumar & Sarvanathan 2004). Although a welcome finding for parents, nurses and infants, there is a wider body of research providing evidence that prone or left lateral positioning in infants is a risk factor for sudden infant death syndrome (Kumar & Sarvanathan 2004). Such evidence needs to be taken into consideration if parents are to be offered sensible, safe advice. Similarly, the results and conclusions of one study need to be considered in the light of other similar studies, as they may differ markedly, depending on the nature of the study design and sample. An oft-quoted example is that of corticosteroids given to women expected to deliver prematurely. A number of individual trials did not identify clear-cut benefits to the treatment; however, when data from all trials were combined in a meta-analysis (see Chapter 7), it became clear that corticosteroids are effective in reducing the risk of death in babies born prematurely (Mulrow 1995).

A wide range of evidence bases relevant to nursing practice

We have mentioned several times that because of the range of settings and people with whom nurses work, the concept of evidence-based practice is particularly challenging for nurses. Nursing care needs to draw on a wide range of evidence bases, within and beyond the 'medical' sciences, including behavioural and social sciences. In assessing these different kinds of evidence, it is important that nurses can appraise the quality of the research critically, and are able to respect and assess different methodologies.

Public health interventions

Nurses working in public health need to be aware of the evidence about effective interventions in other spheres which can have a beneficial impact on health. Perhaps the best such example is the introduction of legislation to make the wearing of seatbelts compulsory, based on epidemiological evidence of reductions in mortality. There is emerging evidence of the reduction in mortality from road traffic accidents as a result of traffic-calming schemes (Bunn et al 2003), and the evidence that the use of smoke detectors (DiGuiseppi et al 1998, Marshall et al 1998) and thermostat controls for tap water (NHS CRD 1996) can reduce the risk of home injuries is already well established. There is good evidence that patient reminder and recall systems are effective in improving immunisation uptake (Jacobson & Szilagyi 2005). Nurses working in public health roles, including health visiting, may be in a key position to advocate such schemes.

Health-related behaviours

The example of smoking illustrates why nurses need to be able to draw on evidence from a range of knowledge domains to inform their work. In the UK, smoking is the single greatest cause of preventable illness and death, with

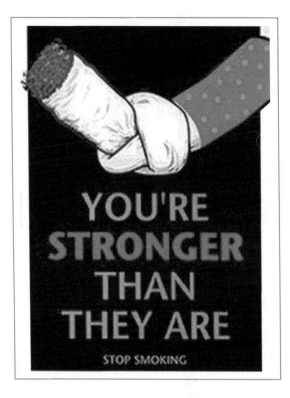

Figure 1.2 Health authorities, health promotion specialists, education authorities and the news media use posters produced by organisations such as GASP Smoke Free Solutions to discourage smoking. Reproduced with permission from GASP, www.gasp.org.uk/gasp.htm

more than 120,000 people per year dying from smoking. There is compelling evidence of the health risks associated with direct and passive smoking (Department of Health 1998a). Smoking cessation strategies are therefore a key aspect of current health policy, with investment in smoking cessation clinics in primary care totalling £60 million over 3 years (Figure 1.2). Smoking hits poorer people harder, widening inequalities in health among social groups. To be effective in reducing smoking rates, nurses working with local communities need to understand the role that smoking plays in some people's lives, and why it is that some people smoke although fully cognisant of the health risks to them and their families. Detailed qualitative work with lone mothers living in poverty illuminated the 'protective' role which smoking played in enabling mothers to cope in very difficult circumstances (Graham 1987, 1988): they balanced smoking's long-term risks against its short-term benefits in enabling them to alleviate the day-to-day stress and flashpoints of caring for young children on very low incomes. The crucial point from this is that any evidence-based anti-smoking strategies must consider alternative supports which would need to be in place to enable such mothers to cope without smoking: to do so would be to truly encapsulate the 'patients' perspectives' as espoused by Sackett et al (2000) as a key dimension of EBM.

Nursing care interventions

In making decisions about interventions (such as drug and other therapies, observations, investigations, etc.), nurses will draw on evidence from multiple sources. Concordance with drug therapy can be influenced by factors ranging from unpleasant side effects of the drug to issues such as perceived recovery from illness, a denial of the illness or its significance (Beers & Berkow 1999), or presence of depression or cognitive impairment (Osterberg & Blaschke 2005). The approach to the problem of poor concordance with treatment therefore requires knowledge from the psychosocial domain, as well as pharmacological knowledge. Where nurses are required to make decisions about costly interventions such as the use of air fluidised beds (see Chapter 2) or establishing a new post, they will no doubt be obliged to present evidence on the financial costs (cost effectiveness) as well as the increased clinical effectiveness compared with other methods to the management team, as well as details of the clinical efficacy of the intervention.

Communication

We have already argued that nursing care is more than a set of investigations and treatment interventions. As for other professionals, effective communication with communities, clients and patients is a key aspect of high-quality nursing care. Again, this means drawing on a range of bodies of knowledge traditionally conceived of as being outside 'nursing', including communication studies and psychology. Indeed, well-intentioned efforts to implement evidence-based practice may be thwarted and subverted if effective communication is not a feature of the clinical encounter. Psychological research has shown that on receiving bad news, recipients can only retain a limited amount of information from the first conversation. It is crucial that nurses understand this, so that they do not overload people when they have bad news to give, they keep their first message simple and focused on the key points they need to impart, and they understand the need for ongoing support and repeated conversations to enable information to be given at a pace with which recipients can cope.

Management evidence

As nursing roles develop, in the context of a greater emphasis on interprofessional teams in all settings, many will find themselves managing teams, which in some cases may include professions who have traditionally thought of themselves as of higher status than nurses. Again, there is a wide evidence base within management sciences on which nurses can draw to make themselves more effective in those roles. Because of the complexity of organisations and of management (including change management), the research methods employed in management sciences are often more qualitative than those employed in the study of highly focused clinical interventions. The research task is often to understand the organisation and how change is perceived, as much as to study the effectiveness of a complex process of change. Compared with the wealth of research evidence on clinical interventions, organisational change and management issues are under-researched (Iles & Sutherland 2001). In the UK, a national NHS R&D programme on Service Delivery and Organisation (SDO) has been set up to fill the yawning gap in organisational and management research in the health sector. Within this programme, a stream of funding has been made available to support SDO research into nursing, mid-wifery and health-visiting services (www.sdo.lshtm.ac.uk/nursingandmid-wifery.htm).

The problem of generalisability

One of the concerns often cited by critics of EBM (as they understand it) relates to the perceived generalisability of published research studies. There are clear dangers with this critique. When proponents argue that unless the evidence was gathered 'here' it is not relevant, this may be a smokescreen to avoid changing practice. However, it is important that the research undertaken has credibility with its potential users: study population samples need to reflect the composition of target populations for the intervention, and the settings and context in which the research is undertaken need to be as 'real life' as possible. In short, it is vital that evidence-based practice is able to draw on practice-based evidence (Hogue 2001, personal communication). For a long time, concerns have been expressed that the distance between academic nursing and the clinical arena has resulted in research that does not relate to the 'reality' of everyday nursing practice (Pearson 2000). Indeed, the key question of how best to generate the evidence base for nursing and ensure its implementation has been around for a long time (Department of Health 1993, 1994, 1995, 1996, 1998b). We all know the perils of developing a research base which is divorced from everyday professional practice. Doctors have wisely avoided that separation, although the combination of academic and professional practice is not without its challenges (Richards 1997).

A study of nursing research outputs between 1988 and 1995 found that although the topics addressed were wide ranging, research concerned with issues relating to the nursing profession (e.g. theory, models, education, research methods, etc.) grew far more rapidly and appeared to be more highly valued than research relating to the care of patients (Traynor et al 2001). The authors postulate that the lower costs and time commitments associated with the former type of research studies, together with the desire to 'self-define' the profession of nursing, may in part account for this difference. This trend in research, of prioritising professional issues over patient care issues, has important ramifications for nurses trying to make informed decisions about aspects of clinical care, particularly with the current and long overdue emphasis given to the patient experience.

When will we get there?

We have demonstrated that the concept of evidence-based practice is not new, but it is reassuring that the commitment to the concept is so firmly stated in recent policies. It is less than 40 years since the first academic departments of nursing were established in the UK, and there has been a phenomenal achievement in terms of nursing's integration (and retention) into higher education. But to what extent have we ensured that vibrant R&D activity around nursing issues and perspectives (whether or not it is undertaken by nurses) is really embedded in nursing practice, and the results implemented?

A number of strategies have been implemented and some are starting to pay dividends. For example, nursing (or practice) development units (NDU) were set up as 'hot-houses for innovation and change in nursing practice' (Redfern et al 1997). The staff of these units are ideally placed to take a leading role in establishing evidence-based practice for nursing; in addition, several of the units have been awarded research grants. Urinary catheterisation is just one topic that has been explored in the light of Sackett and colleagues' (1997) definition of evidence-based practice and the organisational infrastructure required for achieving desired outcomes (Adams & Cooke 1998).

The benchmarking process outlined in *The Essence of Care* (Department of Health 2003b) is another development that has the potential to increase an evidence-based approach to nursing care. Different types of evidence have been used to establish benchmark standards which can be used as a starting point for comparing practice, identifying optimum practice and seeking methods to remedy poor practice. To illustrate, following the launch of the paediatric continence services benchmark in 2001, a participating organisation identified a number of shortfalls in their service: inconsistencies in provision of care across the district; poorly defined patient pathways and discrepancies in information giving. Subsequent collaboration with a neighbouring health-care provider with an excellent paediatric continence service is now under way and aims to improve referral routes, integrate the service across all sectors and develop training programmes that facilitate an evidence-based approach to care (NHS Modernisation Agency 2004).

So what else do we need to do to achieve the shift required to make the vision of evidence-based nursing a reality? Some would argue that it is all a matter of money, of ring-fenced budgets for nursing research and research capacity development, to create a safe haven for nurses to develop their skills and evidence base without the risk of medical domination. Certainly profession-specific funding schemes have made a difference and are a necessary component, but they are insufficient to fulfil what is required.

In terms of developing a cadre of nurse researchers, there are key issues concerning the availability of career paths that enable a combination of research and everyday practice, organisational culture and management support for the research ethos in clinical areas, and colleagues' disdain for or downright jealousy about the research role as they witness it. For example, the potential profile of nurses' involvement in R&D is not enhanced by the experience of some research nurses, employed on short-term contracts, collecting data for medical colleagues in clinical trials, but without any tangible development of personal research potential or acknowledgement in publications (Department of Health 1998b).

The health-care research strategy within the UK is undergoing a fundamental revision in recognition of the role that research can play in improving the health and well-being of the population. The overall aims are for the system to be more responsive to the research needs of patients, the public, health-care professionals and policy makers; for world-class support to be available to researchers; and for health-care organisations to develop the infrastructure required for high-quality research (Department of Health 2006). Research in all health-care areas, including prevention of ill health, promotion of health, disease management, patient care, delivery of health-care and its organisation, public health and social care, is included in the strategy.

The welcome commitment to leadership and R&D within the nursing, midwifery and health-visiting professions surely presents us with a golden opportunity. We now need to get on with it, and work to ensure that the next generation of nurses, and those from previous generations who stay (or return), take it for granted that they should seek out and appraise research findings and apply them. This is not always easy, but we owe it to the public to apply our imagination and enthusiasm to make sure that the care they receive is based on the best available evidence.

References

Adams F, Cooke M 1998 Implementing evidence-based practice for urinary catheterisation. British Journal of Nursing 7(22):1393–1399

Australian Government Department of Health and Ageing 2006 Australian Better Health Initiative. Available online at: www.health.gov.au/internet/wcms/publishing.nsf February 2006

Beers M H, Berkow R (eds) 1999 Factors affecting drug response. In: Merck manual of diagnosis and therapy, 17th edn. Merck Research Laboratories, New Jersey

Bunn F, Collier T, Frost C et al 2003 Area-wide traffic calming for preventing traffic related injuries. Cochrane Database of Systematic Reviews 2003, Issue 1. Art. No.: CD003110. DOI: 10.1002/14651858. CD003110

Bury T J, Mead J M (eds) 1998 Evidence-based healthcare: a practical guide for therapists. Butterworth-Heinemann, Oxford

Cullum N, Nelson E, Fletcher A, Sheldon T 2001 Compression for venous leg ulcers (Cochrane Review). Cochrane Library, Disk Issue 2, 2001. Update Software, Oxford

Cullum N, McInnes E, Bell-Syer S E M, Legood R 2004 Support surfaces for pressure ulcer prevention. Cochrane Database of Systematic Reviews 2004, Issue 3. Art. No.: CD001735. DOI: 10.1002/14651858.CD001735.pub2

Department of Health 1993 Report of the Task Force on the Strategy for Research in Nursing, Midwifery and Health Visiting. Department of Health, London

Department of Health 1994 Supporting research and development in the NHS: report of the R&D Task Force (Culyer Report). Department of Health, London

Department of Health 1995 A research workforce strategy. Paper to Central Research and Development Committee, July 1995 (CRDCP95–22). Department of Health, London

Department of Health 1996 Research capacity strategy for the Department of Health and the NHS. A first statement. Department of Health, London

Department of Health 1997 The new NHS: modern, dependable. Department of Health, London

Department of Health 1998a Smoking kills. Department of Health, London

Department of Health 1998b Developing human resources for health related R&D: next steps. Report of the R&D Workforce Capacity Development Group (Pearson Report). Department of Health, London

Department of Health 1999 Making a difference: strengthening the nursing, midwifery and health visiting contribution to health and health care. Department of Health, London

Department of Health 2000 Towards a strategy for nursing research and development: proposals for action. Department of Health, London

Department of Health 2001 Working together – learning together: a framework for lifelong learning for the NHS. Department of Health, London

Department of Health 2003a Winning ways. Working together to reduce healthcare associated infection in England. Department of Health, London

Department of Health/NHS Modernisation Agency 2003b The essence of care. Patient-focused benchmarks for clinical governance. Department of Health, London

Department of Health 2004 The NHS improvement plan: putting people at the heart of public services. Department of Health, London

Department of Health 2006 Best research for best health. A new national research health strategy. Department of Health, London

DiCenso A, Cullum N, Ciliska D 1998 Implementing evidence based nursing: some misconceptions (editorial). Evidence Based Nursing 1:38–40

DiGuiseppi C, Roberts I, Li L 1998 Smoke alarm ownership and house fire death rates in children. Journal of Epidemiology and Community Health 52:760–761

Fibrinolytic Therapy Trialists (FTT) Collaborative Group 1994 Indications for fibrinolytic therapy in suspected acute myocardial infarction: collaborative overview of early mortality and major morbidity results from all randomised trials of over 1000 patients. Lancet 343:311–322

Graham H 1987 Women's smoking and family health. Social Science and Medicine 25:47–56

Graham H 1988 Women and smoking in the United Kingdom: implications for health promotion. Health Promotion Journal 3(4):371–382

Grahame Smith D 1998 Evidence based medicine: challenging the authority. Journal of the Royal Society of Medicine 35(suppl):7–11

Harrison J E 2000 Evidence-based orthodontics – how do I assess the evidence? Journal of Orthodontics 27(2):189–197

Iles V, Sutherland K 2001 Organisational change: a review for health care managers, professionals and researchers. NCCSDO, School of Hygiene and Tropical Medicine, London

Jacobson J C, Szilagyi P 2005 Patient reminder and patient recall systems to improve immunization rates. Cochrane Database of Systematic Reviews 2005, Issue 3. Art. No.: CD003941. DOI: 10.1002/14651858.CD003941. pub2

Kumar Y, Sarvanathan R 2004 Gastro-oesophageal reflux in children. Clinical Evidence. Available online at: www.clinicalevidence.com

Le Quintrec J L, Bussy C, Golmard J L, Hervé C, Baulon A, Piette F 2005 Randomized controlled drug trials on very elderly subjects: descriptive and methodological analysis of trials published between 1990 and 2002 and comparison with trials on adults. Journals of Gerontology Series A: Biological Sciences and Medical Sciences 60:340–344

Marshall S W, Runyan C W, Bangdiwala S I, Linzer M A, Sacks J J, Butts J D 1998 Fatal residential fires: who dies and who survives? JAMA 279: 1633–1637

Muir Gray J A 1997 Evidence-based health care: how to make health policy and management decisions. Churchill Livingstone, New York

Mulrow C D 1995 Rationale for systematic reviews. In: Chalmers I, Altman D G (eds) Systematic reviews. BMJ Publishing Group, London

National Institutes of Health, US Department of Health and Human Services 2005

About NIH Available online at: www.nih.gov/about/ January 2006

NHS CRD (NHS Centre for Reviews and Dissemination) 1996 Preventing unintentional injuries in children and young adolescents. Effective Health Care 2(5):1–16

NHS Modernisation Agency 2004 Good practice in paediatric continence services – benchmarking in action. Available online at: www.cgsupport.nhs. uk/PDFs/articles/good_practice_paediatric_continence_services.pdf

Osterberg L, Blaschke T 2005 Adherence to medication. New England Journal of Medicine 353:487–497

Pearson M 2000 Making a difference through research: how nurses can turn the vision into reality (editorial). NT Research 5(2):85–86

Plowman R, Graves N, Griffin M et al 1999 The socio-economic burden of hospital-acquired infection. Public Health Laboratory Service, London

Plowman R, Graves N, Griffin M et al 2001 The rate and cost of hospital acquired infections occurring in patients admitted to selected specialties of a district general hospital in England and the national burden imposed. Journal of Hospital Infection 47(3):198–209

Pursey A, Quinney D, Pearson M 1997 Concepts of care in primary health care nursing. In: Hugman R, Peelo M, Soothill K (eds) Concepts of care. Edward Arnold, London

Redfern S, Norman I, Murrells T et al 1997 External review of the Department of Health-funded nursing development units. Executive Summary. Available from Nursing Research Unit, King's College London, Cornwall House, Waterloo Road, London SE1 8WA

Richards R 1997 Clinical academic careers: report of an independent task force. Wellcome Trust, London

Rotter M L 1997 150 years of hand disinfection. Semmelweis' heritage. Hygiene und Medizin 22:332–339

Sackett D, Richardson W S, Rosenberg W, Haynes R B 1997 Evidence based medicine: how to practice and teach EBM. Churchill Livingstone, New York

Sackett D, Strauss S E, Richardson W S, Rosenberg W, Haynes R B 2000 Evidence-based medicine. How to practise and teach EBM, 2nd edn. Churchill Livingstone, London

Traynor M, Rafferty A M, Lewison G 2001 Endogenous and exogenous research? Findings from a bibliometric study of UK nursing research. Journal of Advanced Nursing 34(2):212–222

Tully M P, Cantrill J 1999 Role of the pharmacist in evidence-based prescribing in primary care. In: Gabbay M (ed) The evidence-based primary care handbook. Royal Society of Medicine, London, pp.183–193

Wellcome Trust 2001 Putting NHS research on the map: an analysis of scientific publications in England, 1990–97. Wellcome Trust, London

2 SECTION

Skills for evidence-based practice

2

CHAPTER

How to ask the right question

Jean V Craig

KEY POINTS

- Clinical decisions should take account of best available evidence.
- The process of achieving this entails a number of steps.
- A starting point is to formulate a clearly defined question. The question drives each step of the process and should therefore be carefully considered at the outset.
- A well-formulated question maximises the potential of finding relevant evidence that can be applied to a specific patient in a specific setting.

Introduction

The process for ensuring that clinical decisions are, as far as possible, informed by current research evidence has been described by Sackett et al (2000). This approach entails:

1 converting information needs into clear questions
2 seeking evidence to answer those questions
3 evaluating (critically appraising) the evidence for its validity (truthfulness) and usefulness
4 integrating findings with clinical expertise, patient needs and patient preferences to reach a decision as to the optimum course of action, and then applying this decision
5 evaluating our performance (and the outcome of our decision).

This approach is driven by the belief that up-to-date, well-conducted research, when used judiciously to inform clinical decisions, can help to improve patients' outcomes.

An important first step of the process is to clarify what information is needed to inform a particular aspect of nursing care, and to translate that information need into an explicit and succinct question that will drive the subsequent steps of the process. A carefully formulated question maximises the likelihood that relevant, high-quality evidence is identified and incorporated appropriately into the decision-making process. Where questions are poorly defined or where a haphazard approach is used to find papers, the likely result is hours of non-focused reading of literature that may or may not be relevant or applicable to the topic of interest. Developing 'answerable' clinical questions is thus an invaluable skill for nurses aiming to integrate best research evidence with other key elements of decision making (such as clinical expertise, patient preferences and values, resource availability) when caring for patients.

This chapter describes how to frame questions for interrogating the research evidence. It presents a standardised format for question formulation (as suggested by Sackett et al 1997), and uses clinical examples to illustrate its use. A number of exercises are included at the end of the chapter.

Information for effective nursing care

Nurses, along with other health-care practitioners, are required to make numerous decisions when caring for their patients. Consider the following examples of nursing care/interventions carried out during the course of a morning by a nurse working in a general practice:

- syringing the ears of an elderly gentleman complaining of increasing deafness due to wax build-up
- discussing asthma preventive measures with a teenager who has frequent episodes of asthma
- performing a cervical smear test
- advising a young man on interventions to alleviate acute lower back pain
- running a clinic for patients with type 2 diabetes mellitus.

The information that the nurse needs for managing each of these clinical episodes is extensive and varied. To successfully care for the patient presenting with wax build-up in his ears, the nurse might need an understanding of the purpose of ear wax and of the anatomy of the external auditory canal and tympanic membrane (think of these as foundational or background information needs), as well as knowledge of the effectiveness and comparative benefits and harms of each of the available interventions, and how well they are tolerated by patients (think of these as more specific, foreground information needs). Foundational (background) information, whilst not static, does not always change rapidly, so textbooks might be a suitable resource for accessing such information. In contrast, foreground information is best obtained from up-to-date research articles. The starting point for successfully tracking down such research articles is the focused 'answerable' question. Before looking at methods for focusing questions, briefly consider some of the foreground information that our practice nurse might need when caring for his or her patients. Examples are presented in Box 2.1.

Let's consider the available research evidence for the first question in Box 2.1: 'Which method should I use to remove ear wax?'. Various mechanical methods of wax removal are available including ear curettes, probes or forceps, microsuction, and ear syringing or irrigation in which wax is washed out of the ear canal (Burton & Doree 2003). Many practitioners consider these to be standard treatments. Browning (2004) looked for randomised controlled trials investigating these interventions but found no studies comparing mechanical methods alone with no treatment or alternative treatment. There are reports of harm occurring with ear syringing. Damage to the external auditory canal, perforation of the tympanic membrane, otitis externa, pain and vertigo have all been reported (Sharp et al 1990). Burton & Doree (2003) cite bleeding, infection and disturbance in balance causing nausea and vomiting. In patients with previous tympanic membrane

---

BOX 2.1 Examples of information needs

- Which method should I use to remove ear wax?
- How can I persuade this patient to take his asthma treatments regularly?
- Why does this patient have so many asthma attacks?
- What is the best method of delivering the asthma drugs?
- Do cervical smear tests with normal results accurately exclude cervical cancer?
- Should I test for chlamydia at the time of cervical smear?
- What advice should I give to this young man with back pain?
- What is the best way of monitoring for complications of diabetes?

---

perforation or grommets, the risk of complications may be increased, and ear syringing is contraindicated in patients with a history of mastoid surgery, chronic middle ear disease, a perforated ear drum or where the ear in question is the person's only hearing ear. In a review conducted by the Medical Defence Union (MDU), ear syringing was shown to account for 19% of claims involving general practice procedures, and in more than half of the claims it was the practice nurse who performed the procedure (Price 1997). Complications appeared to be related to poor technique, faulty equipment, exertion of excess pressure and failure to examine the ear (Price 1997). Although modern, electronic pulsed syringes are available, metal syringes, for which the rate of irrigation has to be manually controlled, are still used in some practices (Stubbs 2001). Given the potential for excessive pressure to be exerted on the plunger of the metal syringes, the risk of ear injury is greater with these devices.

Ear drops, in the form of either oil- or water-based solvents, are an alternative to mechanical methods of wax removal. A systematic review reports that the evidence for the effectiveness of ear drops as a stand-alone treatment is inconclusive, but that ear drops are likely to be better than no treatment (Burton & Doree 2003). The trials included in the review were generally of poor quality. The evidence for using ear drops prior to ear syringing is also inconclusive (Browning 2004). From a harm point of view, pruritus and dermatitis have been reported following use of ear drops.

How does this evidence help our practice nurse? When discussing treatment options with the patient, the nurse can draw on this information to explain that it is not yet known which method of wax removal is the most effective, but that ear syringing is likely to carry a greater risk than ear drops. Using this information, the nurse and patient can reach a decision that is right for the patient.

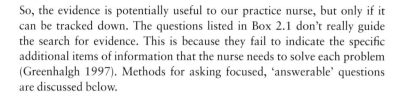

So, the evidence is potentially useful to our practice nurse, but only if it can be tracked down. The questions listed in Box 2.1 don't really guide the search for evidence. This is because they fail to indicate the specific additional items of information that the nurse needs to solve each problem (Greenhalgh 1997). Methods for asking focused, 'answerable' questions are discussed below.

Turning information needs into focused questions

There is an art to phrasing questions in such a way as to elicit a meaningful answer, whether these are questions directed at people or questions asked of the research literature.

As with the research process, the evidence-based process flows from the question. In research, the study design and methods are determined by what the researcher wants to know, i.e. by the research question. Similarly, in an approach that aims to incorporate best evidence in clinical decision making, it is the clinical question that drives each step of the process, in particular searching for relevant evidence, sorting best evidence from weaker, less valid evidence, and ascertaining whether the evidence is applicable to the patients and setting in which it is to be used. Let's look at this in more detail.

Searching for evidence

The more explicit the question, the easier it is to develop a search strategy to interrogate the electronic databases containing health-care publications (such as CINAHL (Cumulative Index of Allied Health and Nursing Literature), MEDLINE, EMBASE or the databases contained within the Cochrane Library). Search strategies generally aim to yield a manageable number of relevant research studies, whilst at the same time not missing too many relevant studies. The key components of the clinical question inform the search strategy. The less focused the question, the larger the numbers of non-relevant studies that will be identified, and the more time wasted by having to sift through unnecessarily long lists of references looking for relevant studies.

To illustrate, the practice nurse wants to know what advice to give to a young man with back pain (Box 2.1). If she or he searched the MEDLINE database from 2000 to 2006, using the phrase 'back pain', this would yield almost 8000 references. Even limiting the search to the most recent year would result in an unmanageable number of references (more than 1600) (search carried out 7/2/06). A quick glance at the references retrieved by this search shows that many of the articles relate to pregnancy and child-birth and are therefore unlikely to be of relevance to the male patient who presented with the complaint. A focused question would help to overcome this problem by providing guidance to the search strategy.

Selecting the best evidence

Once the question has been formulated, the type of study design that will best answer that question becomes clear (Logan & Gilbert 2000). Chapter 4 discusses study designs and their 'hierarchy' in terms of producing valid evidence for particular research questions. For the moment, it is sufficient to have a broad understanding of which study design best addresses a particular question. A question about the effectiveness of a treatment is best addressed by a well-conducted systematic review of randomised controlled trials, or by a randomised controlled trial (RCT) in which participants are randomly allocated to receive or not receive an intervention, and the groups followed up for the outcome event of interest. The point of randomisation is that it avoids the possibility of selection bias (i.e. bias due to systematic differences between the groups in their prognosis or responsiveness to the treatment) (*Bandolier* 2004).

Where information about the prognosis of a disease is required, the best evidence would be provided by a good-quality cohort study. Prognosis refers to the possible outcomes of an illness, and the frequency with which these outcomes occur (Laupacis et al 1994). Patient characteristics that are strongly associated with a particular outcome are called prognostic factors. It is usually impossible (and indeed unethical) to randomise patients to different prognostic factors, and so the RCT is not an appropriate study design for investigating prognosis (Laupacis et al 1994). Instead, a cohort study is conducted where one or more groups (cohorts) who have not yet developed the specified outcome event are followed forward in time and the number of events recorded for each cohort.

A less robust study design for prognostic studies is the case–control study where 'cases' who have already developed the specified outcome event are compared with 'controls' who do not have the same outcomes. The researchers look back in time to see what percentage of participants in each group has the prognostic factor. Case–control studies are particularly useful where the outcome is rare or where a long follow-up is required (Laupacis et al 1994). Case–control studies can also be used to investigate aetiology (the cause) of disease. Here researchers look back in time to establish the percentage of 'cases' and 'controls' that have experienced the exposure of interest.

For a question relating to patients' understanding of their condition or perceptions of an intervention, the best evidence would be a well-conducted qualitative study, of which there are numerous approaches. Regardless of the approach, qualitative research is committed to viewing the phenomenon of interest from the perspective of the people being studied (Bryman 1988), and thus aims to give insight into the different meanings and values that people may attribute to 'events'. Further information on qualitative research is given in Chapter 6.

A search of electronic databases may yield a large number of research studies that appear to be relevant to the clinical question. Knowing which type of study design would best answer the question enables rapid sorting of the retrieved studies such that studies with the most appropriate study design take precedence. It is worth remembering that the preferred study design (summarised in Box 2.2) is not always feasible in terms of costs, time or ethical considerations, and researchers might have to resort to less than optimal study designs. Box 2.2 is certainly not comprehensive. For further information on other types of studies, consult the User's Guides for Evidence-Based Practice (Centre for Health Evidence) at www.cche.net/usersguides/main.asp.

BOX 2.2 Optimal study designs according to clinical question

Questions about effectiveness of an intervention
Systematic review of randomised controlled trial
Randomised controlled trial

Questions about the accuracy of a diagnostic test
Studies that compare the new test against a reference standard test

Questions about prognosis
Cohort studies or, when the outcome is rare or the required duration of follow-up is long, case–control studies

Questions about aetiology (causation)
Case–control or cohort study

Questions about perceptions, attitudes, beliefs
Qualitative research (numerous approaches)

Applying the evidence

When a well-conducted study has been located, a judgement has to be made as to whether the results from the research would be achieved if they were applied to a specific patient in your setting. It is unlikely that the circumstances in which the research study was undertaken will exactly match your clinical situation, and this might affect the applicability or transferability of the study results. When reading a research study, it is important to decide whether the participants included in the study are so dissimilar from your patient/setting that the results cannot be applied. Is it appropriate, for example, to apply the findings of a study that looked at methods for improving compliance with drug treatment in the elderly to a population of teenagers? Methods that are effective in the elderly, such as the dispensing of tablets into individual containers labelled with the days of the week, may be seen by adolescents as embarrassing and may in fact result in reduced compliance. Similarly, a judgement must be made as to whether a similar, but not identical, intervention or test will be likely to produce the same result as that achieved in the study. As shown below, the carefully formulated question usually includes a description of the patient group of interest, the planned treatment(s) or investigation(s), and the key outcomes that the patient hopes to achieve. It is therefore a useful tool for screening out those research studies that are not applicable to the clinical situation or for helping to ensure that differences between the patient and the research population are transparent.

A framework for formulating questions

The PICO (population, intervention, comparison intervention, outcome) framework, devised by Sackett et al (1997), is a useful method for making questions more focused. The question is built in four (or three) parts (Box 2.3). Careful thought is required when deciding how specific each part of the question should be. For **population,** it may be necessary to specify age, gender, disease type, disease severity or co-morbidity. This will depend on whether or not the results of a very broad, inclusive research population could be applied to your specific patient group. If, for example, there are good clinical reasons for suspecting that the results from studies conducted in hospitalised patients are unlikely to be applicable to patients in primary are settings, then the population part of the question should include details of the setting. The **intervention** (or test or exposure) and **comparison intervention** (if any) may need to be described in some detail to ensure clarity. This is especially important for multifaceted interventions (such as

---

BOX 2.3 The four (or three)-part question (PICO)

Patient or problem:	Define who or what the question is about. *Tip: describe a group of patients similar to yours*
Intervention:	Define which intervention, test or exposure you are interested in. An intervention is a planned course of action. An exposure is something that happens such as a fall, anxiety, exposure to house dust mites, etc. (Bury & Mead 1998). *Tip: describe what it is you are considering doing or what it is that has happened to the patient*
Comparison intervention (if any):	Define the alternative intervention. *Tip: describe the alternative that can be compared with the intervention*
Outcomes:	Define the important outcomes, beneficial or harmful. *Tip: Define what you are hoping to achieve or avoid*

---

asthma clinics, nurse development units, etc.) where any number of factors may be responsible for the outcome of interest. Deciding on the most important **outcomes** is not always straightforward, but can be facilitated by considering the patient's perspective. Very general outcomes may be difficult to measure, and details of how outcomes can be objectively measured may need to be specified.

The PICO formula cannot always be easily applied, but nevertheless it is a useful tool. The Scenarios below illustrate the use of this formula.

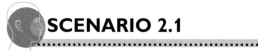

SCENARIO 2.1

A 10-year-old girl who has had open-heart surgery has been very ill for 2 days, requiring artificial ventilation and a number of support drugs to maintain her blood pressure. She has developed a small pressure sore at the back of her head.

The nurse asks the following question:
How can I prevent further pressure sores from developing in this child?

This general question may be difficult to answer. Many factors contribute to tissue breakdown, including poor nutrition, poor circulation, immobility and type of mattress. The nurse decides to focus on the mattress. The child is currently being nursed on a high-specification foam mattress.

At this stage, further defining each component of the question will yield dividends when searching for, and sorting through, relevant research studies.

Population

The nurse must decide whether research carried out in the adult population could be applied to children. The decision of whether to exclude specific age groups is usually based on the known differences in the response to disease, treatments and tests, by each age group, or on the inferred differences which might arise from the above. If the differences are such that the results of a research study will not be generalisable from one age group to another, then age groups should be defined within the question.

In addition, it is important to consider whether, and how specifically, to define the condition. Is there any reason for restricting the question to patients who have had cardiac surgery? Critically ill cardiac patients may have poor circulation and therefore be at increased risk of developing pressure sores; however, other groups of critically ill children (for example children with septicaemia) might also have poor perfusion. One could argue that all critically ill children are probably at similar risk of developing pressure sores, and research carried out in these patients, regardless of their diagnosis, would help to answer the question.

Intervention (or test or exposure)

A variety of mattresses and beds are available on the market, ranging from standard hospital foam or high-specification foam to constant low-pressure devices or alternating pressure devices. Some of these devices may be more effective than others. Depending on the device under consideration, there could be major cost implications. In the year 2000, costs of pressure-relieving devices were found to range from £100 to £30,000 (Cullum et al 2000). The nurse does not want to overly restrict the question, thereby limiting the chance of finding any relevant evidence, but by clarifying what pressure-relieving device could be used for the 10-year-old patient (we will assume this to be the constant low-pressure bed), the search for information is made easier.

Comparison intervention

It is not always necessary to define a comparison intervention, but in this case the intervention against which the proposed device could be compared is the method currently in use. In this scenario, this is the high-specification foam mattress.

Outcome

Outcomes may need to be carefully defined. The nurse wants to prevent further pressure sores but what does she or he mean by pressure sore? The results of studies in which a pressure sore is described as 'full-thickness skin loss' might differ from those of studies that include in their definition 'persistent discoloration of the skin, or partial-thickness skin loss'. Ideally, the identified research would provide data on the outcome that is of interest to the nurse.

In summary:

* *Population*: Critically ill children
* *Intervention*: Constant low-pressure beds
* *Comparison*: High-specification foam mattresses
* *Outcome*: Pressure sores at any stage: constant discoloration of skin, or partial- or full-thickness skin loss.

Our more focused question could therefore be:
In critically ill children, are constant low-pressure beds more effective than high-specification foam mattresses in preventing pressure sores (defined here as constant discoloration of the skin, or partial- or full-thickness skin loss)?

At this stage it is useful to identify which type of *study design* is most likely to provide a valid (believable) answer to the question. As this is a question about effectiveness of a therapy, the study design of choice is a systematic review of randomised controlled trials or a randomised controlled trial (see Chapter 4 for more information). Retrieved studies can be sorted accordingly, with studies of the above design being given highest priority.

Searching for research evidence is covered in detail in Chapter 3, but it is worth briefly mentioning here that all four parts of the question are not always used when developing a search strategy. The nurse could run a preliminary search using terms relating to the *population* (in this case, terms such as 'child', 'paediatric', 'critically ill', etc.) and *intervention* ('low-pressure bed', etc.) parts of the question. If this resulted in an unmanageable number of references, terms relating to the *comparison intervention* or even the *outcome* could also be added. This should further restrict the number of references identified, and should enhance the likelihood of these references being relevant to the question. In addition, a filter could be added to the search so that only studies of a particular design are retrieved. Search filters are discussed in Chapter 3.

The nurse will be able to check the retrieved articles against the focused question. Those that are found to be less applicable (for example, studies that have focused on obese adults) can be set aside in favour of the more applicable studies, i.e. those that are generalisable to the 10-year-old child.

We have looked at one question in detail, but the nurse may have a number of information needs relating to this patient. Some of the questions arising from these information needs are highlighted in Table 2.1.

TABLE 2.1 OTHER QUESTIONS ABOUT PREVENTION OR TREATMENT OF PRESSURE SORES

Population or problem	Intervention (or test or exposure)	Comparison intervention (if any)	Outcome
Patients with pressure sores (partial- or full-thickness skin loss)	Application of hydrocolloids	Application of gauze dressings	Reduced time to healing Faster shrinkage of the pressure sore
Patients with pressure sores (partial- or full-thickness skin loss)	Ascorbic acid supplementation	Usual diet with no additional supplements	Reduced time to healing Faster shrinkage of the pressure sore
Critically ill children	Constant low-pressure devices or alternating pressure devices	Three-hourly lifting or turning	Prevention of pressure sores, defined here as discoloration of the skin, or partial- or full-thickness skin loss Risk of destabilising the patient, poor cardiac output Costs

SCENARIO 2.2

Alison, a 2-year-old infant, presented at the local accident and emergency department with fever and vomiting. In line with departmental policy, urine was collected in a bag (which had been applied to her perineum according to the manufacturer's instructions), then sent for microscopy and culture. The white cell count was found to be high and Alison was started on a course of antibiotics. She was asked to return in 5 days, by which time the urine culture results would be available. At her follow-up appointment, the attending physician was frustrated to note that the culture results showed a mixed growth. It was not clear whether Alison had indeed suffered a urinary tract infection (UTI) or whether the urine sample had simply been contaminated. In view of the risk of underlying urinary tract abnormalities and potential upper urinary tract damage, children with UTI are investigated carefully. Concerned that the methods used for obtaining urine samples were inappropriate, the physician suggested that, in future, bag-catch urine sampling should be abandoned in favour of clean-catch urine sampling. This method requires that the infant's nappy is removed and their carer provided with a sterile container and instructed to watch for the opportunity to catch the urine. The nurses on the unit were worried about the implications of changing practice. They felt that carers might not be successful in capturing urine specimens, and that this would cause delays for patients and their families.

The nurses want to know:
What is the best way of obtaining a urine specimen for culture, from a child?

We can check how focused the question is, by examining each component individually.

Population

The population of interest is children suspected of having UTI; however, the nurses may want to consider further defining the population. The results of a study carried out in older children (who may be able to obtain the urine specimen themselves) are likely to be different from those from a study carried out in children still wearing nappies.

Comparison intervention

Next we will look at the comparison intervention. Comparing two methods is a useful way of reaching a decision about a practice change. When investigating the accuracy of a (new) diagnostic test, the new test is compared against a reference standard test to see how well the two tests agree. A reference standard test is considered to be 'the best available method for establishing the presence or absence of the condition of interest' and can be a single method or a combination of methods (Bossuyt et al 2003). Alternatives to reference standard tests are often sought where the reference standard tests are difficult to perform, invasive, costly, inconvenient or unacceptable to the patient.

The reference standard method for obtaining urine from infants and babies is suprapubic aspiration of urine directly from the bladder (Downs 1999). The procedure is invasive, uncomfortable for the infant, and can be tricky where infants are unco-operative. Alternative methods include bag-catch or clean-catch urine collection methods.

Intervention (or test or exposure)

In this case, there are two interventions of interest: the method of urine sampling which is currently used (i.e. urine bag sampling) and the proposed method of 'clean-catch' sampling. It may be useful to include brief details of the exact methods used when obtaining bag-catch and clean-catch urine specimens, as these may differ from those used by researchers and this could affect the applicability of study results.

Outcome

The key outcome of interest is contamination of the culture specimen. Other outcomes that the nurses may wish to consider are time taken to obtain specimen, acceptability to patient and family, and ease of use.

In summary:

- *Population*: Children suspected of having UTI, who are not yet toilet trained
- *Interventions*: Bag-catch urine specimens
             Clean-catch urine specimens
- *Comparison*: Suprapubic aspiration
- *Outcome*: Contaminated culture specimen, as indicated by bacterial growth in either the bag-catch or clean-catch specimens, not found in the suprapubic aspiration.

The revised question is:
In children suspected of having UTI, who are not yet toilet trained, what is the risk of culture contamination when urine is obtained by (i) bag-catch or (ii) clean-catch, as compared with urine obtained by suprapubic aspiration directly from the bladder?

TABLE 2.2 OTHER QUESTIONS ABOUT DIAGNOSIS OF URINARY TRACT INFECTION

Population or problem	Intervention (or test or exposure)	Comparison intervention (if any)	Outcome
Children suspected of having UTI, who are not yet toilet trained	Clean-catch urine sampling using a sterile container	Suprapubic aspiration directly from bladder	Culture contamination
Obtaining urine samples from children who are not yet toilet trained	Clean-catch method	Bag-catch method	Time taken to successfully obtain urine sample, cost, parent satisfaction, nurse satisfaction

The optimal *study design* for this question would be studies assessing diagnostic test accuracy. Examples of additional questions relating to this scenario are given in Table 2.2.

SCENARIO 2.3

A recent public health report shows that despite national initiatives to promote breastfeeding, uptake is poor. A health visitor who works in a deprived, inner-city community and visits mothers from day 10 after delivery has noticed that many of the mothers feed their babies with infant milk formula rather than breast milk. The health visitor wants to gain a better understanding of the factors that influence mothers to bottlefeed with infant milk formula. This information may help to inform future educational programmes aimed at promoting breastfeeding.

The health visitor asks:
Why do mothers not breastfeed?

The question does not easily fit the PICO formula, but it is nevertheless useful to consider each component of the question. It may be possible to further refine the question, thereby improving the chance of finding relevant research evidence.

Population

The health visitor works with mothers who live in a deprived area of the city, a population that has different needs and different experiences to those of women in more affluent areas. In this case, the health visitor is interested in the views of mothers of all ages. If the problem were specific to very young, first-time mothers, the question would need to reflect this. The health visitor may find it useful to examine the views of both breastfeeding and bottlefeeding mothers in order to obtain information about the factors that influence mothers in their decision to breast- or bottlefeed.

Intervention (or test or exposure)

Unlike questions relating to test accuracy or effectiveness of a treatment, there is no intervention for this type of question.

Outcomes

The health visitor is interested in mothers' perceptions, attitudes, values or beliefs relating to breastfeeding and/or to bottlefeeding with infant formula.

The revised question is as follows:

What are the factors, identified by mothers who live in deprived inner city areas, that influence them to breastfeed or to bottlefeed using infant milk formula?

The *type of research* that is most likely to provide an in-depth understanding of the views of the mothers is qualitative research (discussed in Chapter 6).

Becoming proficient in asking questions

Asking the right question is a skill that requires practice. The following exercises are a useful starting point for practising this skill but are no substitute for the real-life problems encountered in day-to-day practice. To become adept at this skill, nurses will need to practise translating real-life information needs into focused questions on a daily basis.

EXERCISES

Try to formulate focused questions from the following case studies. You may want to think about the study design that is most likely to provide valid results for each of the questions. Some suggestions for focused questions that might arise from these case studies are given in Appendix 2.1.

Exercise 2.1

Mrs York, a 52-year-old woman, sustained a severe wrist fracture following a fall. She was subsequently investigated for, and found to have, osteoporosis. Her doctor discussed the potential benefits and harms of hormone replacement therapy (HRT) with her and together they decided that she should start the treatment. Mrs York has since spoken to family and friends about the potential risks of HRT and has become increasingly concerned that HRT increases her risk of breast cancer. During a well woman clinic, she tells the practice nurse that she is thinking of stopping the treatment.

Exercise 2.2

Mrs Hardy, the mother of a young infant, is trying to decide whether to give up smoking. Her infant has recently had episodes of wheezing and breathlessness, requiring admission to hospital for a couple of nights. Mrs Hardy has been warned about the risks of respiratory problems in children who are exposed to cigarette smoke, but she wants to know if there really is a link between the two.

Exercise 2.3

Jennifer is attending her general practice for a cervical smear test. She has read in the newspaper that a number of women who underwent cervical smear tests, and had negative test results, were later found to have cervical cancer. Jennifer is very nervous about having any tests at all, and is tempted to cancel the smear test in view of the possibility of the results being inaccurate.

Exercise 2.4

A practice nurse has advised Mr Reynolds, a 60-year-old man who is overweight and has hypertension, to reduce weight and to cut down on the amount of salt in his diet. Mr Reynolds is very sceptical that this course of action will help him. The nurse would like to find some evidence that supports her recommendation.

Specific prompts for accessing research evidence

Health-care practitioners should constantly evaluate their practice. New technologies (for example drugs, blood pressure monitoring devices, wound dressings) are introduced on a regular basis, different processes of care (case management, patient-held records, home care of long-term ventilated patients, etc.) are explored and new information (for example, factors associated with sudden infant death syndrome, literacy figures for the adult population, etc.) is published at regular intervals. A questioning approach to health care is important if such 'innovations' are to be identified in the first place and, secondly, if they are to be considered for inclusion in the management of patients. An attitude of 'research mindedness' (Perkins et al 1999, p.4) is needed, asking questions such as 'Which is best?', 'Who should do this?', 'Where should this patient be treated?'. Blind acceptance of a technology that is skilfully marketed by a company representative, or outright rejection of change to an existing practice could potentially impact negatively on patient outcome, resources and cost.

Although nurses would agree with the above, the need to access research evidence in the context of the clinical setting is not always apparent. One of the challenges for nurses and other health-care professionals is to recognise the importance of asking questions about their practice.

Prompts for consulting scientific evidence include:

- uncertainty as to the best course of action
- controversy regarding the way a procedure or therapy should be carried out
- lack of knowledge about the effectiveness of one therapy or test over another
- unexpected patient outcomes
- the introduction of new therapies or technologies
- practices based on tradition
- 'novel' suggestions by patients.

For those aspects of care that are already entrenched in day-to-day practice, a questioning approach is equally important, but perhaps more difficult to achieve. Where a method of care delivery (for example, the 'drugs round' where drugs are dispensed to all ward patients at set times by a designated nurse) has become entrenched as routine practice, practitioners may accept it as the right or only method, and alternatives may not be considered. In addition, 'ritualistic' practices must be examined for clinical and cost effectiveness.

It may be helpful for the nurse to consider whether 'the right person is doing the right thing, in the right way, in the right place, at the right time, with the right result' (Graham 1996). By asking this question, any information gaps will be highlighted. Finally, reflection, a strategy used within nursing to encourage learning from practical experiences (Boud et al 1985), can be used as another method for identifying information needs. By reflecting on 'critical incidents', gaps in knowledge of current research findings can be identified.

Prioritising questions

The volume of decisions and related information needs that arise each day can be overwhelming. It may be necessary to prioritise the questions for which best evidence is to be sought. Questions that are most important to the patient's well-being, that arise repeatedly (Sackett et al 1997) or that have potentially important consequences (such as risk or cost reductions) could be considered high-priority questions. At the Evidence-Based Child Health Unit in Liverpool, topics are prioritised according to the following criteria:

- relevant to the hospital and to NHS priorities
- affects a significant number of patients
- potential to implement change in practice
- demand for the topic from a number of independent sources
- wide variations in practice
- genuine uncertainty or controversy as to best practice.

Questions for research

In the spirit of evidence-based practice, this chapter has focused on questions that nurses in the clinical field are asking; questions which they hope can be answered to some extent by previously published research evidence. However, the same PICO formula can be applied to many research questions (that may or may not arise directly from an interaction with a patient or clinical problem). In research, as with evidence-based practice, the question drives the research project. Asking a general, unfocused question will lead to difficulties at each step of the research process.

Questions and research evidence aren't enough

Our day-to-day clinical decisions are influenced (consciously or unconsciously) by a number of factors (Box 2.4). Although each of these factors is influential in its own right, when used in isolation, they may result in inappropriate decisions. The application of scientific evidence without considered judgement results in a 'cookbook' approach to health care, with nurses following 'recipes' for care regardless of the patient's specific needs. In contrast, over-reliance on personal experience when making

---

BOX 2.4 Factors influencing the decision-making process

Up-to-date research evidence
Clinical expertise:
- formal education
- accumulated knowledge (journal articles, textbooks, press reports, expert opinion, advice from colleagues, clinical audit)
- past experience built on a case-by-case basis
- pattern recognition, intuition
- most recent experience
- skill level
Beliefs, attitudes, values, tradition
Routine, 'the way things are done around here'
Factors relating to the patient and their family:
- clinical circumstances, co-morbid conditions
- preferences, values, beliefs, attitudes, expectations, concerns
- needs
Organisational factors
- national and local policies
- service/resource availability
- funding
- equipment
- time

decisions can be equally damaging. For example, if practice nurses continue to recommend bed rest to people with acute lower back pain because it appears to have worked in the past, they will be ignoring evidence that bed rest is less effective in reducing pain and improving an individual's ability to perform everyday activities than advice to stay active (Hagen et al 2004). In people with type 2 diabetes mellitus, one-off routine annual testing of urine may be the usual practice; however, recent evidence indicates that a single annual near-patient test is not sufficiently sensitive in identifying people with renal disease. Instead urine should be tested at least annually and on more than one occasion for proteinuria and, if found to be negative, it should subsequently be tested for microalbuminuria (NHS CRD 2000).

Up-to-date, valid evidence, directly relevant to the situation at hand, needs to be integrated together with the other influencing factors in order to maximise the likelihood of the expected outcome being achieved.

Summary

The success or failure of explicitly basing nursing practice on best evidence relies on nurses challenging both new and established methods of caring for patients. The skills provided in this chapter, summarised in Box 2.5, provide a starting point for seeking out good-quality evidence to support current practice or a change in practice. This first step in the evidence-based process is an important one, and nurses who take the time to develop carefully worded questions will be well rewarded at each stage in the process.

BOX 2.5 Quick reference: applying your new skills in clinical practice

- Consider what additional information is required when making a health care decision.
- Prioritise which information you need to address.
- Formulate a question.
- Focus the question using the PICO formula.
- Decide how specific or how general each part of the question needs to be.
- Decide which study design is most likely to provide valid results.
- Refer to the focused question at each stage of the evidence-based process, i.e. when searching for or appraising evidence, and when applying the evidence to your situation.

References

Bandolier Glossary 2004. Selection bias. Available online at: www.jr2.ox.ac. uk/bandolier/glossary.html

Bossuyt P M, Reitsma J B, Bruns D E et al 2003 Towards complete and accurate reporting of studies of diagnostic accuracy: the STARD Initiative. Radiology 226:24–28

Boud D, Keogh R, Walker D 1985 Reflection: turning experience into learning. Kogan Page, London

Browning G 2004 Ear wax. Clinical Evidence. Available online at: www.clinicalevidence.com 7 Feb 2006

Bryman A 1988 Quantity and quality in social research. Unwin Hyman, London

Burton M J, Doree C J 2003 Ear drops for the removal of ear wax. Cochrane Database of Systematic Reviews 2003, Issue 3. Art. No.: CD004326. DOI: 10.1002/14651858.CD004326

Bury T J, Mead J M (eds) 1998 Evidence based healthcare: a practical guide for therapists. Butterworth-Heinemann, Oxford

Cullum N, Deeks J, Sheldon T A, Song F, Fletcher A W 2000 Beds, mattresses and cushions for pressure sore prevention and treatment (Cochrane Review). Cochrane Library, Issue 3, 2000. Update Software, Oxford

Downs S M 1999 Technical report: urinary tract infections in febrile infants and young children. Pediatrics 103(4):e54

Graham G 1996 Clinically effective medicine in a rational health service. Health Director June:11–12

Greenhalgh T 1997 How to read a paper – the basics of evidence based medicine. BMJ Publishing, London

Hagen K, Hilde G, Jamtvedt G, Winnem M 2004 Bedrest for acute low back pain and sciatica. Cochrane Database of Systematic Reviews 2004, Issue 4. Art. No.: CD001254. DOI: 10.1002/14651858.CD001254.pub2

Laupacis A, Wells G, Scott Richardson W, Tugwell P, for the Evidence-Based Medicine Working Group 1994 Users' guides to the medical literature. How to use an article about prognosis. Journal of the American Medical Association 272(3):234–237. Available online at: www.cche.net/ usersguides/prognosis.asp

Logan S, Gilbert R 2000 Framing questions. In: Moyer V A, Elliot E J, Davis R L et al (eds) Evidence based paediatrics and child health. BMJ Books, London

NHS CRD (Centre for Reviews and Dissemination) 2000 Complications of diabetes: renal disease and promotion of self-management. Effective Health Care Bulletin 6(1):1–12

Perkins E R, Simnett I, Wright L 1999 Creative tensions in evidence-based practice. In: Perkins E R, Simnett I, Wright L (eds) Evidence based health promotion. Wiley, New York

Price J 1997 Problems of ear syringing. Practice Nurse 14(2):126–127

Sackett D L, Richardson W S, Rosenberg W, Haynes R B 1997 Evidence based medicine: how to practice and teach EBM. Churchill Livingstone, New York

Sackett D L, Strauss S E, Richardson W S, Rosenberg W, Haynes R B 2000 Evidence-based medicine: how to practise and teach EBM, 2nd edn. Churchill Livingstone, London

Sharp J F, Wilson J A, Ross L, Barr-Hamilton R M 1990 Ear wax removal: a survey of current practice. British Medical Journal 301:1251–1252

Stubbs G 2001 Getting to grips with the metal ear syringe. Nursing Times 97(20):40

APPENDIX 2.1

Possible solutions to exercises

Exercise 2.1 – Mrs York

Question 1

Population:	In postmenopausal women with no family history of breast cancer,
Intervention (exposure):	how much does hormone replacement therapy
Outcomes:	increase the risk of breast cancer?
Optimal study design:	Cohort study

Question 2

Population:	In postmenopausal women with osteoporosis,
Intervention:	does hormone replacement therapy
Comparison:	compared with no hormone replacement therapy
Outcome:	reduce the risk of fractures?
Optimal study design:	Systematic review of randomised controlled trials or a randomised controlled trial

Exercise 2.2 – Mrs Hardy and her infant

Population:	In children
Exposure:	who are exposed to passive smoking
Outcome:	what is the risk of respiratory disease?
Optimal study design:	Cohort study

Exercise 2.3 – Jennifer

Population:	In women
Intervention:	who have cervical smear tests
Outcome:	what is the risk of failing to identify cervical cancer in affected women and what is the risk of falsely identifying cervical cancer in non-affected women?
Optimal study design:	Blinded comparison of test and reference standard test

Exercise 2.4 – Mr Reynolds

Question 1

Population:	In men over 50 years of age who are hypertensive
Intervention:	does a weight-reducing diet (or replace this with 'does limiting dietary salt intake')

Outcome:	lower blood pressure and reduce the risk of stroke and cardiovascular mortality?
Optimal study design:	Systematic review of randomised controlled trials or randomised controlled trial

Question 2

Population:	In middle-aged men who have a health condition related to being overweight (the population has been restricted to middle-aged men as their attitudes and perceptions of factors such as body image, their cooking abilities, choice of food, etc. may differ from those of younger men)
Intervention:	(there is no intervention in this case)
Outcome:	what are their perceptions/attitudes towards weight-reducing diets?
Optimal study design:	Qualitative research

3
CHAPTER

Searching the literature

Olwen Beaven and Jean V Craig

KEY POINTS

• Identifying best evidence requires an understanding of basic search
  principles. More advanced techniques will help to
  enhance a search.

• To maximise use of time, resources can be searched in order
  of usefulness.

• Techniques to limit the number of irrelevant articles retrieved (such as
  searching using index terms only) can be used.

• Systematic reviews require extensive searching.

• The internet can be a valuable source of information, especially if reliable/
  quality-assessed resources are used.

Introduction

The purpose of this chapter is to provide a beginner's guide to the principles and practice of searching the research literature. Whilst it is unrealistic to teach the art of searching within the constraints of the printed page, it is possible to pass on a basic understanding of the search process and the core competencies needed to enable readers to progress and develop their searching skills. Whilst this chapter is primarily aimed at novice searchers, it will be useful revision for those who feel more confident and there are also some sections targeted specifically at the advanced searcher. The importance of searching the literature to find information is often overlooked in the hurry to develop new ideas, try new approaches or to get research under way. However, a good literature search can underpin the whole problem-solving process; if key information is missing, it is much harder to identify an appropriate solution. This is particularly true when searching the research literature to try to answer specific clinical questions.

Where is research information found?

The large number of general and specialist journals produced around the world precludes searching for individual articles by hand. Journal indexes have therefore been converted onto electronic databases to facilitate the process of finding research studies. These bibliographic databases gather together articles within a particular subject category such as engineering, biology, sociology, history, medicine or agriculture. Most databases provide similar information about each included article. This is usually the title, author, where it was published (the journal, year, volume, issue and page numbers) and the short abstract/summary if available. Databases do not normally contain the full text of the whole article, although increasingly, free full-text articles are becoming available electronically.

Journal articles in a database are often referred to as 'records'. Each section of an article/record (title, author, abstract, etc.) is called a 'field'. Each new field starts with a two-letter code to make it clearly identifiable. For example, a typical record in a bibliographic database might look something like this (see top of p.53).

Databases are produced in a variety of formats: direct 'online' access, CD-ROM versions or worldwide web/internet options. Increasingly, in many organisations, databases are 'networked' onto all the computers. Databases

TI: The joys of nursing
AU: Anybody G. C., Somebody H. L., Other A. N.
SO: Supernurse, 1997, 15 (2); 378–84
PY: 1997
AB: There have been numerous campaigns over recent years to boost the recruitment of young people into the nursing profession. These have taken a variety of approaches and have focused on different aspects of the job, from how challenging nursing is, to the rewards of watching a patient recover from illness/injury. This paper looks at the positive images of nursing portrayed in these advertising campaigns and compares them with the reality as perceived by nurses currently employed.
UI: SN9725938

are mainly produced by commercial companies and are not usually free of charge. As organisations have to pay for access to databases, this can limit the range made available for searching.

Getting help

Before attempting any literature searching, find out what help is available. Hospital libraries are an obvious port of call for obtaining training, advice, written instructions or self-help tutorials. Librarians will often help you to focus your question, to construct the search and to select which databases to search. Increasingly, librarians are offering an information service whereby they conduct the search for articles relevant to a particular clinical question. Such services are potentially extremely useful, but acquiring the skills to conduct your own searches will prove invaluable in terms of day-to-day clinical decision making.

Basic search principles

Although databases are produced by different companies and vary in terms of subject matter and layout, they all tend to use the same general approach when it comes to searching. This section looks at some basic theory that can be applied to searching most databases. The key principle in searching is to match words that describe your question or topic of interest with journal articles containing the same (or very similar) words, in the hope that

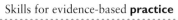

these journal articles will be investigating/discussing your topic/question of interest.

Analysing the question

When starting a literature search, it is important to have a clear question in mind so the exact information required can be identified. The first step in developing a search strategy is to break a question down into its key components (see the PICO question formulation process described in Chapter 2). Think about the population, the interventions/treatments, any comparison interventions and specific outcomes covered by a question. Two examples are given in Box 3.1.

Generating a word list

Having established the key components of a question, generate a word list for each component. All the different synonyms and phrases that could

---

BOX 3.1 Two questions broken down into key components

Question 1: What is the best way to alleviate fear associated with needles and injections?

Population:	People with fear of needles
Intervention(s):	Behavioural
	Relaxation
	Distraction
	Hypnotherapy
	Education
Comparison:	One intervention compared with another
Outcome:	Fear/anxiety reduced

Question 2: Do oral antibiotics/treatments enhance healing or are topical dressings sufficient for treatment of leg ulcers in sickle cell disease?

Population:	People with sickle cell disease leg ulcers
Intervention(s):	Oral treatments in conjunction with topical treatments
Comparison:	Compared to topical treatments alone
Outcome:	Improvement in ulcer (heals, area is reduced)

be used to describe a component, as well as plural and singular words, abbreviations, variations in spellings, possible hyphenation and any regularly used non-English language terms, should be included in the lists. The lists for each component may be fairly comprehensive as shown in Box 3.2.

Be cautious when using abbreviations. Sometimes the same abbreviation is used to represent different terminology. For example, BNF is used for the 'British Nutrition Foundation' as well as the 'British National Formulary', so it may pick up articles on the wrong topic. A search for articles using the abbreviation 'AIDS' will identify articles looking at hearing aids, mobility aids, etc. as well as articles on autoimmune deficiency syndrome. Abbreviations are very useful to include, but a bit of care and thought can help avoid pitfalls.

BOX 3.2 Suggested word lists for questions 1 and 2

Question 1

Population:	Fear of needles, fear of syringes, fear of injection(s), phobia of needles, phobia of syringes, phobia of injection(s), fear of hypodermic(s), phobia of hypodermic(s)
Interventions:	Behavio(u)r(al), education, relaxation, coping skills, psychological, counselling, hypnotherapy, hypnosis, psychotherapy, distraction, divert attention, diversion
Comparison:	(Same as interventions)
Outcomes:	Alleviation or reduction of fear/stress/anxiety, stress relief, calm, relaxed

Question 2

Population:	Sickle cell leg ulcer(s), sickle-cell leg ulcer(s), sickle cell an(a)emia leg ulcer(s), sickle-cell an(a)emia leg ulcer(s), sickle cell disease leg ulcer(s), sickle-cell disease leg ulcer(s)
Interventions:	Ointment, dressing(s), cream(s), topical application, topically applied, oral antibiotic(s), oral drug(s), oral application
Comparison:	(Same as intervention)
Outcomes:	Ulcer reduction, ulcer reduced, area of ulcer reduced, ulcer heals, ulcer healed over, ulcer reduction

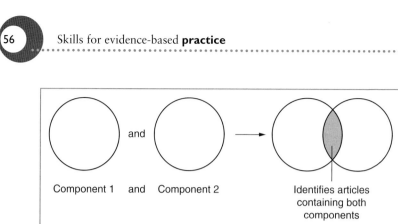

Figure 3.1 The Boolean operator AND only identifies articles containing both specified components

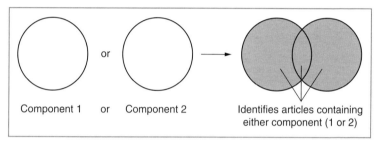

Figure 3.2 The Boolean operator OR identifies articles containing either specified component

Linking word lists (Boolean logic: AND, OR, NOT)

Once separate word lists have been generated, you link them together to get the combination of components needed for a question.

Linking word lists in searching is done using the terms AND and OR. AND combines words/phrases together, so that both must appear within one article to be found by a search (Figure 3.1). For example, for question 1, a search for 'needles AND fear' will find only those articles that contain both the words needles and fear. For question 2, a search for 'sickle cell disease AND leg ulcers' will find only those articles containing both the phrases sickle cell disease and leg ulcers.

OR enables selection of any one of a number of specified words/phrases in a list, so that if either one or another specified word/phrase appears in an article, it will be found in a search (Figure 3.2). For example, for the 'intervention' terms from question 1, a search for 'behavioural OR behavioral

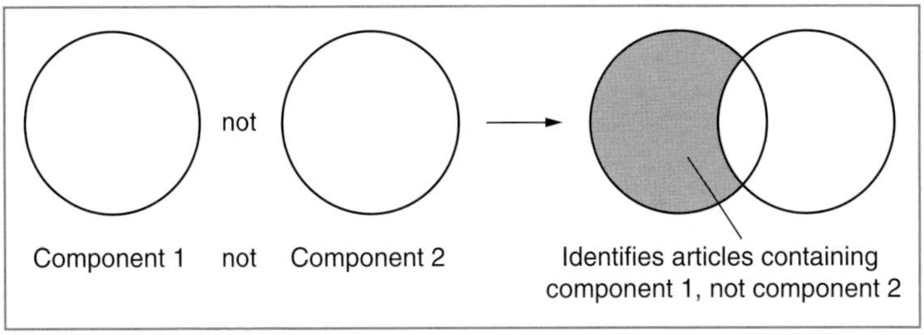

Figure 3.3 The Boolean operator NOT identifies articles containing one specified component but not the other specified component

OR behaviour OR behavior OR education OR relaxation OR hypnotherapy OR hypnosis OR distraction OR diverting attention' will find articles containing at least one of the words/phrases in the list. For question 2, a search for 'ointment OR dressing OR dressings OR cream OR creams OR topical application OR topically applied' will find articles containing at least one of the words/phrases in the list. It is necessary to link all the individual terms/phrases in each word list, using OR, to avoid missing any articles that discuss that specific component.

It is also possible to exclude specific words/phrases from a search, so articles containing them will not be identified. This is done using the term NOT (Figure 3.3). For example, for question 1, a search for 'fear of needles NOT fear of hospitals' will find articles containing the phrase 'fear of needles', which do not also contain the phrase 'fear of hospitals'. For question 2, a search for 'leg ulcer NOT pressure sore' will find articles containing the phrase 'leg ulcer', which do not also contain the phrase 'pressure sore'. Be very cautious when using NOT, as it can inadvertently exclude articles that are relevant to a question.

AND, OR and NOT, in this context, are known as 'Boolean logic operators'.

Additional search tools commonly available

Applying some additional search tools/techniques can help to refine a basic search strategy as developed above.

Truncation

Many databases will retrieve only those records that contain the *exact* word or phrase that you have typed. Truncation is a shortcut device to save time, so that all the different variations of a word do not have to be typed out as part of a search strategy. It works by finding the beginning of a word with any different ending on it. It is often denoted by a * or $ in databases. The 'help' option within the database will explain which symbol should be used for truncation. For example:

- child* would pick up child, children, childhood, etc.
- ulcer$ would pick up ulcer, ulcers, ulceration, ulcerated, etc.

Avoid using truncation after only a few letters at the start of a word – it can pick up more than expected. For example, 'bab*' would pick up baby and babies, but also other words like baboon, babesiosis, babble, babesia, Babinski reflex, etc.

Wildcard

The 'wildcard', available on some databases, allows you to identify alternative spellings of the same word easily. The wildcard is inserted in the middle of a word where an extra letter or alternative letter might be placed. When searched, spellings with any extra letter or different letter in that position will be identified. It is often denoted by a ? in databases. For example:

- an?emia would pick up both anaemia and anemia
- h?emoglobin would pick up both haemoglobin and hemoglobin
- wom?n would pick up both woman and women.

Phrase searching

If, for example, you are looking for articles on *pressure sores*, you will want to avoid retrieving those articles that discuss *pressure* and *sores* separately, as such articles are unlikely to address your information need. In some databases, a search for *pressure sore* will retrieve only those records in which these two words are next to one another (i.e. the database will look for an exact match for the phrase *pressure sore*). However, in other databases, a search for *pressure sore* will retrieve records where the words *pressure* and *sore* appear anywhere in the record, but not necessarily next to each other, thereby increasing the number of irrelevant records retrieved. For these databases, it is necessary to enclose the phrase in quotes ("*pressure sore*") or to use some other technique. The help option within the database will explain which technique to use.

Free text searching

In free text searching, you type words/phrases from your word lists (for one or more components of the question) into the search window, and the database matches these words to records containing the same words anywhere within the abstract, title or author fields (or, in some databases, anywhere within the record). Free text searches usually have a high recall rate (high sensitivity), i.e. large numbers of records are retrieved by the search, but a low precision rate (low specificity), i.e. many of the retrieved records are irrelevant (NHS CRD 2001). This is because any record containing the free text words is retrieved, even if the words are used to discuss a very minor detail within the record.

Index terms

These are keywords that are added onto each journal article, by the database producers, to reflect the main topics covered by that record. Each topic is given just one index term to be used all the time. Index terms are usually quite specific so they accurately reflect the subject matter covered in the record. To illustrate, articles within a specific database that contain the terms breast cancer, breast carcinoma or breast tumour would all be assigned the unique index term: 'breast neoplasm'. It does not matter which words the authors of an article use to describe the topic; if the research investigates breast cancer, it will always be labelled with the index term 'breast neoplasm', within that database. Each journal article will be assigned one or more index terms, to reflect the key topics covered by that article.

This can aid searching, because instead of having to think of every way a component in a search could be described, as with free text searching, the appropriate index term can be used instead. It also means that journal articles that mention a topic only in passing are not identified. This is because index terms are assigned only to those topics which form a large part of the record.

A search that uses just index terms to find articles containing matching index terms is known as a search on 'controlled vocabulary'. A disadvantage of searching on controlled vocabulary is that any records that have not been appropriately indexed might be missed by the search.

Thesaurus

A thesaurus is a collection of all the index terms used by a database producer. It is usually a fairly complex listing, split into different subject areas with a hierarchical structure. A thesaurus can identify index terms of interest and, in some databases, the hierarchy structure can be used to search a range of index terms in one go. More information is given on p.75, under 'Tips for advanced users'.

Combined free text and controlled vocabulary (index) searching

Some databases automatically match free text search terms to appropriate index terms, thereby retrieving records through a combination of free text and controlled vocabulary searching. The help section of the database will clarify whether or not this is done.

Where to search first

Having clarified a question and identified the words necessary to search for relevant information, the next step is to identify the resources most likely to contain relevant articles, and to consider the order in which they should be searched.

In recognition that detailed research publications can be difficult to digest, especially within the context of a busy clinical setting, Haynes (2001) describes a hierarchy of sources of evidence that places publications that 'integrate and concisely summarise all relevant and important research evidence about a clinical problem' at the top. These frequently updated publications should ideally provide exactly enough information (no more, no less) to facilitate clinical decision making (Haynes 2001). The types of resources at this level might include *Clinical Evidence* (see below) and good-quality evidence-based guidelines, i.e. those that have used a systematic approach to identify, appraise and synthesise best evidence and to reach clinical recommendations based on that evidence. In an ideal world, these resources would be linked to the patient's record and would serve as reminders whenever the record was accessed, but we have some way to go before this becomes a reality. At the next level are *synopses of systematic reviews*, reporting only essential information in a format that allows the reader to quickly ascertain the quality of the study (the synopsis includes a quality appraisal) and its key messages. Full-text *systematic reviews*, at the next level in the hierarchy, can be retrieved where more information is required or where there is no relevant synopsis. If, at this stage, no good-quality publications have been found, then *synopses of individual studies* or, failing that, full-text *individual studies* are looked for. Individual studies are at the bottom of the hierarchy because they don't have the 'added value' of the integrated, summarised and critically appraised resources.

The overall aim in searching is to find good-quality, valid evidence to support your clinical decision making, so regardless of the hierarchical level of the retrieved evidence, it will need careful assessing for quality.

Summaries of best available evidence/ evidence-based guidelines

Clinical Evidence provides concise summaries of the best available evidence from systematic reviews, trials and observational studies for a broad array of conditions, and if there is no good evidence, it says so (*Clinical Evidence* 2006). *Clinical Evidence* is produced as a full-text print book and as a concise book (with directions to the internet for full-text access). It is also available in electronic format (for example, via the National Library for Health to NHS Employees in England at www.library.nhs.uk or at www. clinicalevidence.com/ceweb/conditions/index.jsp).

The Joanna Briggs Institute in Australia presents summaries of best practice for a variety of clinical topics relevant to nursing. Its *Best Practice Information Sheets* can be accessed at www.joannabriggs.edu.au/pubs/ best_practice.php

Examples of organisations producing guidelines with explicit, rigorous methods include the Scottish Intercollegiate Guidelines Network (SIGN: www.sign.ac.uk) and the National Institute for Health and Clinical Excellence (NICE: www.nice.org.uk). Guidelines are generated by many different health-care organisations and professional bodies, so use of a guideline searching tool, such as the NLH Guideline Finder (www.library.nhs.uk) or the National Guideline Clearinghouse (from the US Agency for Healthcare Research and Quality: www.guideline.gov) can be extremely helpful in tracking down good-quality guidelines. Guideline resources might have a specialised focus (for example, the PRODIGY guidelines (www.prodigy. nhs.uk/ClinicalGuidance) are aimed at primary health-care professionals) whilst others are more generic (see, for example, *Health Evidence Bulletins Wales* at hebw.cf.ac.uk).

Synopses of evidence

The Knowledge Library within *Bandolier* (www.jr2.ox.ac.uk/Bandolier/ index.html) is a collection of abstracted information from good-quality systematic reviews or individual studies, grouped according to clinical topic. Each report contains additional information, compiled by the team at *Bandolier*, about the importance of the study and/or what it means in terms of clinical practice.

The journal *Evidence-Based Nursing* (ebn.bmjjournals.com) provides research abstracts and expert commentary on the clinical application of research studies that have met certain quality criteria, and that are applicable to nursing practice. Other such journals include *Evidence-Based Medicine*, *Evidence-Based Mental Health* and *Evidence-Based Dentistry*.

To search these resources all in one go, you could use the 'TRIP database', an internet resource discussed on p.84, under 'Search systems on the internet'.

Systematic reviews

Systematic reviews use systematic and explicit methods to identify, select, critically appraise and synthesise the available research evidence pertinent to a specified question (see Chapter 7 for more information). If a systematic review addresses your question, then you are saved the effort of searching for individual studies, ascertaining the quality and findings of those studies, and pulling together (often contradictory) results from the individual studies. If you do find a relevant systematic review, you will of course need to appraise it for methodological quality, clinical importance and applicability, but appraising one systematic review is easier than appraising and assimilating the data from numerous studies.

The Cochrane Library

The first place to check for systematic reviews in health care is in the Cochrane Library. The Cochrane Library is not a standard bibliographic database but is, rather, a collection of separate databases (hence its title 'library'), all of which can be accessed from the opening screen of the Cochrane Library (Figure 3.4). The most useful databases for identifying systematic reviews are the *Cochrane Database of Systematic Reviews (CDSR)* and the *Database of Abstracts of Reviews of Effects (DARE)*. CDSR contains the full text of systematic reviews done through the auspices of the Cochrane Collaboration. These reviews focus on the effectiveness of health-care interventions and so are primarily reviews of studies which are randomised controlled trials (RCTs), the 'gold standard' for ascertaining the effectiveness of an intervention (see Chapters 2 and 4). DARE contains structured abstracts and critical appraisals of systematic reviews, of studies of any design, that are completed by groups outside the Cochrane Collaboration. When searching for a systematic review on the effectiveness of a health-care intervention, it is sensible to search CDSR before searching DARE. Systematic reviews on CDSR, i.e. those carried out by members of the Cochrane Collaboration, are subject to rigorous peer review prior to publication and are updated at intervals to incorporate current research evidence.

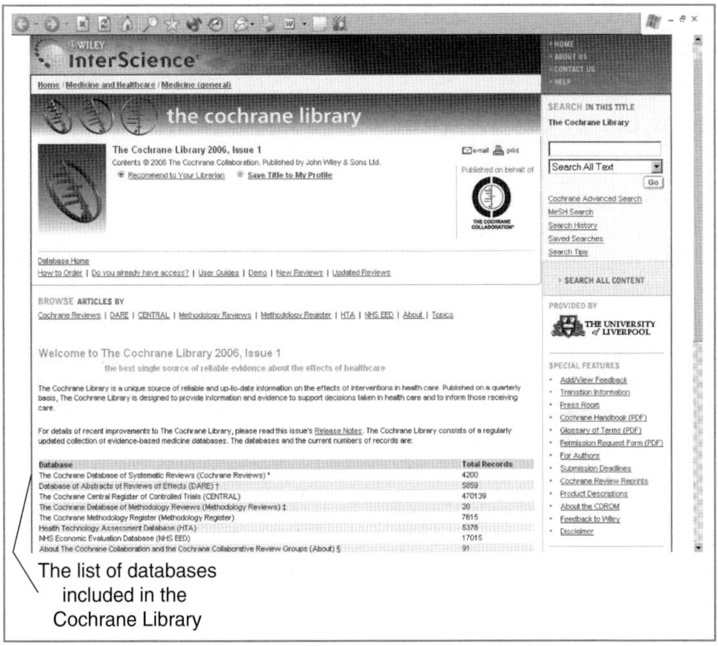

The list of databases
included in the
Cochrane Library

Figure 3.4 The opening screen of the Cochrane Library CD-ROM (from John Wiley & Sons Ltd., reproduced with permission)

The Cochrane Library also includes the *Cochrane Central Register of Controlled Trials (CENTRAL)*. This is not a resource for systematic reviews; rather it is a comprehensive bibliographic database of randomised controlled trials (and possible randomised controlled trials) in health care. If no systematic reviews are found to answer the question of interest, and if the optimum study design for the question is the randomised controlled trial (see Chapters 2 and 4 for more information), then this is an excellent source of evidence. The other databases on the Cochrane Library present information on health technology assessments, economic evaluations of health-care interventions and systematic review methodology.

The Cochrane Library is produced as a CD-ROM and is also available on the internet. Most UK hospitals tend to have access to the internet version via national NHS gateway websites, like the National Library for Health. A detailed user guide and other teaching materials for the internet version are available from the website (www3.interscience.wiley.com/cgi-bin/mrwhome/106568753/userguides.html). Many hospital libraries will also

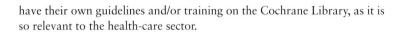

have their own guidelines and/or training on the Cochrane Library, as it is so relevant to the health-care sector.

Bayes Library of Diagnostic Studies and Reviews

The proposed Bayes Library of Diagnostic Studies and Reviews, soon to become available, is composed of two databases: the *Bayes Database of Diagnostic Reviews*, containing structured summaries of systematic reviews of diagnostic studies that have been critically appraised, so a useful first port of call when searching for diagnostic evidence; and the *Bayes Diagnostic Studies Register*, a collection of diagnostic studies identified from other databases such as MEDLINE, EMBASE and specialist databases (Pewsner et al 2002). The Library will cover clinical examinations, medical history taking, X-rays, laboratory tests, ward-based tests and other investigations. It is envisaged that it will be included within the Cochrane Library. Further information about the proposed Library is available at www.medepi.net/meta/guidelines/BAYES_Library.pdf.

The Campbell Collaboration

For evidence-based questions that cross into more social or behavioural oriented interventions, there are the resources of the Campbell Collaboration. This is a 'sister' organisation to the Cochrane Collaboration and its role is very similar, except that it is interested in the effects of interventions that fall into the social, behavioural or educational arenas. The Campbell Collaboration undertakes systematic reviews of studies assessing these sorts of interventions.

The C2 Library refers to the Campbell Collaboration's collection of two databases: the C2 *Reviews of Interventions and Policy Evaluations (C2-RIPE)* database which is the collection of systematic reviews undertaken by the Collaboration, and which places reviews into one of four categories: education, crime and justice, social welfare and methods; and the C2 *Social, Psychological, Education and Criminology Trials Registry (C2-SPECTR)*, a collection of RCTs and possible RCTs on relevant behavioural/educational interventions. Both databases are available via the Campbell Collaboration website (www.campbellcollaboration.org/Fralibrary.html).

Other ways of tracking down this evidence

Additional internet resources, such as TRIP, SUMSearch and OMNI, can be used to find summaries of research evidence for health care. These are described in the section on 'Search systems on the internet' (p.84).

Where to search next

If there are no good-quality summaries of evidence, evidence-based guidelines, synopses or systematic reviews that already answer a question, or if some extra 'top-up' searching is required, the next place to look is in standard bibliographic databases that contain details of a wide range of journal articles.

In the health-care/nursing field there are plenty of databases of interest. For example:

- the Cochrane Central Register of Controlled Trials (CENTRAL) (discussed above)
- MEDLINE (a general medical database, produced in the USA)
- CINAHL (Cumulative Index of Nursing and Allied Health Literature, a general nursing database, produced in the USA)
- EMBASE (a general medical database, produced in Europe; more foreign language material)
- BNI (British Nursing Index, a general nursing database)
- Topic-specific databases such as PsycInfo, a database of abstracts of psychological literature.

See Appendix 3.1 (p.91) for further information.

All these databases are produced by different companies/organisations so they will often look different and contain different information, the specific searching tools available may vary and there will be variation between CD-ROM, internet and 'online' versions.

Which databases you choose to search will depend on factors such as:

- the specific subject of a search
- availability
- how easy/difficult it is to search.

It is helpful to find out as much as possible about any databases that are available (check search tools, etc.) and to do a quick test search to see how useful they are in practice.

Always make a note of which database(s) are searched, the years/date searched, the version(s), and the search terms used, for each question or project that is undertaken. This is particularly useful if, at any time in the future, the search is to be rerun. It also serves as a reminder of how extensive the search was.

An example search on the MEDLINE database (PubMed version)

This next section looks at the process of undertaking a search on the MEDLINE database. MEDLINE is available in a variety of versions including PubMed, OVID, Dialogue and Silver Platter. We have used the PubMed version in our example. PubMed is developed by the National Center for Biotechnology Information at the US National Library of Medicine, and can be accessed free of charge at www.ncbi.nlm.nih.gov/entrez/query.fcgi. PubMed provides numerous methods of searching, only some of which are described below. For further information on using this database, click on the the Help/FAQ (frequently asked questions)/Tutorial links located on the sidebar of the PubMed screen (see Figure 3.5). The tutorial offers

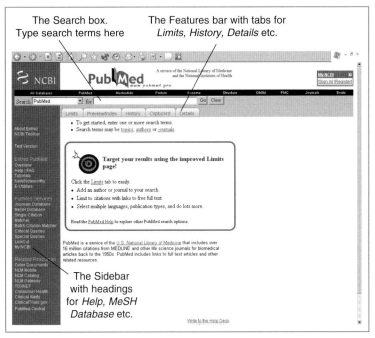

Figure 3.5 The home page for PubMed (from PubMed, US National Library of Medicine)

an interactive training programme. Most health-care databases provide detailed information on search techniques, so you should find it easy to adapt the process described below to any database.

The home page for PubMed is shown in Figure 3.5. Question 1 from the Basic search principles section (Box 3.1) is used in building a search specifically designed for PubMed. Some controlled vocabulary searching, using index terms, as well as free text searching is used.

Step 1: checking what search tools are available

First check the search tools available in the database. This will usually be under the help information in the database (look for a 'help' button or heading). Check which words the database uses for Boolean logic. They are often AND, OR and NOT, but not always. Check also whether they are case sensitive (i.e. whether or not you need to use capital letters). Check for the symbols used for truncation and the wildcard, if available, and check whether a phrase has to be specified in any way, for example by using quotation marks.

In PubMed, the Boolean operators are AND, OR and NOT (upper case); the truncation symbol is *; phrases should be enclosed in double quotes.

Step 2: using the thesaurus

To make use of any indexing terms in a search, it is necessary to identify those terms that correspond to the concepts identified in your question, using the thesaurus.

The thesaurus in PubMed is known as the MeSH® (Medical Subject Headings) thesaurus. MeSH® is a registered trademark of the United States National Library of Medicine. In PubMed, free text terms are automatically matched to appropriate MeSH (index) terms (where available), provided truncation is not used. So, a search using free text terms will automatically retrieve records containing the exact typed words/phrases as well as records containing the relevant MeSH (index) terms. When using truncation, which 'turns off' the automatic matching of MeSH terms to free text terms, you will need to manually select the relevant MeSH terms from the thesaurus, which can be viewed by clicking on MeSH Database in the sidebar (see Step 4 for more information).

In other databases, to view the thesaurus it may be necessary to type the search term into the search box, 'turn on' a matching (mapping) facility by ticking the appropriate box, click on Search or Go and scroll down the displayed list to find relevant index term(s). It is usually possible to click on the index term to get an exact definition/description of that term. If a useful match for a concept is found, make a note of it, so it can be used in the search. Sometimes there will not be a convenient index term available, so stop searching if nothing is identified after looking up a number of different descriptions.

Where time restrictions call for a search with a high precision rate (i.e. with few irrelevant records), and where it is less important that all records are retrieved, then a search using index terms only can be conducted. In PubMed, this is done by building the search in the MeSH Database using the methods described in Step 4.

Step 3: getting a search ready

Having checked through the details of the search tools and found some useful index terms to use, add that information into the written words/phrases list already prepared. It is a good idea to have a written plan to keep track of the search terms that will be typed into the search box, as well as the symbols that will be used. In this way, mistakes are less likely to be made.

The standard way of doing this is to write out the search as a series of steps, each step starting on a new line, with each new line being numbered. The final line of the search should bring together the combination of words you wish to find in the journal articles. This is also the standard format used for entering searches into a database (Boxes 3.3 and 3.4).

In Boxes 3.3 and 3.4, the Boolean operators, and the MeSH terms that were manually selected, have been written in capital letters.

Step 4: entering your search strategy onto the database

At this point the search strategy is ready to be entered. Type the first line of your written strategy into the blank search box (leaving out the line number at the beginning as this will be added automatically). Once it is typed in, click on Go. The database will look for any journal articles containing the words/phrases specified. In PubMed, which automatically maps free text terms to index terms, it is possible to view exactly which terms the database has searched by clicking the Details tab in the features bar (Figure 3.6).

BOX 3.3 Search plan for question 1

#1   fear OR phobia
#2   needles OR syringes OR injections OR injection OR hypodermic OR
      hypodermics
#3   #1 AND #2
#4   hypnotherapy OR hypnosis OR psychotherapy OR behavioural OR
      behavioral
#5   behaviour OR behavior OR education OR coping skills OR
      counselling
#6   relaxation OR distraction OR divert attention OR diversion
#7   #4 OR #5 OR #6
#8   #3 AND #7
#9   stress OR fear OR anxiety
#10   relief OR alleviation OR alleviated OR reduced OR reduction
#11   #9 AND #10
#12   calm OR relaxed
#13   #11 OR #12
#14   #8 AND #13

BOX 3.4 New enhanced search strategy for question 1, specially written for
PubMed

#1   fear or phobi*
#2   PHOBIC DISORDERS
#3   #1 OR #2
#4   syringe* OR needle* OR injection* OR hypodermic*
#5   SYRINGES OR NEEDLES OR INJECTIONS
#6   #4 OR #5
#7   hypnosis OR hypnotherapy OR psychotherapy OR behaviour OR behavior
#8   behavioural OR behavioral OR counsel* OR "coping skills" OR relax*
#9   distract* OR "divert* attention" OR diversion
#10   COUNSELING OR ADAPTATION, PSYCHOLOGICAL
#11   RELAXATION TECHNIQUES OR BEHAVIOR THERAPY
#12   #7 OR #8 OR #9 OR #10 OR #11
#13   stress OR fear OR anxiety
#14   relief OR relieve* OR alleviat* OR reduce* OR reduction
#15   #13 AND #14
#16   calm* OR relax*

#17   #15 OR #16
#18   #3 AND #6
#19   #12 AND #17
#20   #18 AND #19

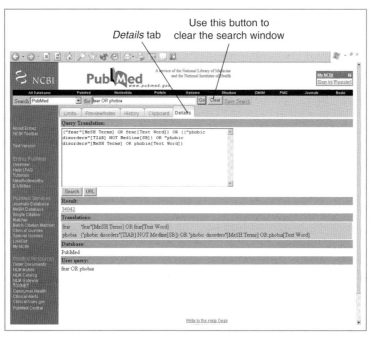

Figure 3.6 The Details tab in the features bar showing exactly which free text and which MeSH terms have been searched (from PubMed, US National Library of Medicine)

You can type the next line of the written search into the search box even if the Details page (or any other page shown on the features bar) is open. First, clear the search box using the Clear button (shown in Figure 3.6). This action does not lose the search: each line of the search will be retained.

To manually add relevant MeSH terms to the search (for example, if you have turned off the automatic matching feature by using truncation), click on the MeSH Database link in the sidebar, type a word/phrase in the search box and click Go, then select the appropriate MeSH term(s) from the terms offered by ticking the relevant boxes (Figure 3.7). Click on Send

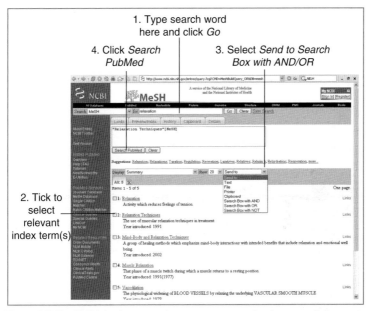

Figure 3.7 The MeSH database is used to construct a search using controlled vocabulary (from PubMed, US National Library of Medicine)

to Search Box with AND or Send to Search Box with OR (depending on which Boolean operator is to be used), then, once all selected terms are in the search box, click on Search PubMed.

To view each line of the search (i.e. the search history), click the History tab in the Features bar (Figure 3.8). As shown in Figure 3.8, each line has automatically been assigned a number (#1, #2, etc.) Don't worry if, as in our search, the numbers are not consecutive or do not start at #1. To combine the lines of the search, type the relevant line numbers, and the appropriate Boolean operators, into the search window (having first clicked the History tab). Continue building the search strategy to replicate, line by line (apart from the numbering), the written search plan. Figure 3.8 shows a completed search. The final line of the search (in this example, line #32) brings together the journal articles that hopefully address the question. Our search has identified 201 articles, some of which might be irrelevant. To view the identified references, click on the final line of the search in the Results column (Figure 3.8).

To restrict the retrieved references to, for example, English language articles and to studies conducted in humans only, click the Limits tab on

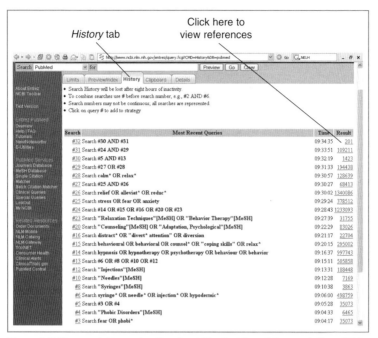

Figure 3.8 The search history for Question 1. The final line of the search (line #32) has retrieved 201 articles (from PubMed, US National Library of Medicine)

the features bar and select the appropriate limits from the available options (Figure 3.9). By applying these limits to our search, the number of identified articles was reduced from 201 to 67. A tick will appear on the Limits tab to remind you that you have limited the search (not shown in Figure 3.9). To remove the limits (for example, to search additional terms for which the limits do not apply), simply delete the tick from the Limits tab.

Depending on how many references are in that final group, they can be viewed, and selected, one by one on screen, but it is often preferable to print them out or to save them to your computer so that you can sift through them at your leisure. Look for a 'print' button or a 'save/download' button to do this. There is usually the choice of which references to print/save and the specific fields to be included.

In PubMed, you can save the identified references in My NCBI (provided you have signed into My NCBI before starting the search). Check the 'help information' for full details. Another option is to save the references directly to your computer as shown in Figure 3.10. Click on the drop-down

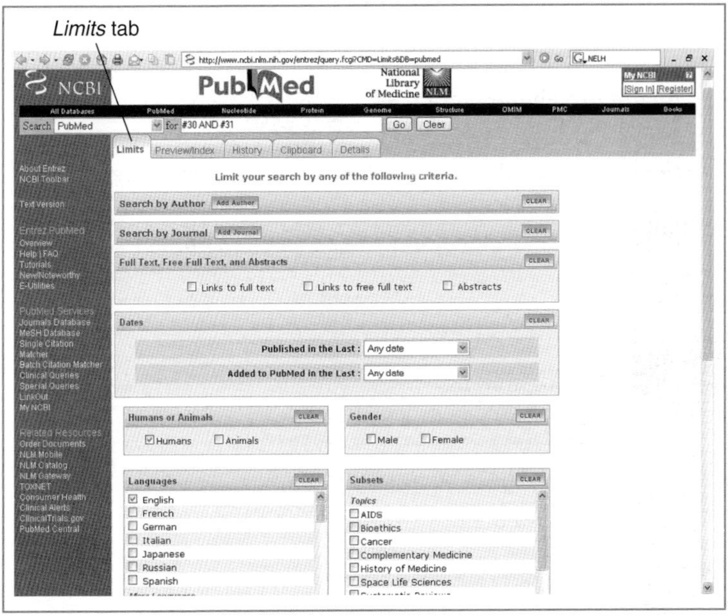

Limits tab

Figure 3.9 The Limits feature (from PubMed, US National Library of Medicine)

box next to the Display button to select the required format (for example, a summary list of references as shown in Figure 3.10 or, preferably, a list of references accompanied by their abstracts). Next, click the Send to box, and select File. You will then be asked where, on your computer, you would like to save the file. To print the references, click the Send to box, then select Printer, having first chosen the required display format.

This completes the procedure for doing a basic search on PubMed.

Common queries regarding searching

In what order should search terms be typed/ listed in a search strategy?

There are no strict rules on how a search should be typed in or written out. Things can be done in any order; words/phrases can be split up, so there are more lines in a search, or lumped together so there are fewer lines overall. As long as the logic of each step is correct and it arrives at the same final combination of words in the last line, the result should be the same.

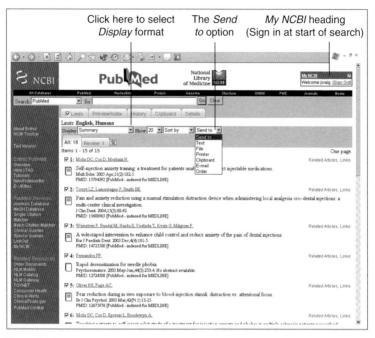

Figure 3.10 Save references in My NCBI, or on your computer using Send to File. To print, select Send to Printer (from PubMed, US National Library of Medicine)

Is it better to use free text or controlled vocabulary (index terms)?

Which should be used depends on the search to be done. Controlled vocabulary using index terms is more accurate, because there is less need to think about all the different terminology that could be used to describe an illness or population, etc. Also, it limits the number of irrelevant articles identified. Where a database has controlled vocabulary, it is best to try and use it if possible. If a more thorough search is required, both types need to be used (as index terms can be assigned incorrectly).

Out of interest, we repeated the search above, but this time we used index terms only where available. Thirty eight articles were identified, compared with the 201 identified when using a combination of free text and index terms. The search using index terms only, yielded the greater proportion of relevant articles.

How do you know when all the relevant journal articles in a database have been found?

Unfortunately, there is no way to know if everything of interest has been found or not. Most bibliographic databases expand very quickly to contain thousands of articles, because there are so many journal papers being published and added to the databases all the time. No one can keep track of precisely the subjects being covered. The idea of searching is to maximise the relevant articles that are found, whilst at the same time minimising the irrelevant material.

Finding 'most' of the useful information in a database is the best that can be hoped for. Searching is a pragmatic exercise and there is always the possibility that something will have been missed unintentionally, regardless of the experience of the searcher.

What do you do if you can't find any relevant articles?

This is often a problem when searching for evidence; there may be no references at all or only items of poor quality. In this situation it can be helpful to go 'back to the beginning' and look at the question and search strategy again. Devising a search strategy is a trial and error process and even experienced searchers will reconsider their approach a number of times, if they struggle to find any useful results. It is not unusual for a 'final' search strategy to require a few attempts before it is generated.

There will be occasions, however, when in spite of trying a range of strategies or resources, no high-quality information is forthcoming and the best available evidence is expert opinion.

Tips for more advanced users

There are a number of further tools and additional ways to prepare a strategy that will help to manage different search results.

Proximity operators

Some database systems have tools available that allow searching for a number of words in the same sentence or paragraph, etc. Some systems allow you to specify exactly how close two words need to be (e.g. within six words of each other). These are called proximity operators.

For example, a database may use WITH to find words/phrases contained in the same sentence and NEAR to find words/phrases contained in the same paragraph. The search 'midwife WITH care team' would find articles containing at least one sentence with both midwife and care team in it, and 'sickle cell NEAR leg ulcer' would find articles containing a paragraph with both sickle cell and leg ulcer in it.

These sorts of tools are most useful in databases where the majority of records have an abstract or summary.

Limiting to specific fields

Most database systems allow searches for information in the specific 'fields' of each journal article. This enables searches for words only in the title, articles by a specific author, or in a certain journal. Most systems tend to give each field in any article an abbreviated code, which can be used when searching. Check the 'help information' in a database to find out about the limiting options and how to select them.

To illustrate, in databases where the codes TI, AU, SO and AB are used to identify the fields Title, Author, Source and Abstract, the search 'injections[TI]' would find articles with the word 'injections' in the title field, 'Bloggs.au' would find articles with the word Bloggs in the author field, and 'nurse in SO' would find articles with the word nurse in the source field.

In PubMed, the search can be limited to a specific field either by adding the code (tag) using square brackets (for example, type 'Bloggs[AU]' in the search box) or by clicking the Limits tab on the features bar and selecting the appropriate Tag Term.

Using the thesaurus

As well as helping to identify index terms of interest, a thesaurus can also allow searching of a group of related index terms in one go. For example, if you were interested in treatments for leg ulcers, you may find a number of indexing terms that are of interest listed in the thesaurus, for example, 'leg ulcers', 'leg pressure sores', 'diabetic foot ulcers', 'foot ulcers', etc. Each of these terms could be added separately into a search strategy, but it would save time if all the indexing terms related to leg ulcers could be added in one step. This is possible in many thesauri because index terms are listed in a hierarchy.

Basic structure of a thesaurus

A thesaurus orders index terms into hierarchical lists, with general terms (like dermatology, surgery, orthopaedics, community care, etc.) at the top and more precise, specific terms (on the same subject) underneath (like psoriasis, keyhole surgery, fractured neck of femur, etc.). When written out, these lists are often called tree structures (the lists 'branch out' rather like a tree). For example, Box 3.5 shows what a section of a medical/health-care thesaurus might look like. Terms at the top of a list are called 'broader terms' and those indented underneath are known as 'narrower' terms. In the example in Box 3.5, 'haemoglobinopathies' is a broader term than 'thalassaemia' and 'sickle cell anaemia', whereas 'thalassaemia' and 'sickle cell anaemia' are narrower terms of 'haemoglobinopathies'. Following the same pattern, 'haemoglobinopathies' is a narrower term of 'blood disorders'.

Exploding index terms

To find all the information related to 'blood', for example, a search should be done on the index term 'blood' and all the other blood-related conditions

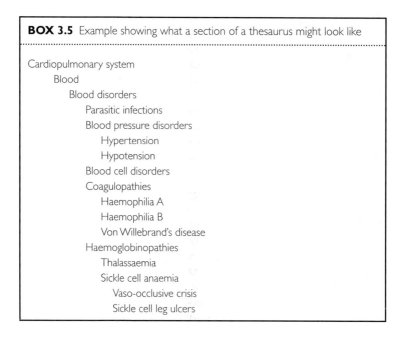

BOX 3.5 Example showing what a section of a thesaurus might look like

```
Cardiopulmonary system
    Blood
        Blood disorders
            Parasitic infections
            Blood pressure disorders
                Hypertension
                Hypotension
            Blood cell disorders
            Coagulopathies
                Haemophilia A
                Haemophilia B
                Von Willebrand's disease
            Haemoglobinopathies
                Thalassaemia
                Sickle cell anaemia
                    Vaso-occlusive crisis
                    Sickle cell leg ulcers
```

or issues in the index as well. This involves searching for blood and all its narrower terms in the thesaurus. To do this in one step is called 'exploding' an index term. By highlighting 'blood' in the thesaurus of the database and then selecting the 'explode' button (before pressing the 'search' button) the search will automatically search 'blood' and all the narrower terms indented underneath it. For example, returning to the section of the thesaurus in the previous example, to search for anything on blood disorders, exploding the index term 'blood disorders' would automatically search the following index terms:

```
Blood disorders
    Parasitic infections
    Blood pressure disorders
        Hypertension
        Hypotension
    Blood cell disorders
    Coagulopathies
        Haemophilia A
        Haemophilia B
        Von Willebrand's disease
    Haemoglobinopathies
        Thalassaemia
        Sickle cell anaemia
            Vaso-occlusive crisis
            Sickle cell leg ulcers
```

The 'explode' function picks up everything *beneath and indented to the right* of the exploded term. Exploding 'blood pressure disorders' would include 'hypertension' and 'hypotension', but would not pick up 'blood cell disorders', 'coagulopathies' or 'haemoglobinopathies'. This is because they are directly under 'blood pressure disorders' and not indented to the right.

In PubMed, MeSH terms are automatically exploded, unless you choose to avoid this option by activating the 'Do not explode this term' button in the MeSH Database (Figure 3.11).

Subheadings

To help make an index term even more precise, or tailored to a specific aspect, some systems include an option to search an index term with certain

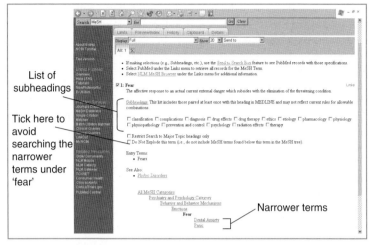

List of subheadings

Tick here to avoid searching the narrower terms under 'fear'

Narrower terms

Figure 3.11 The thesaurus screen showing the tree structure for the MeSH term 'fear' (from PubMed, US National Library of Medicine)

subheadings attached. Subheadings are generally categories such as diagnosis, prevention, adverse reactions, complications, epidemiology, prognosis, surgery, etc. When an index term is assigned to an article, any appropriate subheadings will be linked to the term as well. If it is certain that the search only needs to focus on a narrow aspect of an index term, choosing the appropriate subheading(s) (rather than all of them) will limit the search to just the index term with that subheading attached. In PubMed, the subheadings can be viewed in the MeSH database (Figure 3.11).

Saving search strategies

Many database systems allow a completed search history to be saved, so the search can be run again, without having to type everything out all over again. Whilst this may not be a problem for short searches, once a search builds up a number of lines it can be very helpful to use this facility. In PubMed, the search history can be saved indefinitely using My NCBI. This requires that you sign into My NCBI before constructing the search. Check the 'help information' for more information.

Too many or too few articles

If too many articles are found it may be necessary to narrow down a search to make it more accurate. Use more precise index terms or link them to specific subheadings or perhaps search over a fewer number of years. It may be necessary to break up a broad subject into a series of questions, so the volume of information available can be better managed.

If only a few articles of interest are found, it may be necessary to widen out a search, so it is not so precise. Use broader index terms linked to all subheadings, or more general free text terms. If information is required on a very specific question, a low search result could mean little research has been done on that exact topic. It may be necessary to go back to the original question to see if it can be expanded.

When to stop searching

This very much depends on the objectives of a search. If a comprehensive literature review/survey is required, it needs to be very thorough, so a number of different databases should be searched to get as much useful material as possible. If a few conflicting articles are required on a topic to get an 'evidence base' debate going or to stimulate discussion about treatment options, etc., a quick search on one database may be quite sufficient. If a good-quality, up-to-date evidence-based guideline, synopsis of evidence or a systematic review has been identified, searching may be stopped.

The amount of searching done will also be influenced by the resources that are available: the time and databases available, the number of people involved in searching, etc. If comprehensive searches are done on a number of different databases, there will be gradually diminishing returns. The same journal articles will reappear each time and the volume of new articles identified will decrease. There will come a point when the effort involved in searching is not worth the tiny reward of new material found.

There is no right or wrong answer on when to stop searching. As with many aspects of the search process, it is a pragmatic decision. The main thing is to be explicit about which databases have been searched. This avoids any confusion and allows a search to be accurately updated or expanded by looking in different databases.

Searching for a systematic review

Completing a systematic review is increasingly becoming part of higher degree courses and specialist training programmes. Systematic reviews done in these settings will be restricted by time and the resources available.

This is true for the searching component of the review, as well as the other parts. The searching required to complete a piece of coursework will be a lot less than that required to do a comprehensive systematic review in earnest. However, there are still a few issues to consider that may enhance a standard search.

Unpublished information

There is an increasing awareness that not all good-quality research work is published in professional journals. For various reasons, much interesting research is not reported in this way. In order to try to identify as many relevant studies as possible, there is often a requirement when undertaking a systematic review to go through conference proceedings, theses or project reports, etc. to see if any additional information can be found. Also, many journals are not included in electronic databases. If there is a journal that covers research relevant to a review but that is not included in the databases being searched, it may necessitate going through issues of the journal by hand.

This sort of extra work cannot be done when time is restricted. However, the Cochrane Collaboration has a commitment to try and find unpublished RCTs, so its review groups search conference proceedings and go through journals by hand in an effort to do this. Any extra RCTs found in this way are published on the CCTR/CENTRAL database on the Cochrane Library. This means that searching this database on the Cochrane Library provides a quick and practical solution for finding unpublished information for a review.

Research in progress

Another aspect of searching in a systematic review is the need to identify any research that is in progress or about to be completed that could be relevant to the review. The main resource in this area for UK-based clinical research is the National Research Register (NRR) produced by the Department of Health (DoH). It aims to contain details of all the research being undertaken in the NHS, to help keep track of what is going on and to avoid any unnecessary duplication. Also from the DoH is the Research Findings Register (ReFeR), which provides information on the results of DoH-funded research projects as they are just completed. There are also various lists appearing on the internet covering research in progress, such as the Current Controlled Trials site, which aims to identify RCTs that are under way. Having a quick look at these sorts of resources adds another aspect to a systematic review search.

The NRR can be found at: www.update-software.com/National/
(It is also issued as a CD-ROM, so may be available in hospital libraries or net-worked onto hospital PCs.)
ReFeR can be found at: www.refer.nhs.uk/ViewWebPage.asp?Page=Home
Current Controlled Trials can be found at: http://controlled-trials.com

Searching for an extensive systematic review

Undertaking the search for a fully fledged systematic review (with funding, longer time-scale, etc.) is not something that should be done lightly. It does require a lot of searching experience and knowledge of available resources. Budgeting is necessary to ensure all searching-related activities can be completed (obtaining and translating articles, as well as accessing databases) and the time-scale must allow for searching any conferences or journal titles by hand.

More information on this type of extensive searching can be found in:

- CRD Report 4 – *Undertaking systematic reviews of research on effectiveness. CRD's guidance for those carrying out or commissioning reviews*, 2nd edition 2001. Stage II, Phase 3: Identification of research; Appendix I: Literature searching. www.york.ac.uk/inst/crd/report4.htm
- *Cochrane handbook for systematic reviews of interventions*, Version 1.2.4 (5: Locating and Selecting Studies). Available on the Cochrane Library internet site: www3.interscience.wiley.com/cgi-bin/mrwhome/106568753/HOME (via the Cochrane Handbook (PDF) link, under 'For authors') and also available on the Cochrane Library CD-ROM
- NHS CRD Information Service – *Finding studies for systematic reviews: a checklist for researchers* (updated December 2004). www.york.ac.uk/inst/crd/revs.htm

BOX 3.6 Key points to remember about searching electronic databases

1. Get help
   Attend training sessions in hospital/university libraries. Find out about support for searching in general.
2. Prepare the search
   Sort out the question/topic, generate word lists, have a draft search planned.

3. Find out more
   What database(s) might be useful to search, what tools they have (truncation, thesaurus, etc.), how those tools are used – check the 'help' information
   and any written guidelines.
4. Decide which database to search
   Plan so that you search resources in order of usefulness. Do a brief test
   search, check ease of searching, make sure all useful information is available.
5. Prepare the final search strategy
   Add in index terms, truncation symbols, etc. for the database to be searched.
6. Do the search
   Select index terms, type in free text terms. Get the final set of useful records
   at the end.
7. Print or save the final set of articles
   Print/save the records to look at later on.
8. Keep a record of the resources searched
   Make a note of the database, the version used (Ovid CD-ROM, SilverPlatter
   on the internet, etc.), the years searched and the date the search was done.
9. Keep a record of the search strategy
   Make sure a copy is kept, so the exact details are available for future
   reference.
10. If searching for systematic review, access sources of unpublished and ongoing
    research.

The internet

The internet is often referred to as the 'worldwide web' and it is useful to
think of it in this way to illustrate its positive and negative aspects. Like a
spider on its web, the internet can provide an invisible link between isolated
points, enabling seamless travel to relevant sources without having to follow laborious routes; allowing movement from resource to resource and
back again easily and quickly. However, the internet can also appear to be
an unrelated tangle of too much information – just as a web is a trap for an
unwary fly. There are so many sites of possible interest that it is easy to get
completely lost and overwhelmed. The internet can be a very confusing and
frustrating tool to use, as well as an extremely useful collection of information resources.

The other issue of concern is the lack of quality control. The internet is not
owned or governed by any one company or organisation. Any individual
with the appropriate expertise and equipment can create a 'web page' and

make it available on the internet. There is no registration required, no standards that have to be met and nobody has to be informed. Web pages appear and disappear all the time. People can choose to provide accurate, useful and honest web pages, or not. Hence the concern over offensive, illegal and deliberately misleading information that can appear on the worldwide web. The internet is a vast international collection of information and misinformation that people choose to make available.

Searching the internet

To undertake an organised search for journal articles, use the same sort of bibliographic databases as those discussed in the rest of the chapter. This means using the internet versions of databases (some of which need to be paid for). MEDLINE is the main database that is available free of charge on the internet. PubMed is the version which comes direct from the creators of MEDLINE (the National Library of Medicine in the USA), but there are a number of other versions that are available. Hospital/university libraries should be able to advise about any bibliographic databases they subscribe to on the internet.

Search systems on the internet

In the area of evidence-based health-care information, there are some useful search systems which search websites that list articles and other publications related to evidence-based health care.

TRIP (Turning Research into Practice) database

TRIP searches a broad range of evidence-based health-care related websites including *Effective Healthcare Bulletins*, NHS CRD Reports, *Bandolier*, the Cochrane Library databases, the *Evidence-Based Journals* and many others. The search screen is very simple to use. Just type in the word or phrase to be identified and when the search has been completed, a list of Results by Category (evidence based, guidelines, medical images, etc.) is displayed. Choose a category and a list of relevant items is presented, with the name of the resource in which they were found. Click on items one by one to view them. Users are currently allowed five free searches; for more extensive access, a subscription is required. The TRIP database can be searched at: www.tripdatabase.com/

SUMSearch

This is a search system devised by the University of Texas, Health Science Center at San Antonio. When search term(s) are typed in, this system will automatically check (internet versions of) MEDLINE, DARE, the National Guideline Clearinghouse from the Agency for Health Care Policy and Research (AHCPR), an online textbook (usually the Merck Manual) and a few other databases depending on the topic. It uses the MeSH (MEDLINE) thesaurus, so index terms can be used to search as well as free text. The search screen is straightforward to use and the system makes suggestions to help produce an accurate search. Search results are split into two types: broad/general discussions of the topic, or systematic reviews and original research. SUMSearch can be found at: sumsearch.uthscsa.edu

Searching the internet more generally

To search the internet more generally for sites with any information related to a specific disease/illness or intervention, there are a number of different 'search engines' and 'meta-search engines' that can be used. They tend to use a simple approach, searching for any word or phrase that is specified. Typical search engines include Google, Alta Vista, Yahoo, Lycos, etc. and typical meta-search engines include SavvySearch, MetaCrawler, etc.

These systems trawl through web pages trying to find useful resources. Unfortunately, the result is often a list of thousands of sites to go through. Whilst this can be an interesting way to investigate what is on the internet, it is not the most efficient way to find useful information, especially if you are new to the internet or have limited time available. It is much easier to start off by using sites that give directions to quality-assessed and/or useful information. These usually take the form of recommended lists of 'gateway' sites, which are regularly updated and expanded as required.

Gateway sites

The most obvious sort of 'gateway' point is that provided on the web page of an organisation. Many university and hospital sites (often listed on the library/information service pages) include links to key websites considered reliable and useful to staff and students.

In the UK there are NHS library sites with links to various resources, available to NHS employees. These are the National Library for Health (NLH) (England); Health on the Net Northern Ireland (HONNI); e-Library NHS Scotland; and Health of Wales Information Service (HOWIS) e-Library. These typically provide access to evidence-based resources, guidelines, databases, electronic journals and books, etc. Some items are freely available but others will require passwords, which hospital libraries should be able to provide. These library-style collections of resources, made accessible through one website, are increasingly becoming the best places to start looking for information. Equivalent 'national electronic library sites' are probably available to those working in other countries too. Local hospital libraries should be able to advise on any such resources.

There are also some subject-specific 'gateway' sites, set up to serve groups of academics, researchers, students and others wanting information in that field. These are usually funded through academic research grants or projects and are available for anyone to use (with no charge). A number of these gateways are relevant to the health-care sector.

OMNI (Organising Medical Networked Information)

This gateway is designed to direct viewers to health and medicine web pages that have been assessed and met the desired quality standard. It has a section dedicated to MEDLINE sites on the web, giving an outline of what each site provides and often a review of the site from someone who has recently used it. It also provides some self-help tutorials on searching the internet, as well as links to sites that match its quality criteria. OMNI can be found at: omni.ac.uk

NMAP (Nursing, Midwifery and Allied health Professions)

This gateway is a recent development that focuses specifically on identifying quality websites related to nursing, midwifery and the allied health professions. NMAP can be found at:nmap.ac.uk

Both OMNI and NMAP form part of the BIOME group of gateways, which cover a range of topics in the biological sciences.

SOSIG (Social Science Information Gateway)

This is not part of the BIOME group but aims to provide an equivalent resource for those interested in the social sciences. Of particular relevance to health care is the coverage of psychology (including mental health), social welfare (including community care and carers) and education. SOSIG can be found at: www.sosig.ac.uk

Lists

Some groups provide lists of websites on certain subject areas to help people identify sites of possible interest. For evidence-based health care, there is an excellent list provided by ScHARR (the School of Health and Related

Research), at Sheffield University, known as 'Netting the Evidence – A ScHARR Introduction to Evidence Based Practice on the Internet'. It consists of a list of evidence-based health-care websites, each with an accompanying description, providing very useful background about each site. 'Netting the Evidence' can be found at: www.shef.ac.uk/scharr/ir/netting/

Links

The other approach to finding sites of interest is to go to the sites of organisations you already know about. Most professional bodies, research groups and charities have web pages, usually with a list of links to other websites that they think will be useful and of interest to their members and readers of their web page.

In evidence-based health care there are a number of organisations, such as the NHS Centre for Reviews and Dissemination, the Cochrane Collaboration, the Centre for Evidence Based Nursing, etc., which have web pages. In the nursing field there are sites for the Royal College of Nursing, the Royal College of Midwives, etc. By visiting these organisation web pages, further suggestions of other places to look for relevant information may be found.

See Appendix 3.2 for further information.

Books and journals

There are a variety of publications discussing internet resources on health care and providing guidance for users. Whilst printed resources can become out of date quite quickly (especially when considering an ever-changing environment like the internet), they are another means to get ideas or advice on websites that might be worth investigating. For example:

- Pallen M 1998 Guide to the internet: an introduction for healthcare professionals, 2nd edn. BMJ Publishing, London
- Anon 1999 Health Net: a health and wellness guide to the internet, 2nd edn. McGraw-Hill, London
- Kiley R 1999 Medical information on the internet: a guide for health professionals, 2nd edn. Churchill Livingstone, Edinburgh
- Nicoll L H 1998 Nurses' guide to the internet, 2nd edn. Lippincott, Philadelphia.

A few specialist newsletters/journals are also starting to appear, looking at the internet for health-care professionals. These provide a way to keep track of new websites and developments. Two such publications are *Health on the Internet* and *Internet Medicine*.

Hospital and university libraries are the first place to look for any relevant books and/or journal titles about the internet.

Further information on using the internet

Training and teaching tools available on the internet to help novice users find out more about searching and using internet resources in general include:

- Bare Bones, from the University of South Carolina, Beaufort Library. This provides a basic tutorial on searching the internet. It can be found at: www.sc.edu/beaufort/library/pages/bones/bones.shtml
- Internet for Nursing, Midwifery and Health Visiting. This is a teach-yourself tutorial on information skills for the internet. It can be found at: www.vts.rdn.ac.uk/tutorial/nurse.

There are also a large number of general publications available on how to use the internet (*Idiot's Guides*, etc.). Hospital and university libraries may have a few books like this available to borrow.

BOX 3.7 Key points to remember about searching the internet

1. The internet is a collection of all sorts of information. It has no quality control and no rules or regulations, so as well as extremely useful information, there may also be misleading or incorrect information.
2. To search for journal articles, use internet versions of established bibliographic databases (organisations may have to pay for access).
3. For evidence-based health-care information (articles, reports and other documentation) on the internet, try the search systems TRIP or SUMSearch.
4. For directions to quality-assessed websites or suggestions of particularly useful websites, use 'gateway' sites or subject lists or links compiled by reliable groups/organisations.
5. For other ideas on useful internet resources, check libraries for any publications covering health-care sites on the internet (books or newsletters/journals).
6. To do some very broad searching, probably identifying thousands of websites of variable quality, use general internet search engines or metasearch engines.

References

Clinical Evidence. About us. Available online at: www.clinicalevidence.com/ceweb/about/index.jsp 6 Feb 2006

Haynes R B 2001 Of studies, syntheses, synopses and systems: the "4S" evolution of services for finding current best evidence. Evidence Based Medicine 6:36–38

NHS CRD 2001 Undertaking systematic reviews of research on effectiveness. CRD's guidance for those carrying out or commissioning reviews, 2nd edn. CRD report number 4. Available online at: www.york.ac.uk/inst/crd/report4.htm

Pewsner D, Battaglia M, Bucher H, Egger M, Grossenacher F, Minder C (The Writing Committee) 2002 The Bayes Library of Diagnostic Studies and Reviews, 2nd edn. Available online at: www.medepi.net/meta/guidelines/BAYES_Library.pdf

Further reading

These are general articles about searching the health-care literature aimed at the beginner/intermediate. As far as possible, they are directed at a nursing audience. They should give more advice and ideas on how to approach literature searching in the clinical setting.

Cooke A 1999 Quality of health and medical information on the internet. British Journal of Clinical Governance 4(4):155–160

Cullum N 2000 Users' guides to the nursing literature: an introduction. Evidence-Based Nursing 3:71–72

Glanville J, Haines M, Auston I 1998 Finding information on clinical effectiveness. British Medical Journal 317:200–203

Hendry C, Farley A 1998 Reviewing the literature: a guide for students. Nursing Standard 12(44):46–48

Hunt D L, Haynes R B, Browman G P 1998 Searching the medical literature for the best evidence to solve clinical questions. Annals of Oncology 9(4):377–383

Hunt D L, Jaeschhke R, McKibbon K A 2000 Users' guides to the medical literature: XXI using electronic health information resources in evidence-based practice. Journal of the American Medical Association 283(14):1875–1879

Johnston L 2004 Research matters: searching for evidence to use in the practice setting. Neonatal, Paediatric and Child Health Nursing 7(1):26–28

Lowe H J, Barnett G O 1994 Understanding and using the Medical Subject Headings (MeSH) vocabulary to perform literature searches. Journal of the American Medical Association 271(14):1103–1108

McKibbon K A, Marks S 1998 Searching for the best evidence: part 1: where to look. Evidence-Based Nursing 1(3):68–69

McKibbon K A, Marks S 1998 Searching for the best evidence: part 2: searching CINAHL and Medline. Evidence-Based Nursing 1(4):105–107

NHS Centre for Reviews and Dissemination 2001 Accessing the evidence on clinical effectiveness. Effectiveness Matters 5(1). Available online at: www.york.ac.uk/inst/crd/em.htm

Rau J L 2004 Searching the literature and selecting the right references. Respiratory Care 49(10):1242–1245

Ringler R D 2005 How to use the internet wisely. Nursing Spectrum (Florida Edition) 15(2):26–27. Available online at: community.nursingspectrum.com/MagazineArticles/article.cfm?AID=13487

Sindhu F, Dickson R 1997 The complexity of searching the literature. International Journal of Nursing Practice 3(4):211–217

Sindhu F, Dickson R 1997 Literature searching for systematic reviews. Nursing Standard 11(41):40–42

Thomas B H, Ciliska D, Dobbins M, Micucci S 2004 A process for systematically reviewing the literature: providing the research evidence for public health nursing interventions. Worldviews on Evidence-Based Nursing 1(3):176–184

Thompson C 1999 Searching for the evidence. Nursing Times/Learning Curve 3(3):12–13

Younger P 2004 Using the internet to conduct a literature search. Nursing Standard 19(6):45–51

APPENDIX 3.1

Electronic databases

This is by no means a comprehensive list, but a selection that is most likely to be available on hospital or university computer networks.

General medical

MEDLINE   Produced by the National Library of Medicine (NLM) in the USA. Contains information from 1966 onwards. Uses index terms and has a thesaurus (MeSH). It has a USA and English language bias. Very widely available.

EMBASE   Produced by Elsevier Science, based in The Netherlands. Contains information from 1974 onwards. Uses index terms and a thesaurus (known as Emtree). Has a European bias and more emphasis on pharmaceutical information.

Nursing

CINAHL   Cumulative Index to Nursing and Allied Health Literature, produced in the USA. Contains information from 1982 onwards. Uses index terms and has a thesaurus (called the Subject Heading List). See website: www.cinahl.com

BNI   British Nursing Index, produced in the UK. Contains information from 1994 onwards. Consolidates, from 1994, the British Midwifery Index and Nursing Bibliography and RCN Nurse ROM. Has a UK and English language bias.

Specialist

AIDSLINE   Database of information on HIV and AIDS, produced by the NLM. Contains information from 1980 onwards.

CANCERLIT   Database of information on cancer, produced by the US National Cancer Institute.

CABHealth   Database of information relating to human nutrition; parasitic, communicable (including AIDS/HIV) and tropical diseases; medicinal plants and public health. Contains information from 1973 onwards. Strong international and developing country coverage. Uses index terms and has a thesaurus (CAB thesaurus).

AMED
Allied and Complementary Medicine, produced by the British Library. Contains information from 1985 onwards. Includes physiotherapy, occupational therapy, rehabilitation and palliative care. Uses index terms and a thesaurus (AMED thesaurus, based on MeSH).

PsycINFO
Produced by the American Psychological Association. Contains information from 1887 onwards. Covers all aspects of psychology. Uses index terms and a thesaurus (Thesaurus of Psychological Index Terms) for items dating from 1967 onwards.

LLBA
Linguistics and Language Behavior Abstracts. Contains information from 1981 onwards. Coverage includes speech, language and hearing pathology.

Health management

HealthSTAR
Produced by the NLM and American Hospitals Association (between 1978 and 1999). Contains information from 1975 onwards. Covers health-care planning, policy and administration. Includes effectiveness of procedures, products and services and evaluation of patient outcomes.

HMIC
Health Management Information Consortium database. Produced in the UK, an amalgamation of databases from the Nuffield Institute of Health (University of Leeds), the Department of Health and the King's Fund.

Others

EBM Reviews
Database comprising CDSR, DARE and the *American College of Physicians (ACP) Journal Club* journal.

Science Citation Index
Essentially an electronic version of the *Current Contents* publications covering scientific journals. Aims to add newly published articles on to the database promptly.

Social Science Citation Index
Sister publication to Science Citation Index, covering social science journals.

APPENDIX 3.2

Useful websites

National library sites

A first port of call for nurses employed by the NHS in the UK are the national library websites:

National Library for Health (NLH): www.library.nhs.uk

Health on the Net Northern Ireland (HONNI):
www.honni.qub.ac.uk/OnlineResources/

e-Library NHS Scotland:
www.elib.scot.nhs.uk/portal/elib/pages/index.aspx

Health of Wales Information Service, e-Library (HOWIS):
www.wales.nhs.uk/sites3/home.cfm?OrgID=520

These sites provide access to many of the organisations listed below.

Nursing organisations

For quality-assessed resources go to NMAP: nmap.ac.uk

Royal College of Nursing: www.rcn.org.uk/

Royal College of Midwives: www.rcm.org.uk/

Nursing and Midwifery Council:
www.nmc-uk.org/nmc/main/splash.html

Midwives Information and Resource Service (MIDIRS) – a 'not for profit' organisation: www.midirs.org/

Community Practitioners' and Health Visitors' Association:
www.msfcphva.org/index.htm

Evidence-based practice organisations

For a comprehensive list, go to 'Netting the Evidence – A ScHARR Introduction to Evidence Based Practice on the Internet':
www.shef.ac.uk/scharr/ir/netting/

Centre for Evidence Based Nursing:
www.york.ac.uk/healthsciences/centres/evidence/cebn.htm

Joanna Briggs Institute (Australia): www.joannabriggs.edu.au/about/home.php

NHS Centre for Reviews and Dissemination (includes the publications *Effective Health Bulletins* and *Effectiveness Matters*): www.york.ac.uk/inst/crd/

Cochrane Collaboration: www.cochrane.org/index0.htm

Cochrane Library:
  www3.interscience.wiley.com/cgi-bin/mrwhome/106568753/HOME

Cochrane Library User Guide for the internet:
  www3.interscience.wiley.com/cgi-bin/mrwhome/106568753/userguides.html

Campbell Collaboration: www.campbellcollaboration.org/

Campbell Collaboration databases – C2 Library:
  www.campbellcollaboration.org/Fralibrary.html

Clinical Evidence: www.clinicalevidence.com/ceweb/conditions/index.jsp

Health Evidence Bulletins Wales: www.hebw.uwcm.ac.uk

National Institute for Health and Clinical Excellence (NICE):
  www.nice.org.uk/

NHS Health Technology Assessment Programme: www.hta.nhsweb.nhs.uk

Health-care guidance and guidelines

Scottish Intercollegiate Guidelines Network: www.sign.ac.uk

National Institute for Health and Clinical Excellence: www.nice.org.uk

PRODIGY Guidance: www.prodigy.nhs.uk/ClinicalGuidance/

NLH Guidelines Finder: www.library.nhs.uk

National Guideline Clearinghouse (US guidelines): www.guideline.gov/

Critical appraisal of quantitative studies 1: Is the quality of the study good enough for you to use the findings?

Faith Gibson and Anne-Marie Glenny

KEY POINTS

- Why is critical appraisal necessary?
- The principles of critical appraisal.
- Identifying the appropriate research design for your clinical practice question.

- Assessing the quality of a study that asks a question about the effectiveness of a therapy or intervention.
- Assessing the quality of a study that asks a question about the accuracy of a particular diagnostic test or method of assessment works.
- Assessing the quality of a study that asks a question about finding out the likely pattern and/or outcome of a particular health problem/disease.
- Critical appraisal in practice.

This chapter should be read in conjunction with Chapter 5.

Introduction

On a daily basis nurses and other health-care professionals are faced with a range of important clinical decisions. Practice based on evidence can decrease the uncertainty that patients and health-care professionals experience in a complex and constantly evolving health-care system. Not all published research evidence can be used for making decisions about patient care. Deficiencies in research design can make an intervention look better than it really is (Moher et al 1995). In addition, the location and participants of a particular research study may affect the results in a unique way. It is therefore necessary to assess the quality, importance and applicability of any research evidence that is being consulted to answer a specific clinical question.

The process used to do this is known as critical appraisal and is a core skill for those wanting to use evidence in their practice. Critical appraisal is a discipline for increasing the effectiveness of your reading, by encouraging systematic assessment of reports of research evidence to see which ones can best answer clinical problems and inform 'best practice' (O'Rourke 2005). The meaning of research evidence is most fully appreciated when considered within the context of clinical practice, where it can have a direct impact on clinical decisions. Clinical decisions are influenced not only by research evidence but also by clinical expertise and patient preference (Sackett et al 1996). A variety of appraisal approaches can be used to determine the certainty and applicability of knowledge underpinning each of these three aspects of decision making (Stevens 2005). However, in this chapter, we focus on the appraisal of research evidence only, and specifically, quantitative research evidence. So, how do you critically appraise evidence produced through quantitative research designs? What does it demand of you?

Critical appraisal can be broken down into three distinct but related parts as illustrated in Figure 4.1.

1. Are the results of the study valid? In other words, is the quality of the study good enough to produce results that can be used to inform clinical decisions?
2. What are the results and what do they mean in my context/for my patient?
3. Will the results help locally? Can I apply them in my clinical setting?

Answering 'Yes' or 'No' to these questions can prove a challenge to healthcare practitioners. As Oxman et al (1993) observe, research evidence comes in shades of grey, rather than black and white: results *may* be valid, *might* show clinically important findings, *perhaps* will improve the patient's outcome.

Over the past 20 years or so, researchers and clinicians around the world have been working together to develop standard approaches to addressing these three questions. This work has led to the development of quality criteria for assessing the design of research studies. These criteria have been incorporated into critical appraisal checklists in the form of streamlined guides and toolkits that make the process of assessing studies much easier (see the 'Appraising' section of Netting the Evidence (www.shef. ac.uk/scharr/ir/netting/) for examples of quality appraisal guides/toolkits).

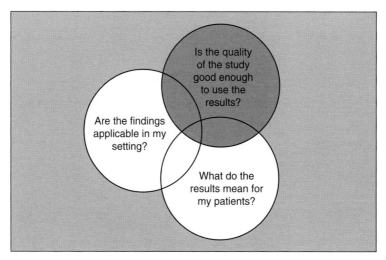

Figure 4.1 The three aspects of critical appraisal for evidence-based practice

This and the next chapter (Chapter 5) provide a set of tools that can be used for critical appraisal. The chapters also provide help in developing the skills and knowledge necessary to use these tools. The remainder of this chapter will consider how to assess whether the quality of the study is good enough for the results to be used (i.e. shading in Figure 4.1). Chapter 5 addresses the other two aspects. Both chapters use practical examples to illustrate the process: clinical scenarios are used to generate clinical questions and the relevant published research papers are then appraised. The same examples are used in both chapters. You will obtain more benefit from the examples if you obtain copies of the published research papers.

Is the quality of the study good enough for me to use the results?

One of the tests that all researchers face in the design and conduct of research in real-world settings is that of minimising bias. Bias refers to any influence or action in a study that distorts the findings or slants them away from the true or expected (Burns & Grove 2001). In other words, any factor (for example, the way the study is conducted, analysed or published) that leads to interventions appearing to be effective when in fact they are not, or vice versa. The critical reader of research must always be aware that there may be multiple explanations for the findings reported in a study (Johnston 2005).

When designing a research study, the researchers have to consider a number of questions (Box 4.1). These questions apply in every type of research

---

BOX 4.1 Questions to be considered in the design of a research study (after Sim & Wright 2000)

What entities or variables to examine
Under what conditions to examine these entities or variables
What type(s) of data to collect
From whom (or what) to collect these data
At what time points to collect the data
What method to employ for data collection
How data will be analysed

design. The decisions made by the researchers in response to each of these questions directly affect the degree to which the results of a study may be affected by bias. The strategies for the minimisation of bias are now well known. Different strategies are required for different research designs and for the different stages of the study (Moore & McQuay 2000). When looked at from the perspective of the research consumer, these bias minimisation strategies become quality criteria that can be used to assess the quality of a study. The strategies adopted by the researchers to minimise bias should be evident in the reporting of the research. Critical appraisal checklists are designed to summarise the bias minimisation strategies and help practitioners to ask the most relevant questions that will lead to a decision about the quality and hence usefulness of a paper. Tables 4.2, 4.3 and 4.4 show worked examples of using quality criteria to assess the worth of three different studies; the quality criteria are explained in detail later in the chapter.

Is the study design appropriate to the question?

As shown in Chapter 2, the process of critical appraisal for evidence-based practice starts with the formulation of a question that arises from clinical practice. For critical appraisal purposes, clinical practice questions can, broadly speaking, be categorised into different types. In this and the following chapter, we focus on clinical questions about:

- the effectiveness of a therapy or intervention
- the accuracy of a diagnostic test or method of assessment, and
- the prognosis of a particular disease or health problem (see Chapter 6 for discussion of critical appraisal of questions requiring qualitative research designs).

For each type of question there is a corresponding 'most appropriate' research design (overall plan or structure used by the researcher) that can be used to answer the question with a known degree of precision and minimal risk of bias (Blaikie 2000). In this chapter we have focused on the optimal study design for three different types of questions, as presented in Table 4.1. However, it is important to remember that there may be good reasons why researchers choose to use study designs that at first appear to be less appropriate for the research question. Each research project presents unique challenges and a certain degree of flexibility is required by the researcher.

TABLE 4.1 MATCHING STUDY DESIGN TO QUESTIONS

Type of question	Example question	Research design
The effectiveness of a therapy or intervention.	Does the wearing of elastic compression stockings prevent deep vein thrombosis in long-haul flights?	Randomised controlled trial.
The performance or accuracy of a particular diagnostic test/method of assessment.	In primary care, does asking patients about feeling depressed, experiencing loss of interest and needing help accurately identify those who are clinically depressed?	Study investigating test accuracy where a new method of assessment is compared with a reference standard test.
Finding out the likely pattern and/ or outcome of a particular health problem or disease (i.e. prognosis).	Are women oral contraceptive users, who smoke, at greater risk of myocardial infarction (MI)?	Cohort study: participants exposed to an agent (contraceptive pill) are followed forward in time to see if they develop an outcome (MI) Case–control study: participants with the condition (MI) are matched with controls (no MI). Study looks back in time to identify exposure to an agent (contraceptive pill).

For each research design, specific criteria need to be considered. These will be explored in more detail later in this chapter.

In the case of questions about whether a particular diagnostic test or method of assessment performs well, a study design that compares the accuracy of a new test when used on people with and without the target condition against a reference standard will be most appropriate (Mant 1999a). Where the question is about the most likely outcome of a particular health problem (i.e. the prognosis), the most appropriate design will be one that measures relevant outcomes in individuals with (and perhaps without) the relevant condition over a sufficient period of time (Mant 1999b). If the clinical question is about whether a particular intervention (e.g. a nurse-led discharge package) produces a certain outcome (e.g. decreased hospital stay), a study that compares length of hospital stay in a group receiving the intervention with length of stay in a group not receiving the intervention is required. There are a number of possible research designs that could be used for such a study but large, multicentred randomised controlled trials (RCTs) are likely to give the best evidence of effectiveness (Gray 1997), provided they are conducted rigorously.

Regardless of the type of study, a rigorous approach to the design, conduct, analysis and reporting stages of the study is important in view of the effect that each of these stages can have on the results. For example, RCTs with methodological shortfalls, such as failure to conceal from the patient and assessor the group to which the patient has been allocated, tend to overestimate treatment effects (Mathews 2000).

Systematic reviews

There has been an explosion in the amount of published research evidence, much of which is not always easily accessible to practitioners. When searching for evidence, it is unlikely that all the studies that address a particular question will be identified. In addition, wading through large numbers of articles can be extremely time consuming and may not be an option for a busy practitioner. Where relevant studies are identified, their conclusions may differ, and this poses a dilemma for the person trying to find a solution to a problem.

These are just some of the reasons for the growing interest in systematic reviews as a form of evidence. A systematic review summarises pertinent research evidence on a defined health question, using explicit and rigorous methods (Cullinan 2005). In contrast to a traditional narrative review, which might simply reflect the findings of a few papers that support an author's particular point of view (Johnston 2005), a systematic review entails systematic and explicit methods for identifying, assessing and synthesising the available research evidence. This is an important distinction and one which highlights the biases associated with traditional, narrative reviews. There are numerous advantages to systematic reviews. For the busy practitioner, the most important advantage would seem to be their potential for aiding translation of research evidence into practice (Evans & Pearson 2001): the well-conducted review offers the clinician a rigorous distillation of the pertinent research evidence and recommendations for clinical practice. Systematic reviews can help to overcome many of the practical and methodological limitations of individual studies (Chalmers & Altman 1995), as discussed in Chapter 7.

To date, the majority of systematic reviews have focused on effectiveness of different interventions, where the study design used by the primary authors was the controlled trial. However, systematic reviews of other types of study designs are also being conducted. In this chapter we have not looked at critical appraisal of systematic reviews; however, critical appraisal checklists specific to systematic reviews are available. Chapter 7 provides more information.

The hierarchy of evidence

When looking for evidence about the effectiveness of interventions, properly conducted systematic reviews of RCTs or properly conducted RCTs provide the most powerful form of evidence. The process of randomisation means that the observed differences between the intervention group and the comparison group are more likely to be due to the intervention and not to other factors such as patient, nurse or doctor preference (Mathews 2000). There will, however, always be circumstances where randomisation may be inappropriate or impossible, particularly in health service research (Bowling 1997). An obvious example is studies about harm or prognosis. It would not be ethical to give subjects a substance that was thought to be hazardous to their health. In circumstances where there are clear reasons for not randomising, studies with other designs have a vital role in providing evidence (Martin 2005).

Evidence that some research designs are more powerful than others has given rise to the notion of a hierarchy of evidence (Summerskill 2000). Figure 4.2 illustrates this hierarchy for studies relating to effectiveness of therapies or interventions. The continuum is used to illustrate the increasing risk of bias inherent in each research design. The higher a methodology appears in the hierarchy, the more likely the results of such methods are to represent objective reality and hence the more certainty the practitioner

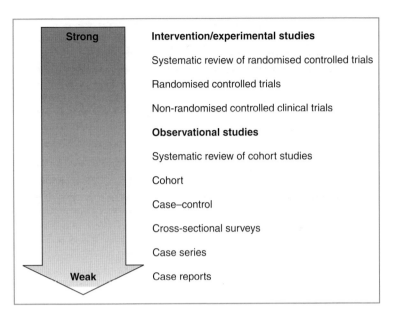

Figure 4.2 The hierarchy of evidence for questions about the effectiveness of an intervention/therapy

has that the intervention will produce the same health outcomes (Johnston 2005). Such hierarchies provide a useful 'rule of thumb' against which to grade studies.

The hierarchy of evidence shown in Figure 4.2 has led some clinicians to expressing concerns that the only questions considered to be important are those about effectiveness of interventions, and that the only valid type of study is the RCT (Evans & Pearson 2001, French 2002). However, it must be emphasised that different research questions have different hierarchies and require evaluation through different study designs. RCTs are the 'gold standard' for primary study design upon which to base decisions on the effectiveness of health-care interventions, but they are not necessarily appropriate, or ethical, to answer other questions. For example, it would be inappropriate to conduct a RCT to answer the question 'How do young people with cancer experience and manage fatigue?'. Given that the researcher would not be intervening in any way, and that the study aims to examine the experience of fatigue, explore influencing factors and management strategies adopted by young people with cancer, a prospective, cohort follow-up design using narrative inquiry would be more appropriate.

Worked example 4.1: Assessing the quality of a study that asks a question about the effectiveness of a therapy or intervention

Scenario

You are part of a nursing team in a children's hospital delivering care to children with complex needs. The philosophy of your team is one that incorporates the whole family: that of family-centred care. The mother of Henry Pink, one of the children receiving respite care in your unit, shares her worries about an upcoming flight she is taking. The family has been given some money from a local charity to visit Disney World in Florida. The whole family, including Grandma and Grandad, is very excited about this visit. Mum's worries centre on a journal article she read in a women's magazine about the risk of deep vein thrombosis and the benefits of wearing elastic stockings. Although all are fit (with no history of thromboembolic problems), Mrs Pink has worries for herself and her parents. You agree to ask one of your colleagues about it, as the colleague recently undertook a long-haul flight to Kenya and investigated this topic prior to flying. Your colleague recalls one particularly helpful paper. You suggest to the child's mum that you will help her to 'make sense' of this paper so that she can reach a decision about any action she might need to take before their holiday.

Your clinical practice question

Does the wearing of elastic compression stockings prevent deep vein thrombosis in passengers undertaking long-haul flights?

Finding the evidence

Your colleague supplies the following paper that looks as though it might be relevant:

Scurr J H, Machin S J, Bailey-King S, Mackie I J, McDonald S, Coleridge Smith D 2001 Frequency and prevention of symptomless deep-vein thrombosis in long-haul flights: a randomized trial. Lancet 357:1485–1489

The paper reports the results of a RCT involving 89 male and 142 female long-haul air passengers, over the age of 50 years, with no history of thromboembolic problems. Passengers were randomised to two groups, with those in the intervention group being issued below-knee graduated elastic compression stockings to be worn for the duration of the flight. The control group did not receive any intervention. The primary outcome was symptomless deep vein thrombosis. Assessments were made of the veins using duplex ultrasonography, and blood samples were taken to measure gene mutations (factor V Leiden and prothrombin), which are known to predispose to venous thromboembolism. In addition, a sensitive D-dimer assay was used to screen for the development of recent thrombosis.

What is the quality of the study?

Table 4.2 shows a worked example of the critical appraisal for the paper referenced above, using the appraisal tool 'Ten questions to help you make sense of randomised controlled trials', published by CASP (2002).

Relevance of criteria in Table 4.2

- The importance of randomisation has already been discussed: the aim is to ensure that, as far as possible, the two groups are similar apart from the intervention. This means that any difference in outcome between the two groups is likely to be due to the intervention. A computer-generated number sequence is one example of an appropriate randomisation method.

- The group to which the patient has been allocated must be concealed from the clinician/researcher until the patient has been accepted into the trial. This is often referred to as allocation concealment and is an important factor in reducing bias. If the clinician believes that the patient may benefit from the treatment, and realises that the patient is due to be allocated to the control group, he or she may consciously or subconsciously dissuade the patient from participating in the trial. Ideally, randomisation should be carried out by someone removed from the project using, for example, sequentially numbered sealed, opaque envelopes. Randomisation based on criteria such as date of birth are not recommended as clinicians are able to work out from the date of birth and the allocation sequence which group the patient is to be allocated to.

- Where possible, patients, clinicians and researchers should be 'blinded' as to whether a patient is in the treatment or control group. If patients know that they are in the control group, they may feel that they have received

TABLE 4.2 ASSESSING THE QUALITY OF A STUDY THAT INVESTIGATES WHETHER A PARTICULAR INTERVENTION IS EFFECTIVE: A WORKED EXAMPLE USING THE CASP CHECKLIST 'TEN QUESTIONS TO HELP YOU MAKE SENSE OF RANDOMISED CONTROLLED TRIALS' (CASP 2002, WITH PERMISSION, © MILTON KEYNES PRIMARY CARE TRUST, 2002)

Type of question	Assessment criteria	Response (Yes / Can't tell / No)	Comment
Screening question	Did the study ask a clearly focused question?	**Yes**	This study sought to determine the frequency of deep vein thrombosis (DVT) in the lower limb in middle-aged men and women during long-haul economy class air travel and the efficacy of elastic compression stockings in its prevention.
	Was this a randomised controlled trial (RCT), and was it appropriately so?	**Yes**	This study compared the frequency and prevention of DVT in two groups randomly allocated to wear or not wear stockings. The study design (RCT) is appropriate for investigating the effectiveness of an intervention.
Detailed questions	Were participants appropriately allocated to intervention and control groups?	**Yes**	The author states that passengers were randomly allocated to receive compression stocking (n=115) or no stockings (n=116); however, the method of randomisation is not described. Sealed envelopes were used to conceal from the investigators and passengers which group the passengers were to be allocated to.

Were participants, staff and study personnel 'blind' to participants' study group?	Can't tell	Not possible to blind the passengers or the staff administering the stockings. They all knew who was receiving treatment. It might have been possible to blind the laboratory staff and the ultrasonographer, but there is a high risk that the patients might have revealed to the ultrasonographer which group they were in.
Were all the participants who entered the trial accounted for at its conclusion?	Yes	Yes, trial profile clearly describes and states intention to treat in the analysis section. Data on all participants originally randomised have been included in the analysis. The authors show the numbers of passengers lost to follow-up for each group. These appear to be equally distributed between groups.
Were the participants in all groups followed up and data collected in the same way?	Can't tell	This is unclear; insufficient information is provided about the actual study procedure. It would be difficult to comment on the influence of performance bias.
Did the study have enough participants to minimise the play of chance?	Can't tell	This was described as a pilot study and therefore no power calculation was undertaken.

(Continued)

TABLE 4.2 (CONTINUED)

Type of question	Assessment criteria	Response (Yes / Can't tell / No)	Comment
	How are the results presented and what is the main result?		Presented as a proportion of participants experiencing DVT after airline travel. None of the participants wearing stockings had a DVT. Although an increased risk of superficial thrombophlebitis in varicose veins if the stockings are worn is reported, the increase is not statistically significant. 10% (n=12/116) of participants not wearing stockings developed a symptomless DVT. The authors conclude that wearing an elasticated stocking during long-haul air travel may be associated with a reduction in symptomless DVT.
	How precise are the results?		Confidence intervals are reported for each group, not between groups, but are indicative of clinical significance.
	Were all the important outcomes considered so the results can be applied?	No	A number of limitations were addressed in the paper that would need to be considered such as in-flight behaviours, e.g. walking, and drinking water and the effect they may have had on the results. The reported risk of thrombophlebitis in varicose veins if the stockings are worn would also need to be taken into consideration.

substandard care and may, as a result, alter their behaviour. Similarly, clinicians may consciously or subconsciously take compensatory measures for patients who are in the control group (for example, by offering alternative therapies or additional support, etc.). Any difference in the treatment effects between the two groups may be due to this additional attention rather than the intervention. The researcher may have preconceived ideas about the treatment and, where the outcomes of interest are fairly subjective, these preconceptions may influence the way in which the researcher interprets and analyses the data. Clearly, blinding is not possible in all studies but attempts should be made to blind one (single-blind) or all (double-blind/treble-blind) of the above groups of people.

- People drop out of studies for all sorts of reasons: death, relocation to another geographical area, treatment found to be too unpleasant, etc. It is important that the researcher tries to identify whether the reasons relate to the outcomes of interest. The analysis should ideally be done on an 'intention to treat' basis: patients are analysed in the groups to which they were randomised regardless of whether they swap from the intervention arm of the trial to the control arm or vice versa. If participants in the treatment group stop taking a drug because they feel worse (and blame the drug), and are then included in the control group, the drug may appear to be more effective than it really is due to exclusion of those patients with poor outcomes from the treatment group.

- Look to see if the investigators estimated how many people needed to be studied in order to answer their research question. Studying more people than is necessary wastes resources, whilst studying too few people might lead to results that reflect chance alone, rather than the real situation. To illustrate, in a trial of 10 participants, where five are randomised to receive drug A and five to receive drug B, and where the outcomes are the same for both groups, this could mean one of two things: either there is no difference between the drugs or one of the drugs is more effective but, because of the small numbers of participants, this difference between the drugs is not shown (Kirkwood 1988). A 'power calculation' will provide an estimation of the required sample size. The power of a study is the probability of obtaining a significant result if the difference between outcomes in two groups is ⩾ the smallest worthwhile clinical difference specified.

- Demographic and health status details for the two groups are of interest. Significant differences between the two groups, for example differences in age, co-morbid conditions, gender or disease severity, could potentially affect the results of the study. The groups should ideally be similar, on average, for any variables that are likely to influence outcome. Similarity between groups is not always achieved by randomisation, even where the methods of randomisation are adequate.

- It is helpful if the intervention is described in sufficient detail to allow clinicians to reproduce it in their own setting. In addition, the primary outcome in which the investigators would expect to see a clinically important difference should be given, along with details of how the outcome was to be measured. Measurement instruments which have been validated outside the study and found to measure what they purport to measure, and which are sensitive, appropriate and acceptable, inspire more confidence than measurement instruments that have not been validated.

The quality assessment bottom line

This study met most of the quality criteria. The main exception is the lack of blinding; however, this is a common feature of studies of non-pharmaceutical interventions as it can be difficult or impossible to conceal from the patient and the clinician what is being done. It is often possible to blind the individual who is measuring or assessing the outcome – in this study, the laboratory staff and the ultrasonographer. There was, however, a risk that passengers might have revealed to the ultrasonographer which group they were in. If this was the case, one could argue that the ultrasonographer may (consciously or subconsciously) have been more vigilant when examining non-stocking passengers, and this could potentially impact on the study results.

Overall, we can conclude that the difference between the outcomes in the two groups was unlikely to be subject to a high level of bias (for the criteria examined), which suggests that we can trust the results of this study. The applicability of the study and what the results mean for our patients are considered in Chapter 5.

Worked example 4.2: Assessing the quality of a study that asks a question about the performance or accuracy of a particular diagnostic test or method of assessment

Scenario

Thomas Davies, a 45-year-old man, has been referred to the practice nurses by his general practitioner who is 'fed up' with seeing him when there is 'nothing wrong with him'. You notice from his records that Mr Davies has been registered with the practice for 5 years. He hardly ever visited the practice until the last 3 months and since then he seems to have visited nearly every week. During your interview Mr Davies tells you that he lost his job as a supervisor in a warehouse 6 months ago and has been unable to find work since. When you question him further, he tells you that he has never had any mental health problems but he says that during the last month he has felt really down. He also feels that he has little interest in anything, so much so that some days he just sits in his armchair all day unless his wife 'nags him, to get out from under her feet'. From the information Mr Davies provides, you think he might have clinical depression. You wonder how accurately a patient's self-reported loss of interest and 'feeling down' diagnoses clinical depression.

Your clinical practice question

In patients with clinical depression, how accurately does patient response to questions about feeling down or depressed and loss of interest diagnose clinical depression?

Finding the evidence

You phone the local hospital library and give them your question to run a systematic search for you. They phone you a few days later and tell you that they have not found any summarised evidence, but the following article may be useful:

Arroll B, Goodyear-Smith F, Kerse N, Fishman T, Gunn J 2005 Effect of the addition of a 'help' question to two screening questions on specificity for diagnosis of depression in general practice: diagnostic validity study. British Medical Journal 331: 884–887

The paper reports the results of a diagnostic accuracy study of 1025 people attending a primary care setting in New Zealand. The study assesses the accuracy of one type of assessment instrument (asking two questions about feeling down and about loss of interest or pleasure in doing things during the past month, and a question as to whether help was needed) compared with a different and longer assessment instrument (the mood module of the Composite International Diagnostic Interview [CIDI]) in diagnosing clinical depression.

What is the quality of the study?

Table 4.3 shows a worked example of the critical appraisal for the paper referenced above, using the appraisal tool 'Twelve questions to help you make sense of a diagnostic test study', published by CASP (1998).

Relevance of criteria in Table 4.3

- The 'new' test should be compared against the method that is currently regarded as 'the best' (i.e. the reference standard) and both tests should be applied in all participants.

- An appropriate spectrum of patients (i.e. patients with mild, moderate and severe forms of the condition) should ideally be included in the study, with details of the proportions of each of these groups given. A test may be able to identify people who are severely ill, but not those with a mild form of the condition.

- Ideally, a consecutive set of participants who fulfil the inclusion criteria should be tested. This ensures that individuals are not inappropriately 'selected out' of the study, thereby affecting the results and conclusions of the study.

- It is recommended that the clinician or investigator is 'blinded' to the results of the test that is carried out first. If the clinician suspects from the initial test that the patient does not have the disease in question, he or she may decide to avoid subjecting the patient to the second test. Blinding also avoids the conscious and unconscious bias of causing the reference standard to be overinterpreted when the diagnostic test is positive and underinterpreted when it is negative (Sackett et al 2000).

- Reliability (reproducibility) of a test needs to be considered: the results of tests carried out by different individuals or by the same individual at different times should remain unchanged, provided the true underlying variable being measured remains the same. Disagreement between two examiners is called interobserver variability, and disagreement within one examiner over time is called intraobserver variability. In tests that are not reproducible, it is difficult to know whether a true measurement is being obtained. This creates problems in research and in clinical practice.

The quality assessment bottom line

This study appears to meet the quality assessment criteria, therefore we can trust the results. The applicability of the study and what the results mean for our patients are considered in Chapter 5.

TABLE 4.3 ASSESSING THE QUALITY OF A STUDY THAT INVESTIGATES THE PERFORMANCE OR ACCURACY OF A PARTICULAR TEST/ METHOD OF ASSESSMENT: A WORKED EXAMPLE USING THE CASP CHECKLIST 'TWELVE QUESTIONS TO HELP YOU MAKE SENSE OF A DIAGNOSTIC TEST STUDY' (CASP 1998, WITH PERMISSION, © MILTON KEYNES PRIMARY CARE TRUST, 1998)

Type of question	Assessment criteria	Response (Yes / Can't tell / No)	Comment
Screening question	Was there a clear question for this study to address?	**Yes**	This study sought to determine the accuracy of an assessment instrument (two written screening questions for depression with the addition of a question asking about whether help is needed) in diagnosing depression.
	Was there a comparison with an appropriate reference– standard?	**Yes**	Responses to two screening questions and a question inquiring about help required were compared to a validated instrument, the CIDI.
Detailed questions	Did all patients get the diagnostic test and the reference standard?	**Yes**	It appears as if all participants entering the study were invited to complete both the CIDI and the other assessment tool.
	Could the results of the test of interest have been influenced by the results of the reference standard?	**No**	The tests were performed independently. The research assistant did not look at the results of the screening questions until after the CIDI was completed and therefore would not have known if the participant had been diagnosed as depressed prior to administering the reference standard.

(Continued)

TABLE 4.3 (CONTINUED)

Type of question	Assessment criteria	Response (Yes / Can't tell / No)	Comment
	Is the disease status of the tested population clearly described?	No	Very limited information is provided about the participants, other than they were attending a general practitioner clinic and were receiving no psychotropic drugs.
	Were the methods for performing the test described in sufficient detail?	No	Very little information is provided about the actual protocol followed.
	What are the results?		When compared with the CIDI, the two screening questions with the help question had a sensitivity of 96% and a specificity of 89%. Overall, the two screening questions with the help question had a good sensitivity and an excellent specificity for screening depression.

How sure are we about these results?		Confidence intervals are included, although they are described for each group rather than between groups.
Can the results be applied to your patient or population of interest?	**Can't tell**	Difficult to say as so little information is provided about the population.
Can the test be applied to your patient or population of interest?	**No**	No intra- or interobserver reliability established for the test, therefore variability of the assessment remains unknown.
Were all outcomes important to the individual population or considered?	**Can't tell**	Although the questions are reported to have good sensitivity and specificity for major depression, limited description of the population does little to establish how far the tests were evaluated in an appropriate spectrum of patients.
What would be the impact of using this test on your patients/population?		Brevity of the questionnaire may be useful to consider in clinical practice; further testing is required.

Worked example 4.3: Assessing the quality of a study that asks a question about the likely pattern and/or outcome of a particular health problem/disease

Scenario

Florence Barrett, a 33-year-old mother of two, has stopped by the doctor's surgery on her way to work to collect a repeat prescription for oral contraception. You look in her case notes and notice that she has not had a pill review check this year and you invite her to return for a review the following week. You also ask her whether she is still smoking and she tells you that she smokes between 25 and 30 cigarettes per day. You note from her records that she has been using oral contraception for just over 1 year since the birth of her second child. You recall reading something about there being a higher risk of myocardial infarction (MI) in pill users who smoke and decide that before her visit you will investigate the following clinical question.

Your clinical question

Are women who smoke and take oral contraception at higher risk of MI than women who smoke but use other forms of contraception?

Finding the evidence

You begin a search on PubMed (MEDLINE via the internet) using the 'clinical queries' function and, selecting the prognosis filter, enter the terms 'myocardial infarction AND oral contraceptives'. Twenty citations are identified, one of which is:

Burkman R T 2000 Cardiovascular issues with oral contraceptives: evidence-based medicine. International Journal of Fertility and Women's Medicine 45(2):166–174

This is a review article but does not meet the criteria of a systematic review. Neither does it provide raw data. One of the references cited is:

> Mant J, Painter R, Vessey M 1998 Risk of myocardial infarction, angina, and stroke in users of oral contraceptives: an updated analysis of a cohort study. British Journal of Obstetrics and Gynaecology 105: 890–896

The paper reports the results of a cohort study involving 17,032 women using contraception who were followed up for 20–26 years. One of the outcome measures used is the rate of MI. This is compared in women who had used oral contraception and those that had not. Subgroup analysis compares the rate of MI in women who smoke and use oral contraception and women who smoke and do not use oral contraception.

What is the quality of the study?

Table 4.4 shows a worked example of the critical appraisal for the paper referenced above that uses the quality criteria from the JAMA guidelines on critical appraisal (Laupacis et al 1994). A brief explanation of why the criteria are important is provided below, but readers are referred to the JAMA guidelines for a more detailed discussion.

Relevance of criteria in Table 4.4

- It is important that the participants in the study truly have the disorder of interest, and that they are entering the study at a common point in the course of their disease. In a study aiming to identify the risk of renal disease in people with diabetes, for example, if some of the participants already have undiagnosed mild kidney damage at the start of the study, this could influence the results in a negative way.

- Length of follow-up should be adequate for all possible outcomes (especially negative outcomes) to become manifest. If participants, for example people who have smoked 20 or more cigarettes a day for 1 year, are followed up for 4 years to establish risk of lung cancer, the conclusions of the study are likely to be different than if followed up for 15 years.

- People are inevitably lost to follow-up and the reasons for this should be explored. If participants are lost to follow-up through death rather than because they feel better, and this information is known to the researcher, he or she can take this into consideration when presenting the results.

TABLE 4.4 ASSESSING THE QUALITY OF A STUDY ABOUT THE LIKELY PATTERN OR OUTCOME OF A PARTICULAR HEALTH PROBLEM OR DISEASE

	Criteria	Quality appraisal question	Worked example
Design	Longitudinal cohort study.	Was a group of participants followed up prospectively over a period of time?	Yes. A cohort of 17,032 women who used contraception were recruited when they were between the ages of 25 and 39 years and followed up for between 20 and 26 years.
Sample	Clearly defined, representative, assembled at a similar point.	Was a defined, representative sample of patients assembled at a common (usually early) point in the course of their life and/or disease?	Yes. 17,032 British, Caucasian, married women, who used contraception and were aged between 25 and 35, were recruited from 17 large family planning clinics in England and Scotland.
Measures	Appropriate endpoints.	Were appropriate endpoints specified in advance of the study?	Yes. The outcome measures used were occurrence of angina, myocardial infarction or stroke that was associated with hospital admission, referral to hospital or death.
Researcher	No dependent relationship between subject and investigator.	What is the researcher/investigator's relation to those being investigated?	The study investigators were academic staff at the University of Oxford. The study was not funded by any manufacturers of contraception.

Data collection	Follow-up of adequate duration.	Were the patients followed up for long enough?	Yes. 17,032 women were enrolled to the study between 1968 and 1974. All women were followed up until age 45. At age 45, 15,292 women were still participating in the study. At age 45 the cohort was divided into three groups: 1. Never used oral contraception (n=5881) 2. Used oral contraception for 8 or more years 3. Remainder. Only those women who had never used the oral contraceptive pill or had used the oral contraceptive pill for 8 or more years were followed up after the age of 45.
	All cases accounted for at end of study.	Were endpoints given for all participants?	No. End measurements were not obtained in women who dropped out of the study. Reasons for their withdrawal are not always given.
Data analysis	Effects of potential confounders accounted for.	Does the data analysis take into consideration the effect of any potentially confounding variables?	Yes. Event rates were adjusted for relevant potential confounders: age, social class, smoking, obesity and parity. In addition, the analysis was carried out twice, the second time excluding women with risk factors for a cardiovascular event (because they were less likely to be prescribed oral contraception).

NB: These questions are specifically for the critical appraisal of cohort studies.

- Outcome measurement can be a source of bias, especially where the outcome is a subjective one, for example quality of life. The outcome should therefore be clearly defined in advance. In addition, where outcome measurement requires a degree of judgement, the person taking the measurement or doing the assessment should be blind to the patient's condition.

- When observing health outcomes over time, it is important to take account of the factors or variables that can affect health. In longitudinal studies, time itself acts as a confounding variable. As people get older they develop more illness regardless of any other factors. The effect of such confounding variables can be taken into account in the process of data analysis.

The quality assessment bottom line

The only area in which the quality of the study is questionable is in respect of the number of women who were lost to follow-up. The loss of patients is often unavoidable in large-scale longitudinal studies such as this one. From our point of view, we are concerned about the effect this loss of patients may have on the validity of the conclusions made in the study. In all, 1740 women were lost to follow-up, which is approximately 10% of the original sample. Is this too many? One way to decide is to use the '5 and 20' rule. Fewer than 5% loss probably leads to little bias, greater than 20% loss seriously threatens validity (Sackett et al 2000).

A second approach is to ask a series of 'what if?' questions, known as sensitivity analysis. We can use different combinations of 'what if' scenarios to examine the possible effects of adding the missing cases back into the data analysis. The key thing here is to consider whether the cases lost to follow-up would have a different pattern of outcomes from those who remained. For our particular clinical question, we would ask ourselves the question of whether the heavy smoking, oral contraception users who dropped out were any more likely to have an adverse outcome than those who remained. The results of the study and its applicability to Mrs Barrett are considered in more detail in Chapter 5.

Critical appraisal in practice

The critical appraisal tools given above are designed to help develop skills and knowledge of critical appraisal. Other tools produced by different organisations are available (see the 'Netting the Evidence' website for more information: www.shef.ac.uk/scharr/ir/netting/).

Although initially it may feel otherwise, critical appraisal gets easier with practice and people quickly become adept at recognising whether they will be able to use a paper or not. Answers to the questions outlined in Tables 4.2–4.4 are often included in the methodology sections. If not, there is a high probability they are not there at all and so it may not be worth bothering to look at the rest of the paper.

It is important to remember that research is a real-world process. This means that researchers are often forced to compromise on certain aspects of the research and to modify the study design for lots of legitimate reasons. There is no such thing as a perfect research study. Similarly, it is also important to recognise that research is done on samples of a population who will never be identical to patients attending a clinic, the patients in a ward, etc. It is unrealistic to search for perfect research studies where the study population exactly matches a patient group. People who are new to critical appraisal may feel that no research is good enough and quickly judge a paper as not being relevant to a particular population. The trick is to identify studies that can be applied to a specific clinical context where the design is *good enough* for the results to be trusted.

The tools in this chapter contain the basic questions necessary for assessing the quality of research studies in the practice environment. More sophisticated critical appraisal tools and techniques are available for people who are becoming more experienced or are doing critical appraisal on questions not covered in this chapter (for example, those published as a series in the Journal of the American Medical Association, the so-called JAMA user guides). Details of where to find these can also be found at the 'Netting the Evidence' website.

If the study is good enough to use and can be applied in the clinical setting of interest, the next step is to work out what to do about it. If a change in practice is required, how should that change be brought about? Simply telling colleagues that the evidence says they should be doing B rather than A has been demonstrated to be a rather ineffective change method (Mulhall 1999). Methods for increasing the chance of successfully changing practice are discussed in Chapters 9–11.

Presenting the results of critical appraisal to colleagues in a systematic way, which makes explicit the process used to come to these conclusions, is an important part of preparing for change (Melnyk 2005). The critical appraisal tools used above provide a method for generating a summary of a study. Another way of doing this is to use CATs or critically appraised topics, which are one-page summaries of research papers. These were developed by the Centre for Evidence-Based Medicine in Oxford and examples of completed CATs can be accessed via their website (cebm.net/cats. asp). They also produce CATmaker software, which is a computer program that can be used to make CATs. Raw data from the study can be entered into the program which will calculate some useful numbers for summarising the results in terms of effects on individual patients, e.g. the number needed to treat (NNT). This is discussed in more detail in Chapter 5.

Summary

This chapter has established why critical appraisal is necessary and important for evidence-based practice. The principles of research design and method underpinning the use of quality criteria to assess studies have been outlined. Critical appraisal for evidence-based practice is a three-part process comprising assessment of the quality of the study, assessment of the applicability of the study and interpretation of the study results for the individual patient. This chapter has focused on the assessment of the quality of a study and provided practical examples of how this can be done for three different types of clinical question that require the use of different research designs.

Scenario 4.1 leads to a clinical question on the effectiveness of elasticated stockings to influence frequency and prevention of DVT after flying long-haul economy class. The most appropriate research design for this question (in the absence of a systematic review) is a randomised controlled trial. Table 4.2 gives an example of the assessment of the quality of a trial investigating this topic.

Scenario 4.2 leads to a clinical question about whether patients' self-reported feelings and a request for help predict clinical depression. The most appropriate study design for this question is a study investigating diagnostic accuracy. Table 4.3 gives an example of the assessment of the quality of a published diagnostic study on this topic.

Scenario 4.3 generates a clinical question about whether users of oral contraception are at greater risk of MI. The most appropriate study design for this question is a cohort study. Table 4.4 gives an example of the assessment of quality of a published cohort study that addresses this question.

Acknowledgements

We give special thanks to Mark Newman and Tony Roberts whose contributions to the previous edition have provided the foundation for this chapter.

References

* Papers used for critical appraisal examples.

* Arroll B, Goodyear-Smith F, Kerse N, Fishman T, Gunn J 2005 Effect of the addition of a "help" question to two screening questions on specificity for diagnosis of depression in general practice: diagnostic validity study. British Medical Journal 331:884–889

Blaikie N 2000 Designing social research. Polity Press, Cambridge

Bowling A 1997 Research methods in health: investigating health and health services. Open University Press, Buckingham

Burkman R T 2000 Cardiovascular issues with oral contraceptives: evidence-based medicine. International Journal of Fertility and Women's Medicine 45(2):166–174

Burns N, Grove S K 2001 The practice of nursing research: conduct, critique and utilization, 4th edn. W B Saunders, Philadelphia

CASP Critical Appraisal Skills Programme 1998 Twelve questions to help you make sense of a diagnostic test study. Available online at: www.phru.nhs. uk/casp/casp_diagnostic_tool.pdf May 2006

CASP Critical Appraisal Skills Programme 2002 Ten questions to help you make sense of randomised controlled trials. Available online at: www.phru. nhs.uk/casp/casp_rct_tool.pdf May 2006

CASP Critical Appraisal Skills Programme 2005. Available online at: www.phru.nhs.uk/casp/casp.htm November 2005

Chalmers I, Altman D G 1995 Systematic reviews. BMJ Publishing, London

Cullinan P 2005 Evidence-based health-care: systematic reviews. In: Bowling A, Ebrahim S (eds) Handbook of health research methods: investigation, measurement and analysis. Open University Press, Buckingham, pp.47–61

Evans D, Pearson A 2001 Systematic reviews: gatekeepers of nursing knowledge. Journal of Clinical Nursing 10:593–599

French P 2002 What is the evidence on evidence-based nursing? An epistemological concern. Journal of Advanced Nursing 37(3):250–257

Gray J A M 1997 Evidence-based health-care: how to make health policy and
    management decisions. Churchill Livingstone, Edinburgh

Johnston L 2005 Critically appraising quantitative evidence. In: Melnyk
    B M, Fineout-Overholt E (eds) Evidence-based practice in nursing and
    health-care: a guide to best practice. Lippincott Williams and Wilkins,
    Philadelphia, pp.79–125

Kirkwood B 1988 Essentials of medical statistics. Blackwell Science, Oxford

Laupacis A, Wells G, Richardson S, Tugwell P 1994 Users' guides to the
    medical literature. V. How to use an article about prognosis. Journal of the
    American Medical Association 272:234–237

Mant J 1999a Studies assessing diagnostic tests. In: Dawes M, Davies P, Gray
    A, Mant J, Seers J, Snowball R (eds) Evidence-based practice: a primer for
    health-care professionals. Churchill Livingstone, London, pp.59–69

Mant J 1999b Case control studies. In: Dawes M, Davies P, Gray A, Mant J,
    Seers J, Snowball R (eds) Evidence-based practice: a primer for health-care
    professionals. Churchill Livingstone, London, pp.73–85

*Mant J, Painter R, Vessey M 1998 Risk of myocardial infarction, angina,
    and stroke in users of oral contraceptives: an updated analysis of a cohort
    study. British Journal of Obstetrics and Gynaecology 105:890–896

Martin R M 2005 Epidemiological study designs for health-care research and
    evaluation. In: Bowling A, Ebrahim S (eds) Handbook of health research
    methods: investigation, measurement and analysis. Open University Press,
    Buckingham, pp.98–163

Mathews J N S 2000 An introduction to randomized controlled clinical trials.
    Arnold, London

Melnyk B M 2005 Creating a vision: motivating a change to evidence-based
    practice in individuals and organizations. In: Melnyk B M, Fineout-Over-
    holt E (eds) Evidence-based practice in nursing and health-care: a guide to
    best practice. Lippincott Williams and Wilkins, Philadelphia, pp.443–455

Moher D, Jadad E R, Nichol G, Penman M, Tugwell P, Walsh S 1995 Assess-
    ing the quality of randomised controlled trials: an annotated bibliography
    of scales and checklists. Controlled Clinical Trials 16:62–73

Moore A, McQuay H 2000 Bias. Bandolier 7(10):1–5

Mulhall A 1999 Creating change in practice. In: Mulhall A, Le May A.
    Nursing research: dissemination and implementation. Churchill Living-
    stone, Edinburgh, pp.151–175

O'Rourke A 2005 Critical appraisal. In: Bowling A, Ebrahim S (eds) Hand-
    book of health research methods: investigation, measurement and analysis.
    Open University Press, Buckingham, pp.62–84

Oxman A D, Sackett D L, Guyatt G H and the Evidence-Based Medicine
    Working Group 1993 How to get started. Based on the Users' Guides to

Evidence-Based Medicine and reproduced with permission from Journal of the American Medical Association 270(17):2093–2095. Available online at: www.cche.net/usersguides/start.asp 29 Jan 2006

Sackett D L, Rosenberg W M C, Muir Gray J A, Haynes R B, Richardson W S 1996 Evidence based medicine: what it is and what it isn't. British Medical Journal 312:71–72

Sackett D, Strauss S, Scott Richardson W, Rosenberg W, Haynes R 2000 Evidence-based medicine: how to practise and teach evidence-based medicine, 2nd edn. Churchill Livingstone, Edinburgh

*Scurr J H, Machin S J, Bailey-King S, Mackie I J, McDonald S, Coleridge Smith P D 2001 Frequency and prevention of symptomless deep-vein thrombosis in long-haul flights: a randomized trial. Lancet 357: 1485–1489

Sim J, Wright C 2000 Basic elements of research design. In: Sim J, Wright C (eds) Research in health-care: concepts, designs and methods. Nelson Thornes, Cheltenham

Stevens K R 2005 Critically appraising knowledge for clinical decision making. In: Melnyk B M, Fineout-Overholt E (eds) Evidence-based practice in nursing and health-care: a guide to best practice. Lippincott Williams and Wilkins, Philadelphia, pp.73–78

Summerskill W S M 2000 Hierarchy of evidence. In: McGovern D B P, Valori R M, Summerskill W S M, Levi M (eds) Evidence-based medicine. BIOS Scientific Publishers, Oxford, pp.14–16

Further reading

Internet resources

There are numerous websites that contain materials for critical appraisal. However, these sites often change their website address and new sites are opening up all the time. We have therefore provided you with the address for the most comprehensive and up-to-date information about evidence-based practice on the web, 'Netting the Evidence'. This site was established and is maintained by Andrew Booth at Sheffield University. www.shef.ac.uk/~scharr/ir/netting/

Books

Crombie I K 1996 The pocket guide to critical appraisal. BMJ Publishing, London

Greenhalgh T 2006 How to read a paper, 3rd edn. BMJ Books, Blackwell Publishing, London

Melnyk B M, Fineout-Overholt E 2005 Evidence-based practice in nursing and health-care: a guide to best practice. Lippincott Williams and Wilkins, Philadelphia

Ogier M E 1998 Reading research – how to make research more approachable, 2nd edn. Baillière Tindall, London

Sackett D, Strauss S, Scott Richardson W, Rosenberg W, Haynes R 2000 Evidence-based medicine: how to practise and teach evidence-based medicine, 2nd edn. Churchill Livingstone, Edinburgh

5

Critical appraisal of quantitative studies 2: Can the evidence be applied in your clinical setting?

Anne-Marie Glenny and Faith Gibson

KEY POINTS

- How to decide whether the results of a study can be applied to your patients/clinical setting.
- Using confidence intervals instead of '*p*-values'.
- Developing a clinically useful interpretation of study results:
  - Interpreting results from a study about the effectiveness of therapies: calculating odds ratios, risk ratios, relative risk reductions, absolute risk reductions and the number needed to treat (NNT)

- Interpreting results from a study about the accuracy of a diagnostic test or assessment: calculating likelihood ratios, pre- and post-test odds
- Interpreting results from a study about prognosis or harm: calculating the number needed to harm (NNH).

Introduction

In Chapter 4 the need for research users to critically appraise published research was established. The three aspects of critical appraisal were outlined (Figure 5.1) and the methods used to assess the quality of studies examined. This chapter describes in detail the skills and knowledge required for the other two aspects of the critical appraisal process. The first section will discuss how to decide whether the results from a study can be applied to your patients and/or in your clinical setting. The second section will demonstrate how you can translate the results given for a study sample into clinically meaningful results for an individual patient. The three scenarios developed in Chapter 4, and their respective pieces of evidence, will be used to illustrate this process.

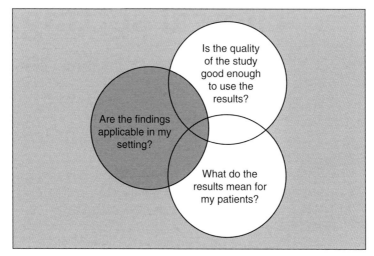

Figure 5.1 Aspects of the critical appraisal process. 2: Assessing applicability

Deciding whether the results can be applied in your clinical setting

Chapter 4 has dealt with the quality of health-related research studies. How well has a study been conducted for the research question being asked? Can we trust the study's results? What needs to be recognised, however, is that not all high-quality studies are applicable to all patients or all clinical settings. Health-related research takes place all over the world, in settings that may be very different from the one in which your patients are found. In addition, there is a tendency for studies to include 'scientifically clean' populations (Greenhalgh 1997), excluding patients who have co-existing illnesses or additional risk factors. This can mean that patients included in health-related research are often very different from those seen in everyday clinical practice. The context in which you practise and/or the context of each patient's consultation are, to some degree, unique. Alongside the assessment of a study's quality, it is important to consider whether the results obtained can be applied to your patients and your clinical setting. Can the results of a trial recruiting patients aged 18–50 years be applied to patients over 60 years of age? If a study has been conducted in Brazil, what do the results mean with regard to patients being treated in the UK?

It is unlikely that the patients and settings used in a research study will ever be identical to yours. When addressing the issue of applicability, we need to consider the extent to which differences in patients and settings might affect the results. Are the differences so great that we might expect the direction of effect to alter? If the differences would only change the size or extent of the effect of the treatment, rather than changing the effect from one of benefit to one of harm, then it may be possible to adjust the result to reflect the impact in your patients. For example, if a treatment has been shown to be effective on a relatively fit study population, we might expect a greater effect to be observed on a very sick patient seen in practice.

These issues are illustrated in the discussions of the interpretations of the results for each scenario under the heading 'The clinical bottom line'.

Questions for assessing applicability

Although the assessment of quality (Chapter 4) and the assessment of applicability have been addressed separately in this book, in practice they are likely to occur simultaneously in the critical appraisal process. The assessment of both quality and applicability can be used to determine whether a study is worth reading in full. If a fundamental flaw is identified in the study design which means the results of the study cannot be trusted, there is little point in reading the full article. Similarly, if it is clear from the details presented in the study that the results cannot be applied to your patient population and/or the clinical setting, then there is no need to read further.

The assessment of applicability is not an exact science and requires some degree of subjectivity. Specific questions can help to ascertain the applicability of a study's results (CASP 2005). Unlike the quality assessment, the same questions can be used whatever the type of question or study design being appraised. Questions to consider when assessing applicability include the following.

- **What are the characteristics of the participants in the study?** Do they differ from the patients you see in practice? If so, do they differ on factors that could potentially affect the outcome of interest (consider age, co-morbidity, severity of condition, gender, etc.). Are the differences likely to affect the direction of the effect seen in the study or just the size of the effect?

- **Where has the study been conducted?** Is the study setting so different from yours that the results achieved in the study are unlikely to be achieved in your clinical setting? Again, are the differences likely to affect the direction of the effect seen in the study or just the magnitude of the effect?

- **Is it feasible to introduce the intervention or test described in the study?** Suppose the results of a research study into the care of patients with stroke suggest that patient outcomes are better when they are looked after in a specialist unit (i.e. one that requires certain types of equipment and staff with specialist training) rather than in a general ward. Such a change may not be possible on your unit. This does not mean that you should give up altogether (the issue should perhaps be referred to your unit manager); however, it does mean that you will need to look at other aspects of stroke management that are within the capacity of your team to deliver.

- **Have all the important outcomes been considered?** Have the researchers considered all the outcomes that are truly important to the patient and all those involved in their care and treatment planning? If important outcomes have not been considered, how does this affect the interpretation of the results presented? Researchers often focus on outcome measures that are relatively quick and easy to measure, rather than those that are of practical importance. For example, surrogate outcomes, such as blood pressure, are often used to reflect the more clinically important outcomes, such as risk of heart attack. Surrogate outcomes are often used when the observation of a clinical outcome would require a long follow-up. However, when interpreting the findings from surrogate outcomes we have to be certain of the link between the surrogate and clinical outcome. Is the utility of the surrogate well established?

- **Do any reported benefits outweigh the costs?** When thinking of the costs and benefits of the intervention or test, think beyond purely financial terms. In most situations doing something new or in a different way will involve stopping doing something else. The costs of 'stopping' need to be weighed up against the benefits of the proposed change. Where the costs are perceived by the patient and/or staff as being too high, the proposed change is unlikely to be accepted.

- **What are your patient's preferences?** Incorporating research evidence into practice should not mean ignoring patient preference. All patients are different and what one patient considers to be a reasonable intervention, treatment plan or outcome may be unacceptable to another. Forcing a patient to use the intervention indicated by evidence would be unethical and may be counterproductive.

Table 5.1 works through these questions and provides answers for the example of the case of Florence Barrett (see Chapter 4, Worked example 4.3, p.116). The relevant aspects of the scenario have been reproduced in Box 5.1.

What do the results of this study mean in my context/for my patients?

Once you have decided the quality of the study is good enough and the results can be applied in your setting, the next stage is to interpret what the results of the study mean for your individual patient. This is the third aspect of critical appraisal highlighted in Figure 5.2. It is a common misperception that evidence-based practice is all about statistics. We hope that it is already clear that this is not the case. The evidence-based practice approach is that the statistical analyses carried out in a study are not the most important consideration when critically appraising a paper. Most important is the choice and quality of the study design. If a study was well designed for the research question being asked, then there is a high probability that the researchers' interpretation of the results can be trusted (Sackett et al 2000). Even well-done statistical analysis cannot compensate for bias caused by deficiencies in the study design. When critically appraising

> **BOX 5.1** Information from the scenario in Worked example 4.3 relevant to the assessment of applicability
>
> *Patient:* Florence Barrett, 33 years old, mother of two, used oral contraception for just over a year, smokes 25–30 cigarettes per day.
>
> *Clinical question:* Is Florence, a heavy smoker using the oral contraceptive pill, at higher risk of myocardial infarction than women who smoke but use other forms of contraception?
>
> *Evidence:* Mant J, Painter R, Vessey M 1998 Risk of myocardial infarction, angina, and stroke in users of oral contraceptives: an updated analysis of a cohort study. British Journal of Obstetrics and Gynaecology 105:890–896

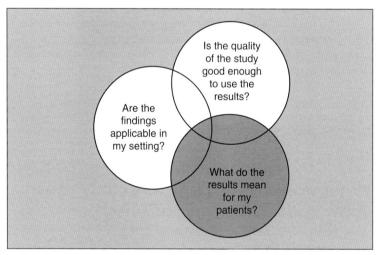

Figure 5.2 Aspects of the critical appraisal process. 3: Interpreting results

a research study, the reader does not have to be an expert in statistics. However, it is useful if the reader is able to calculate and interpret different effect measures, taking into account both the statistical significance and clinical importance of the results.

p-values and confidence intervals

The way the results of research are reported can often make it difficult to apply them in daily clinical practice. One reason for this is that one of the

TABLE 5.1 QUESTIONS FOR ASSESSING THE APPLICABILITY OF A STUDY

Question	Example: Scenario 4.3
What is the study about?	The study investigated the risk of myocardial infarction, angina and stroke in users of oral contraceptives compared with users of other methods of contraception
What are the characteristics of the participants in the study?	The study included women aged 25–39 who attended 17 family planning clinics in England and Scotland. Both smokers and non-smokers were included. All women were British, married and Caucasian. Those study participants who smoke can be assumed to be similar to Florence Barrett
Where has the study been conducted?	Participants in the study were recruited from family planning clinics in England and Scotland
Is it feasible to introduce the intervention or test described in the study?	As this was a study about prognosis or outcomes, this question is less relevant. However, if the results suggested that Florence was at greater risk of an MI if she continued to use oral contraception there are no impediments to changing the method of contraception Florence uses apart from her own preferences
Have all the important outcomes been considered?	The research paper focuses on the risk of myocardial infarction, angina and stroke. The original cohort study has been used to explore other outcomes such as fractures, spinal osteo-arthritis, eye disease and hepatic problems. These outcomes are published in separate papers (Hannaford et al 1997,

(Continued)

Table 5.1 (CONTINUED)

Question	Example: Scenario 4.3
	Vessey et al 1998a, b, 1999). A discussion with Florence would help identify the outcomes most important to her
Do any reported benefits outweigh the costs?	The potential benefit to Florence is a reduction in her risk of MI. This has potential knock-on benefits for members of her family and the health services. Potential costs to Florence and her family include increased risk of unwanted pregnancy and increased inconvenience that other suitable methods of contraception might entail. These costs may be hidden from the view of health professionals but should not be underestimated
What are your patient's preferences?	No information is given about Florence's preferred method of contraception. Her visit to the surgery was not prompted by a desire to change methods, suggesting she is happy enough with the oral contraceptive pill. The results about her level of risk of myocardial infarction (her overall risk can be calculated using CHD risk calculators) should be discussed with her to allow her to come to her own decision after weighing up the relative benefits and costs of any change

major concerns of researchers is to establish the likelihood of their result being caused by chance. The p-value is frequently presented to illustrate this likelihood. Its value always lies between zero and one. A p-value of 0.5 would tell us that there is a 1 in 2 (50%) probability of the result being due to chance. If this were the case, we would be unlikely to accept the results of the study as being significant. Conventionally, we accept a p-value of 0.05 or below as being statistically significant. That means a probability of 1 in 20 that the result is due to chance. Some papers may use a more rigorous cut-off point of p equal to 0.01 or below as statistically significant (a 1 in 100 probability that the result is due to chance). The p-value alone does not give any indication of the size or direction of the difference (or treatment effect) (Gardner & Altman 1986). Therefore, it does not help you assess what the likely effect will be on your patient.

Health-related research studies may present results accompanied by confidence intervals, which provide more information than the p-value alone. A formal definition of a confidence interval is 'a range of values for a variable of interest constructed so that this range has a specified probability of including the true value of the variable' (Last 1988). The accepted convention is to use the 95% confidence interval. This means that you can be 95% certain that the true value of the variable of interest lies within the 95% confidence intervals.

Confidence intervals are a clinically useful way of measuring the precision of an estimate of effect size. When evaluating the effect of an intervention, a confidence interval not only provides us with information on statistical significance, but also indicates the range within which the true treatment effect is likely to lie. If, when comparing interventions, the confidence interval includes the value of 'no effect', then the difference between the interventions is not statistically significant. The narrower the gap between the upper and lower 95% confidence intervals, the more certain we will be about the precision of the estimate. The 95% confidence intervals can be calculated for most common statistical estimates or comparisons, examples of which will be presented below under 'Developing a clinically meaningful result'.

Effect measures

A number of clinically meaningful effect measures have been developed for different types of question/study designs. These include measures such as odds ratios (OR), risks ratios (RR), relative risk reductions (RRR) and absolute risk reduction (ARR). One increasingly popular measure is the number needed to treat (NNT), which is useful for interpreting results from studies about the effectiveness of a therapy or intervention (Laupacis et al 1988). NNT shows how many patients have to be given the intervention for one extra person to benefit who would not have done so if given the comparison treatment. Studies that look at whether a particular method of diagnosis or assessment works often give results as the sensitivity (proportion of people with a condition who test positive) and specificity (proportion of people without the condition who test negative) of the test. These can be converted (using likelihood ratios) into probabilities that express how likely the diagnosis is for a particular patient.

More studies are being published which use these types of measures to report their results but health-care practitioners still need to understand how to calculate these themselves. At first some of the calculations may seem a bit intimidating. However, despite their apparent complexity, they usually only involve some simple arithmetic that can, if necessary, be done with pencil and paper. The most effective way of learning these techniques is by working through real examples. The following sections will describe how these measures are calculated and interpreted, along with associated confidence intervals, using as examples the results given in the papers we have already critically appraised in Chapter 4.

Interpreting the results of studies about the effectiveness of a particular therapy or intervention

This section will describe how the data from a study can be used to calculate the number needed to treat (NNT). The results from the paper referenced in Worked example 4.1 (Chapter 4, p.104) will be used (Box 5.2).

BOX 5.2 Information from the scenario in Worked example 4.1 relevant to an assessment of the effectiveness of an intervention

Patient: Mrs Pink and her parents, who have booked a long-haul flight.

EBP question: Do compression stockings prevent deep vein thrombosis in the lower limb during long-haul air travel?

Evidence: Scurr J H, Machin S J, Bailey-King S, Mackie I J, McDonald S, Coleridge Smith P D 2001 Frequency and prevention of symptomless deep-vein thrombosis in long-haul flights: a randomized trial. Lancet 357:1485–1489

Results reported in the study: The results for deep vein thrombosis (DVT) and superficial thrombophlebitis (SVT), assessed within 48 hours of the passengers' return flight, are presented. For those passengers allocated to the stocking group, 0 out of 115 had DVT compared to 12 out of 116 passengers not wearing compression stockings. With regard to SVT, 4 out of 115 passengers wearing stockings developed SVT compared to 0 out of 116 in the no-stocking group.

Developing a clinically meaningful result

A 2 × 2 table like the one shown in Figure 5.3 is a standard tool for calculating clinically meaningful results and will be used in each example in this chapter. Each cell in the table contains a number and is labelled with a letter – a, b, c and d. In a comparative study participants are divided into two groups: the group which received the 'new' or experimental therapy (cells a and b) and the group which did not (cells c and d). The presence (cells a and c) or absence (cells b and d) of the outcome of interest is reported for both groups. The letters in the cells are used in the formulae for calculating summary measures like the odds ratios (OR), risks ratios (RR), relative risk reductions (RRR), absolute risk reduction (ARR) and the number needed to treat (NNT) (Table 5.2). The numbers to go in each cell are obtained from the study results. It is often possible to calculate the numbers if they are not given.

Figure 5.3 uses the results from the study conducted by Scurr and colleagues (2001), the study being used in this scenario.

Calculating effect measures

The formulae for calculating different effect measures are given in Table 5.2. In this section we will focus specifically on the ARR and the NNT, an increasingly popular way of presenting the results of controlled clinical trials. In a trial comparing an experimental treatment with a control treatment, the NNT is the estimated number of patients who need to be treated

		Outcome: Deep vein thrombosis		Totals	
		Present	Absent		
Study groups	Experimental group (compression stockings)	a 0	b 115	a + b 115	
	Control group (no compression stockings)	c 12	d 104	c + d 116	
Totals		a + c 12	b + d 219	a + b + c + d 231	

Figure 5.3 A 2 × 2 table for interpreting results of a study on the effectiveness of an intervention with data from the study by Scurr and colleagues (2001)

TABLE 5.2 CALCULATING EFFECTS MEASURES

Measure	Description	Formula	Example (see Figure 5.3)
Odds ratio (OR)	The odds of an event (outcome) in the experimental group divided by the odds of an event in the control group. Usually expressed as a decimal proportion. An OR of 1 indicates no difference between the two groups (value of 'no effect')	$(a/b)/(c/d) = ad/bc$	$(0/115)/(12/104)$ $= (0 \times 104)/(115 \times 12)$ $= 0$
Risk ratio (RR) Also known as relative risk or rate ratio	The risk of an event in the experimental group (known as the experimental event rate (EER)) divided by the risk of an event in the control group (known as the control event rate (CER)). Usually expressed as a percentage. A RR of 1 indicates no difference between the two groups	$(a/(a + b))/(c/(c + d))$	$(0/115)/(12/116)$ $= 0/0.1$ $= 0 (0\%)$

Absolute risk reduction (ARR) Also known as risk difference or rate difference	The risk of an event in the control group (the control event rate (CER)) minus the risk of an event in the experimental group (the experimental event rate (EER)). Usually expressed as a percentage. An ARR of 0% indicates no difference between the two groups	$c/(c + d) - a/(a + b)$ $= 0.1 - 0$ $= 0.1$ (10%)
Relative risk reduction (RRR)	The ARR divided by the risk of an event in the control group. Can also be calculated as $1 - RR$. Usually expressed as a percentage. A RRR of 0% indicates no difference between the two groups	$ARR/(c/(c + d))$ also $1 - RR$ $0.1/(12/116)$ or $1 - 0 = 1$ (100%)
Number needed to treat (NNT)	The reciprocal of the ARR. Usually expressed as a whole number	$NNT = 1/ARR$ $1/0.1 = 10$

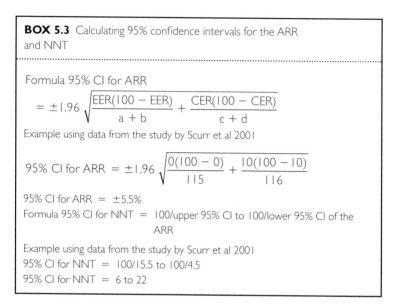

BOX 5.3 Calculating 95% confidence intervals for the ARR and NNT

Formula 95% CI for ARR

$$= \pm 1.96 \sqrt{\frac{EER(100 - EER)}{a + b} + \frac{CER(100 - CER)}{c + d}}$$

Example using data from the study by Scurr et al 2001

$$95\% \text{ CI for ARR} = \pm 1.96 \sqrt{\frac{0(100 - 0)}{115} + \frac{10(100 - 10)}{116}}$$

95% CI for ARR = ±5.5%
Formula 95% CI for NNT = 100/upper 95% CI to 100/lower 95% CI of the ARR

Example using data from the study by Scurr et al 2001
95% CI for NNT = 100/15.5 to 100/4.5
95% CI for NNT = 6 to 22

with the experimental treatment for one additional patient to benefit (Altman 1998). The smaller the NNT, the more important the treatment effect. In this example (Table 5.2) the ARR is 10%, indicating that the absolute benefit of stockings is a 10% reduction in DVT rate. The NNT is 10 (the figure is typically rounded up toward the more conservative whole number). This means that 10 long-haul flight passengers need to wear compression stockings to prevent one extra passenger from developing symptomless DVT. When presenting any measure of effect, the 95% confidence intervals should also be presented. Box 5.3 demonstrates how the confidence intervals can be calculated for both the ARR and NNT. For the ARR the 95% confidence intervals are 4.5% to 15.5%, indicating that 95% of the time the absolute benefit may be as low as 4.5% or as high as 15.5%. Given that the confidence intervals do not capture the value of 'no effect', 0% (see Table 5.2), we can see that the results are statistically significant. The 95% confidence intervals for NNT are 6 to 22.

The clinical bottom line

The clinical bottom line refers to what the results actually mean for clinical practice. The clinical bottom line for the study in this example could be described as follows. In long-haul flight passengers, compression stockings prevent one symptomless DVT for every 10 passengers who wear them.

BOX 5.4 Information from the scenario in Worked example 4.2 relevant to an assessment of a diagnostic test

Scenario: Thomas Davies, a 45-year-old frequent attender, visits practice nurse. He is unemployed, no mental health problems, self-reported 'feeling down and loss of interest'. Nurse feels that he has a 50% chance of having clinical depression (which means he has 50% chance of not having clinical depression).

Clinical question: In patients with clinical depression, how accurately does patient response to two screening questions and a question relating to help diagnose clinical depression?

Evidence: Arroll B, Goodyear-Smith F, Kerse N, Fishman T, Gunn J 2005 Effect of the addition of a 'help' question to two screening questions on specificity for diagnosis of depression in general practice: diagnostic validity study. British Medical Journal 331: 884–889

Results: A positive response to either screening question and help question had a sensitivity of 96% (95% CI 86–99%) and a specificity of 89% (95% CI 87–91%).

Mrs Pink and her parents, being fit and with no history of thrombo-embolic problems, would have been eligible for the study, age permitting. There is no reason to suppose that she would not have benefited from the intervention. A potential harm presented in the study is an increased risk of superficial thrombophlebitis in varicose veins if the stockings are worn, although the increase was not statistically significant.

Interpreting the results of studies that investigate the performance or accuracy of a particular diagnostic test/method of assessment

This section will focus on calculating and understanding some clinically useful measures for interpreting the results of studies that measure how good a test or method of assessment is at finding a target condition. These include sensitivity, specificity, positive and negative likelihood ratios and pre- and post-test probabilities. The results from the paper referenced in Worked example 4.2 will be used as an example (see Chapter 4, p.111). The relevant details from the paper and scenario are given in Box 5.4.

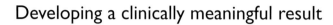

Developing a clinically meaningful result

The results of diagnostic studies are usually reported in terms of sensitivity (in our example, this would be the chance of having a positive result using 'either screening question plus help questions' if you have depression) and specificity (the chance of having a negative result using 'either screening question plus help questions' if you do not have depression). These figures are given in the example paper (Box 5.4). A high sensitivity is a useful result because the presence of a negative test result in a patient virtually rules out a positive diagnosis. In this example (sensitivity 96%), we could say that if Mr Davies answers 'no' to the screening questions plus help question, we can be fairly sure that he does not have depression (we would only be wrong in four patients out of 100).

A high specificity is a useful result because a positive test result in an individual patient effectively rules in a positive diagnosis. In this example (specificity 89%), if Mr Davies answers 'yes' to either screening question plus the help question, we could be reasonably sure that he had clinical depression. Eleven patients in 100 answer 'yes' to one of the questions but do not have clinical depression. Whilst the sensitivity and specificity are useful when they are high, it is rare for both the sensitivity and specificity to be high on the same test as there is nearly always a trade-off between the two.

In addition, the performance of a test is affected by the prevalence of the condition in the underlying population. In an individual patient, this is referred to as the pre-test probability of an individual having the condition. In our scenario the nurse thought that Mr Davies had a pre-test probability of 50% of having clinical depression (which means he has 50% probability of not having clinical depression). What the nurse wants the test to do is to increase this probability to as near 100% as possible, either that he does or does not have depression. This is called the post-test probability.

In a study which tests whether a diagnostic test or assessment works, the new test is compared to an existing 'gold standard'. This is a method that is assumed to diagnose the target condition with certainty. All patients with and without the condition receive both tests. The results of the study can be reported in a 2 × 2 table. Figure 5.4 shows a 2 × 2 table complete with data from the study on the 'screening questions plus help question' (Arroll et al 2005). In this study the gold standard is the score obtained using the Composite International Diagnostic Interview (CIDI).

		Target disorder: Depression as diagnosed by CIDI		Totals
		Present	Absent	
New test: 'two screening questions plus help question'	Positive	a 45	b 94	a + b 139
	Negative	c 2	d 795	c + d 797
Totals		a + c 47	b + d 889	a + b + c + d 936*

* 1025 patients agreed to participate; 936 completed the CIDI.

Figure 5.4 A 2 × 2 table for interpreting results of the 'two screening questions plus help question' study on the diagnosis of depression by Arroll and colleagues (2005)

Calculating the difference between the pre- and post-test probability

What the nurse and Mr Davies need to know is, does answering 'yes' or 'no' to the screening questions plus help question mean that Mr Davies does or does not have clinical depression? Technically this is the likelihood that a positive test result is a true positive and that a negative test result is a true negative. The ratio of true-positive results to false-positive results is known as the positive likelihood ratio. The ratio of true-negative results to false-negative results is known as the negative likelihood ratio. We can calculate these from the sensitivity and specificity respectively. The formulae for calculating these measures are given in Table 5.3. Using the data from the study by Arroll et al, the positive likelihood ratio is 8.7. This means that a positive result to the 'screening questions plus help question' is nearly nine times as likely in someone who has clinical depression than in someone who does not (i.e. a true positive rather than a false positive).

However, this is still not a very helpful result. The question arises: nine times as likely as what? If Mr Davies was very unlikely to be clinically depressed before taking the test then being nine times as likely does not necessarily mean that he is clinically depressed. The interpretation of likelihood ratios depends partly on the underlying prevalence (Mant 1999). As mentioned previously, in our scenario the nurse thought that Mr Davies had a pre-test probability of 50% of having clinical depression (and a 50%

TABLE 5.3 FORMULAE FOR CALCULATING USEFUL CLINICAL MEASURES FOR ANSWERING QUESTIONS ABOUT WHETHER A PARTICULAR DIAGNOSTIC TEST OR METHOD OF ASSESSMENT WORKS

Measure	Formula	Example (Worked example 4.2 data)
Sensitivity	a/a + c	45/47 = 0.96 or 96%
Specificity	d/b + d	795/889 = 0.89 or 89%
Positive likelihood ratio	Sensitivity/ (100 − specificity)	96/(100 − 89) = 8.7
Negative likelihood ratio	(100 − sensitivity)/ specificity	(100 − 96)/89 = 0.04
Pre-test odds	Prevalence/ 100 − prevalence	50/(100 − 50) = 1
Post-test odds	Pre-test odds × likelihood ratio	1 × 8.7 = 8.7
Post-test probability	Post-test odds/ (post-test odds + 1)	8.7/(8.7 + 1) = 89.7%

probability of not having clinical depression). The pre-test probability of 50:50, which is the same as pre-test odds of 1:1, can be combined with the likelihood ratio to give us the post-test odds or probability. In this example 1:1 can be multiplied with the likelihood ratio 8.7, giving post-test odds of 8.7:1 in favour of clinical depression. If, like us, you are more comfortable with probability than odds, post-test odds of 8.7:1 converts to a more useful, but not diagnostic, post-test probability of 89.7%.

Calculating post-test probability using the nomogram

Another simpler way of calculating Mr Davies' chance of having depression given a result from the 'two questions' method is to use the nomogram shown in Figure 5.5. Find 50% on the left-hand column, then find 8.7 in the middle column (the positive likelihood ratio) and read off the post-test probability on the right hand column (about 90%). This means that there is still a 10% chance that, even given a positive result using the screening questions plus help question method, Mr Davies does not have depression. For a negative result, find 50% on the left-hand column again, then find 0.04 (the negative likelihood ratio) in the middle column and read off the post-test probability (about 3%). This means that if Mr Davies answers no

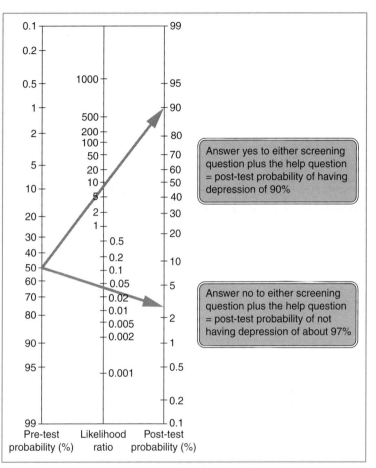

Figure 5.5 Likelihood ratio nomogram showing interpretation of data from the study by Arroll et al (2005) applied to the scenario in Worked example 4.2 (Chapter 4, p.110). (From Sackett et al 2000, with permission)

to the screening questions plus the help question, there is a 97% chance that he does not have clinical depression.

The clinical bottom line

The clinical bottom line in our example study could be as follows. Using a quick assessment tool can rule out depression in primary care settings. This allows more detailed assessment to be targeted at cases where the assessment is positive. The results of the study suggest that a negative result using the two questions plus help question indicates that it is very unlikely that Mr Davies is clinically depressed. A positive result does not provide us with a certain diagnosis of clinical depression. In our scenario Mr Davies is positive for the two questions plus help question. He may well have clinical depression but a more detailed assessment, perhaps by a psychologist or counsellor, may be necessary to firmly establish the correct diagnosis.

Interpreting the results of studies about prognosis or outcome of a particular condition and/or harm

If we are satisfied that the evidence from a study can be applied and is of good enough quality to use, then we need to decide if the association between exposure and outcome is sufficiently strong and convincing for us to have to do something about it. Worked example 4.3 can be used to illustrate this (see Chapter 4, p.116). Relevant details from the paper and scenario are given in Box 5.5. Studies of prognosis/harm usually report results in terms of proportions or rates of events in the two groups being

---

BOX 5.5 Information from the scenario in Worked example 4.3 relevant to the assessment of association between exposure and outcome

Patient: Florence Barrett, 33 years old, mother of two, used oral contraception for just over a year, smokes 25–30 cigarettes per day.

Clinical question: Are women who smoke and take oral contraception at higher risk of myocardial infarction than women who smoke but use other forms of contraception?

Evidence: Mant J, Painter R, Vessey M 1998 Risk of myocardial infarction, angina, and stroke in users of oral contraceptives: an updated analysis of a cohort study. British Journal of Obstetrics and Gynaecology 105:890–896

Results: In heavy smokers there is a fourfold increase in the risk of myocardial infarction if the oral contraceptive pill is taken, from 0.24 per 1000 woman-years in heavy smokers who have never used oral contraception to 1.18 per 1000 woman-years at risk in current users of oral contraception. In heavy smokers (15+) the relative risk is 4.0 for ex-users of the oral contraceptive pill, 4.2 for ever-users of the oral contraceptive pill and 4.9 for current users.

compared. In this scenario the result of interest is the difference between the rate of myocardial infarction in women who smoke more than 15 cigarettes a day and use the oral contraceptive pill and women who smoke more than 15 cigarettes a day but have never used the oral contraceptive pill. For the clinical question in the scenario, the results of interest can be found in the text that describes Table 2 and in Table 2 itself in the paper by Mant et al (1998). In this study the researchers have quite appropriately adjusted the results for other potential confounding variables such as age, parity, social class and obesity.

Developing a clinically meaningful result

The outcome of interest is the difference between the rate in the YES (heavy smoker, user of the oral contraceptive pill) group and the rate in the NO (heavy smoker, never used the oral contraceptive pill) group. There are several different ways in which we can interpret this difference, some of which are reported in the paper. A 2 × 2 table can be used to aid interpretation of the study results. A 2 × 2 table using the headings from the study by Mant and colleagues is given in Figure 5.6. The raw data are not reported in the paper, only the resulting rates.

Relative risk and its limitations

One of the results reported in the study by Mant et al (1998) is the relative risk (RR). Researchers often report the RR as a measure of effect size. This measures the relative difference in the percentage affected in each group. For example, where the results of a study show that the percentage affected in one group is 0.0025 and in the other 0.01, this can legitimately

		Adverse outcome: Myocardial infarction		Rates
		Present	Absent	
Exposed to the treatment (oral contraception)	Yes: Heavy smokers, use oral contraceptives	a	b	a/(a + b) = rate in Yes group
	No: Heavy smokers, never used oral contraceptives	c	d	c/(c + d) = rate in No group

Figure 5.6 A 2 × 2 table for prognostic/harm studies (scenario in Worked example 4.3 from Chapter 4, p.116)

be presented as a fourfold difference in the risk between groups. However, in this example the absolute difference between the two groups is less than 1%. Depending on the question or the study, different measures will be important. For example, if the outcome is mortality, a difference of 0.75% may be considered sufficient to change practice. If the outcome is benefit obtained by using a very expensive drug with unpleasant side effects, a difference of 0.75% may not be considered sufficient to change practice.

In this example the RR tells us that the rate of myocardial infarction per 1000 woman-years is 4.9 times greater amongst women who smoke heavily and use oral contraception compared with women who smoke heavily and have never used oral contraception. As a general rule of thumb, in cohort studies we can say that a RR increase of more than 3 is unlikely to be the result of bias (Sackett et al 2000). From the results of the paper we can deduce that there is a difference in rates between the two groups and that this difference is unlikely to be the result of bias. But is the difference big enough to recommend a change of contraception method for Mrs Barrett?

Calculating the number needed to harm (NNH)

There are a number of other measures we can calculate to help Mrs Barrett make that decision. Table 5.4 shows the formulae for these calculations with completed examples using data from the study by Mant et al. In order to calculate the number needed to harm (NNH), we first need to calculate the absolute risk increase (ARI). The ARI tells us the size of the difference between the two groups. The ARI in this example tells that the difference between the groups is equivalent to less than 1 event per 1000 woman-years. Florence Barrett is not going to live for 1000 years so what does this result mean to her? Another way of presenting this result is to use the number needed to harm. The NNH tells us the number of women who smoke heavily that would have to take oral contraception for 1 year to cause one extra myocardial infarction. In the example, the NNH = 1063 (for some reason this figure is given as 1060 in the abstract of the paper by Mant et al 1998).

The clinical bottom line

The clinical bottom line for this study might be as follows. There is an increased risk of myocardial infarction in heavy smokers who use oral contraception. This increased risk is very small. A total of 1063 heavy smokers would need to take oral contraception for 1 year for one extra woman to experience a myocardial infarction. As a heavy smoker, Mrs Barrett is at greater risk of having a myocardial infarction if she continues

TABLE 5.4 FORMULAE FOR CALCULATING USEFUL CLINICAL MEASURES FOR ANSWERING QUESTIONS ABOUT PROGNOSIS/HARM

Measure	Formula	Example
Relative risk (RR)	$(a/(a + b))/(c/(c + d))$	$1.18/0.24 = 0.49$
Absolute risk increase (ARI)	$(a/(a + b)) - (c/(c + d))$	$1.18 - 0.24 = 0.94$ per 1000
Number needed to harm (NNH)	$1/ARI$	$1/0.00094^a = 1063$

[a]Rate per 1000 converted to percentage by dividing by 1000.

to use oral contraception. This increase in risk is comparatively small. The benefit she might gain from switching methods of contraception is probably even smaller than the results given here suggest, as she will not return to the level of risk of a person who has never used oral contraception. The possible benefits in terms of a small reduction in risk of myocardial infarction have to be weighed up against a possibly larger increase in risk of unwanted pregnancy.

The best advice that the nurse could give Florence is to stop smoking as this would reduce her lifetime risk of myocardial infarction (regardless of whether she uses oral contraception or not).

Summary

This chapter has described how you can decide whether the results of a study can be applied in your setting and how you can calculate clinically useful measures to interpret the results given in studies for your patients/ setting. These two processes, combined with the process used to assess the quality of studies described in Chapter 4, make up the critical appraisal process. It is important to recognise that all three aspects of the critical appraisal process are interlinked. The quality and applicability aspects are probably the most important parts of critical appraisal to learn. Only you know the setting in which you wish to apply the results and published studies very rarely assess their own quality, whereas it is becoming more common to publish study results in clinically useful forms.

The information obtained in the process of deciding on the applicability of a study and the clinically useful measures can be combined with the quality assessment results in a critically appraised topic (CAT), which can then be shared with your colleagues and patients. However, it is important to recognise that critical appraisal is only one part of the EBP process and on its own will not result in improvements in the quality of care that you might want to achieve. It is therefore important that you take equal care to learn and practise the other stages in the EBP process described in the other chapters of this manual.

Acknowledgements

We give special thanks to Mark Newman and Tony Roberts whose contributions to the previous edition have provided the foundation for this chapter.

References

* Papers used for critical appraisal examples.

Altman D G 1998 Confidence intervals for the number needed to treat. British Medical Journal 317:1309–1312

***Arroll B, Goodyear-Smith F, Kerse N, Fishman T, Gunn J 2005** Effect of the addition of a "help" question to two screening questions on specificity for diagnosis of depression in general practice: diagnostic validity study. British Medical Journal 331:884–889

CASP Critical Appraisal Skills Programme 2005 Available online at: www. phru.nhs.uk/casp/casp.htm November 2005

Gardner M, Altman D G 1986 Confidence intervals rather than P values: estimation rather than hypothesis testing. British Medical Journal 292:746–750

Greenhalgh T 1997 How to read a paper: assessing the methodological quality of published papers. British Medical Journal 315:305–308

Hannaford P C, Kay C R, Vessey M P, Painter R, Mant J 1997 Combined oral contraceptives and liver disease. Contraception 55(3):145–151

Last J M 1988 A dictionary of epidemiology. Oxford University Press, Oxford

Laupacis A, Sackett D L, Roberts R S 1988 An assessment of clinically useful measures of the consequences of treatment. New England Journal of Medicine 318(26):1728–1733

Mant J 1999 Is this test effective? In: Dawes M, Davies P, Gray A, Mant J, Seers J, Snowball R (eds) Evidence-based practice: a primer for health care professionals. Churchill Livingstone, London, pp.133–157

***Mant J, Painter R, Vessey M 1998** Risk of myocardial infarction, angina, and stroke in users of oral contraceptives: an updated analysis of a cohort study. British Journal of Obstetrics and Gynaecology 105:890–896

Sackett D, Strauss S, Scott Richardson W, Rosenberg W, Haynes R 2000 Evidence-based medicine: how to practise and teach evidence-based medicine, 2nd edn. Churchill Livingstone, Edinburgh

*Scurr J H, Machin S J, Bailey-King S, Mackie I J, McDonald S, Coleridge Smith P D 2001 Frequency and prevention of symptomless deep-vein thrombosis in long-haul flights: a randomized trial. Lancet 357:1485–1489

Vessey M, Mant J, Painter R 1998a Oral contraception and other factors in relation to hospital referral for fracture. Findings in a large cohort study. Contraception 57(4):231–235

Vessey M, Hannaford P, Mant J, Painter R, Frith P, Chappel D 1998b Oral contraception and eye disease: findings in two large cohort studies. British Journal of Ophthalmology 82(5):538–542

Vessey M, Painter R, Mant J 1999 Oral contraception and other factors in relation to back disorders in women: findings in a large cohort study. Contraception 60(6):331–335

Whooley M A, Avins A, Miranda J, Browner W S 1997 Case-finding instruments for depression: two questions are as good as many. Journal of General Internal Medicine 12:439–445

Further reading

See Chapter 4, p.125.

6

CHAPTER

Qualitative research: critical appraisal

Andrea Litva and Ann Jacoby

KEY POINTS

- Describe the nature of qualitative inquiry.
- Explain the different types of qualitative data collection.
- Discuss how to appraise qualitative research.
- Consider how qualitative research can inform clinical practice.

Introduction

There is a growing awareness among medical disciplines of the need to extend the boundaries in the types of research used to contribute to the practice of evidence-based medicine (Black 1994, Popay & Williams 1998, Pope & Mays 1995). Muir Gray (1997) asserts that the practice of evidence-based medicine requires information obtained using a range of research methods, thus moving beyond the discipline of clinical epidemiology which currently underpins it (Barbour 2000, Green & Britten 1998). This requires the practitioner to engage with qualitative methods, which are best suited to investigating the beliefs, attitudes and preferences of practitioners and patients and so can aid understanding of how evidence is turned into practice.

This chapter begins with an outline of the nature of qualitative research, providing a brief summary of different types of research methods used. We then describe the various ways in which the quality of research using qualitative methods can be assessed. The chapter concludes by exploring how a qualitative approach can inform clinical practice. This includes both the production and application of clinical evidence. Throughout the chapter, examples of qualitative studies are used to demonstrate how different methods can produce findings to inform clinical practice.

What is qualitative research?

A central feature of qualitative research is that it does not seek to produce quantified answers to research questions (Pope & Mays 1995). The goal of qualitative research is to produce insights on the social world, within natural settings, by giving emphasis to the meanings, experiences, practices and views of those involved. Qualitative research is non-positivistic, meaning that insights are 'interpreted' rather than 'uncovered'. 'Truth' is considered to be relative to its context, not absolute. It may appear in the first instance that qualitative research shares certain qualities with personal anecdotes or journalism, but it is vastly different in practice. While stories are told for their dramatic or other informative qualities, this takes place without analysis or critical evaluation. Whether we believe these stories is usually based upon who is telling them. In contrast, good qualitative research requires such elements as explicit sampling strategies and detailed explanations of how data have been systematically collected and analysed to give the reader confidence in the conclusions drawn.

In this section, the features that are characteristic of all qualitative research are described. While they can be found in all examples of qualitative research, it is important to recognise that there can be great variability in practice, in relation to each of the characteristics.

Naturalistic inquiry

There is no standard approach in qualitative research (Silverman 1993). However, Marshall & Rossman (1989) have demonstrated that the various strands in qualitative research have in common a commitment to naturally occurring data or naturalistic inquiry; that is, to studying phenomena within their natural setting rather than within an artificial or controlled one. Naturalistic inquiry has been described by Guba (1981) as a 'discovery-oriented' approach that minimises investigator manipulation of the study setting and places no prior constraint on what the outcomes will be. Qualitative research is committed to understanding real-world situations as they unfold, from the point of view of the people who live in these worlds. This involves entering their worlds and trying to see things from their point of view. The researcher makes no attempt to manipulate the research setting, but at the same time is aware of the impact they can have upon it. This is different from experimental research, where the investigator usually attempts to control study conditions by manipulating, changing or holding constant external influences, so that a limited set of measurable outcome variables are produced.

Emphasis on the meanings, views, experiences and practices of the informants

Bryman (1988) states that the profound commitment to viewing any phenomenon from the perspective of the people being studied is one of the most fundamental features of any qualitative inquiry. Silverman (1993) broadens this point to include a focus upon uncovering the behaviours or practices of informants. The emphasis is upon making sense of settings and human actions by letting the researcher get as close to the informants as possible. In doing so, the researcher, in effect, becomes the research instrument and the quality of the research is greatly dependent upon the researcher's ability to develop rapport with informants, collect data systematically and interpret them (Guba & Lincoln 1981). In qualitative research, there is clear acknowledgement that observer bias cannot be avoided. Instead, open disclosure of preconceptions and assumptions that can influence data collection and analysis becomes part of the conduct of inquiry. It is therefore not uncommon for a qualitative researcher to provide a brief account of their personal bias (disclosure) in order to encourage informants' voices to be the ones that ultimately emerge.

An inductive process

Qualitative research is inductive as opposed to deductive: the research proceeds from the ground up. It begins with observations of phenomena, constructs, explanations or understandings, building towards generating theories. In some instances, qualitative researchers opt for an open and unstructured strategy, refusing to impose preformulated theoretical frameworks and concepts in advance of the study (Bryman 1988, Glaser & Strauss 1967). Alternatively, qualitative research may be influenced by a particular theory that informs the questions asked and of whom (e.g. feminist research), but still allows data to emerge in such a way as to explore the extent to which the theoretical framework is supported by the research findings.

Context and holism

Central to qualitative research is the importance of context and understanding phenomena holistically. Rather than seeking to isolate and manipulate variables, qualitative research seeks to study a phenomenon in context and to reach an understanding of the social, historical, economic and political contexts from which it has emerged. Therefore, the whole phenomenon is under study and approached holistically as a complex system.

For qualitative researchers, the social world cannot be simplified without missing important factors that are not easily quantifiable. Using a holistic approach, qualitative researchers gather data on multiple aspects of a setting under study, in order to assemble a comprehensive and complete picture of the social dynamic, of a particular situation or programme under study. This differs from the logic and procedures of many quantitative approaches where 'independent' and 'dependent' variables are identified and isolated, and then statistically manipulated. The statistical findings are then used to draw inferences about relationships between these measured variables.

Types of qualitative methods

Qualitative methods can be divided into two types: human-to-human and 'artefactual' methods (Guba & Lincoln 1981, Lincoln 1992). Human-to-human methods include interviewing, participant and non-participant observation, and focus groups. Artefactual methods include the use of documents such as letters, memoranda, reports and diaries. The following is a brief discussion of the different methods used in qualitative inquiry.

Interviews

Interviews are often used in health research to explore how users feel about services they are offered or to understand attitudes and perceptions underlying certain health and illness behaviours. They are used to gain knowledge about how different people interpret and experience the world around them, allowing researchers to gain access to these views, and to find out why they have emerged. In this situation the researcher is interactive and sensitive to the language and concepts used by an informant. They aim to explore what the informant says in order to uncover new areas or ideas often inaccessible by quantitative methods.

For example, interviews can be useful for exploring patients' and carers' experiences of particular treatments. In a study by Davies et al (1996), semi-structured interviews were used to explore patients' and relatives' perspectives of the value of radiotherapy for malignant cerebral glioma. By using the semi-structured approach, the researchers were able to expand on specific issues, while allowing patients and relatives to speak about any matters that affected them. The interviews revealed that relatives were much more likely to be aware of poor prognosis than were patients themselves, who were generally unaware of it. This lack of awareness made it difficult to discuss the issue of satisfaction with some patients. Of the patients who were aware, while they made negative comments about the use of radiotherapy, they were generally not dissatisfied with it. The authors concluded that patients' perceptions of the value of radiotherapy were closely tied to their understanding of their condition.

While the distinction is often made between interviews that are structured and those that are unstructured, it is generally accepted that it is impossible to carry out any interview without having some degree of structure. Therefore, qualitative interviews are distinguished by the degree to which they are standardised. Denzin (1970) identified three different types of interviews: standard schedules, non-schedule standardised and non-standardised interviews (Box 6.1).

Focus groups

A focus group is a group interview that uses the communication *between* informants to generate data (Kitzinger 1995). It is important to note that

---

BOX 6.1 Three types of interview identified by Denzin (1970)

- *Standard schedule* The wording and order of all questions are exactly the same for each respondent. These are also referred to as 'structured' interviews and the research instrument is administered in the same way each time. The use of standardised questions raises issues about whether the research is truly qualitative. However, structured interviewing using open-ended questions does allow informants some flexibility in how they respond. Consequently it can fall (just!) within the domain of qualitative research.

- *Non-schedule standardised* The researcher begins with a list of pre-identified themes or information required, but the actual phrasing and order of the questioning are determined by the flow of the conversation. In this way, the research attempts to maintain a 'conversation-like' tone but also gains answers to very particular questions. For example, Litva (1997) wanted to explore lay perceptions of health, illness and disease. A list of predetermined themes was used to ensure that all the informants were asked about the same issues.

- *Non-standardised interviews* There is no specific set of questions or themes and questions are not asked in any particular order. Usually a researcher covers only one or two issues and questions asked are driven by what an informant says in the interview and consist mostly of probing for clarification (Britten 1995).

---

with focus group research, a researcher is interested in the interaction as well as what is actually said.

Focus groups can be useful when a researcher wants to explore something that may not be very clear in informants' minds. Focus groups can allow informants to express and clarify their views in ways that are not easily accomplished in one-to-one interviews. They are recommended for use with informants who feel that they have nothing to say or are deemed 'unresponsive'. By participating in a discussion, these particular informants may find it easier to uncover how they really feel about something.

Using open-ended questions, the researcher allows the group to identify and pursue their own priorities using their own vocabulary. People use many forms of expression – sarcasm, joking, anecdotes, arguing – and focus groups enable the researcher to access these different forms of discourse. This method has been used to explore the experiences of different groups of people in relation to disease, treatment and use of health services. Because focus groups can be culturally sensitive, they are ideal for exploring the perceptions held by various ethnic groups. Farooqi et al

(2000) used focus groups with randomly selected South Asians living in Leicester to explore their perceptions of the risks of lifestyle factors for coronary heart disease. A range of views were uncovered that included varying levels of understanding of risk factors for coronary heart disease. For example, many of the informants perceived stress to be a major risk factor, and identified barriers to improving lifestyle, such as how to cook traditional Indian food more 'healthily'. The group also revealed that language difficulties were a barrier to accessing health services.

Focus groups can be useful for exploring attitudes and needs of health professionals, as well as exploring how clinical evidence is translated into practice. For example, Coenen et al (2000) used focus groups to explore general practitioners' diagnostic and therapeutic decisions regarding adult patients presenting with complaints of coughing. They found that decisions to prescribe antibiotics for coughing were often weighed against and influenced by the perceived effect that not prescribing treatment might have on the doctor–patient relationship. This led Coenen et al (2000) to conclude that clinical indicators play only one part in therapeutic decision making.

Observational methods

Observational methods are used by qualitative researchers in order to develop a systematic, detailed observation of behaviour and talk, by watching and recording what people say (Mays & Pope 1995). The researcher enters the social world or contexts in which informants exist (as opposed to bringing them to another environment) and attempts to collect data systematically in an unobtrusive manner. In this way, observational methods are said to occur in a naturalistic setting. The goal of participant observation is to grasp the informant's 'point of view, their relation to life, to realise their vision of the world' (Malinowski 1922). The decision to use observational methods is influenced by the extent to which the activities and interactions of a setting are felt to give meaning to the phenomena being investigated (Bogdewic 1992). Gold (1958) and Junker (1960) identify four different types of observational roles defined by the amount of researcher participation: participant, participant observer, observing participant and observer (Box 6.2).

The data obtained from observational methods are usually in the form of 'thick descriptions' of the people, contexts, conversations, sounds and smells, in the form of detailed fieldnotes, often supplemented by audio/video recording or photographs. Observational methods are particularly well suited for the study of organisations and how people within them perform their functions. They can uncover behaviours or routines of which

---

BOX 6.2 Four types of observational role

- *Participant* The researcher often hides their identity and attempts to become immersed in the day-to-day activities and the setting of the informants. There is often the danger of becoming too immersed in the community under investigation and losing one's critical standpoint. At this point the researcher begins to identify completely with the group being studied and completely loses their critical stance.

- *Participant observer* The researcher overtly observes the informants and there is prolonged engagement with the informants but at the same time restricting involvement in the informants' daily activities. The researcher's critical stance is maintained but less so than for observing participation.

- *Observing participant* This relationship is more formal than the previous one. The researcher is overt and known to the informants but there is usually no prolonged engagement and contact is likely to be briefer than for participating observers.

- *Observer* This is similar to experimental designs. The researcher only observes and does not become involved in the informants' activities.

---

informants themselves may be unaware. This method has been used to explore the role that clinical evidence plays in some surgical decision making. Bloor (1976) observed at an ENT outpatient clinic to uncover how decisions to admit children for tonsillectomy were made. By observing how surgeons made decisions to operate, Bloor found that clinical research evidence was not the only factor used when making a decision to perform a tonsillectomy. While some surgeons would wait for clinical signs as the chief indicator for surgery, others would operate if there was evidence that tonsillitis was severely disrupting a child's daily activities, particularly school.

In order to understand the role of pharmaceutical consultation in patient health-seeking behaviour, Hassell et al (1997) combined participant observation with in-depth interviews to study advice giving in community pharmacies. The authors found that patients use pharmacies as the first 'port of call' for many minor ailments, often preferring the pharmacist's advice to that of their GP. The study findings highlighted the role that pharmacies play in keeping certain disorders from the doctor's surgery. They also demonstrated the potential value of closer partnerships between the community pharmacy and general practice.

BOX 6.3 Three types of document used in qualitative research

- *Informal*: includes naturally occurring written accounts of everyday life such as unstructured diaries, autobiographical accounts and letters.

- *Formal*: includes documents constructed about everyday life such as death certificates, structured diaries, medical notes, various public records, time-tables or work rosters.

- *Visual*: documents with a visual quality such as photographs, advertisements, posters, films, map charts or video.

Methods based on texts

Qualitative methods based on texts depend on the collection and analysis of different types of documents. The use of textual sources or documents has been a relatively neglected method in qualitative research (Atkinson & Coffey 1997). There are three categories of documents commonly used: informal, formal and visual (Box 6.3).

It may be difficult to understand the contribution that artefacts or document analysis can make to evidence-based medicine. However, in a study by Miller et al (1999), diaries were used to collect the illness experiences of patients suffering from lower back pain. The authors found that diaries elicited useful and diverse information about their illness experiences, supporting the relevance of a biopsychosocial approach to management of their condition. In addition, they concluded that there was some evidence of benefit to the patient from having written down and expressed their illness experiences.

A well-known study by Bloor (1994) combined document analysis with interviews to explore the level of consistency in the death certification process. Drawing on a sample of doctors responsible for a higher than average number of death certificates, Bloor asked them to fill in a dummy death certificate, based upon a short summary which described the circumstances of death of a patient. Bloor asserts that it was the combination of interviews and document analysis that helped reveal the inconsistencies arising in what doctors listed as the cause of death, even when all were provided with the same information.

Many written or visual documents can form the basis for a textual analysis. For example, the personal account by Rier (2000) of being in an intensive care unit was based upon a notebook he used to communicate with others while he was intubated. This was complemented by faxes sent by his partner to his parents living overseas, his medical notes and, later on, speaking with nurses and people who had visited him. Inadvertently, these documents allowed him to reconstruct an experience usually unavailable to researchers, but also inaccessible to himself, as many of his memories about the event were lost. The result of Rier's work is a detailed and illuminating account of being a critically ill patient in an intensive care unit.

Appraising qualitative research

Within qualitative research there is much debate around the issue of the need for criteria to assess qualitative research. This debate is complicated by the diversity of opinion between qualitative researchers from different traditions as to the aims of qualitative research, and hence what constitutes good practice (Sandelowski 1986). While some feel that the search for standard criteria is misconceived (Smith 1984), the majority recognise the importance of establishing appropriate criteria to assess the quality of qualitative research proposals and findings generated from qualitative data (Denzin & Lincoln 1994, Hammersley 1990, Lincoln & Guba 1985, Murphy et al 1998). Although there is contention (Kirk & Miller 1986), it is well recognised that, as qualitative research emerges from a methodological paradigm distinct from quantitative research, a specific and relevant set of criteria needs to be developed (Lincoln & Guba 1985).

Within health research, there have been several attempts to develop checklists, guidelines or sets of criteria (Dingwall et al 1998, Mays & Pope 1995, Murphy et al 1998, Seale & Silverman 1997). Depending upon the author, particular criteria have received more or less emphasis than others. There is always a risk that the content of these sets of guidelines, criteria or checklists serves simply to discourage potential researchers from trying to conduct qualitative research (Chapple & Rogers 1998). Barbour (2000) stated that the uncritical adoption of different 'qualitative techniques' (such as triangulation, respondent checking, thick description) is likely to result in a case of 'the tail wagging the dog' and in itself does not create rigorous qualitative research.

It is important to recognise that the techniques we present are not exhaustive and that there is disagreement within the qualitative research community (see Smith 1984). There can be no algorithmic criteria produced that can unproblematically judge the quality of qualitative research (Hammersley 1992). Box 6.4 provides a simple overview of the criteria that are covered in the following section but we emphasise that it cannot be treated as a rigid checklist. Instead we present the criteria in the form of critical questions that

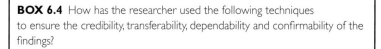

BOX 6.4 How has the researcher used the following techniques
to ensure the credibility, transferability, dependability and confirmability of the
findings?

Credibility
Respondent/member checking
Negative case analysis
Triangulation (source/data, methods, investigator, theoretical)
Constant comparative analysis

Transferability
Thick description
Theoretical triangulation

Dependability
Flexibility in research design
Mechanical recording devices
Verbatim transcription
Researcher triangulation
Respondent/member checking

Confirmability
Thick description
Reflexivity

should be considered when appraising a piece of qualitative research. Each criterion is explained before describing the techniques used to address it. It is common to find that the same technique is often used to satisfy two or more criteria (e.g. thick descriptions). There may be an inclination to turn this into a 'checklist' approach to assessing qualitative research. The assessment of qualitative research – indeed, any research – requires judgement and a good understanding of the method and what it is trying to accomplish. In order to educate the readers' judgement, in the following section we propose that the quality of qualitative research is determined based upon a critical assessment of how well the issues of credibility, transferability, dependability and confirmability are addressed.

Appraising credibility: would those having the experience recognise the researchers' account of it?

In quantitative research, validity is the extent to which a proposition is generated, refined, tested and matches what occurs in human life. However, this concept rests upon the assumption that there is a single reality. Qualitative research embraces the notion of multiple, constructed realities. Therefore, it is difficult to develop a single benchmark against which the truth-value of its claims can be judged. Consequently, Lincoln & Guba (1985) and Hammersley (1990) suggest that validity in qualitative research should be assessed by the extent to which an account accurately and plausibly represents the social phenomena under scrutiny. Key to this is the question of how well a description of a phenomenon under study is recognised by both those who have experienced it and those outside the experience (Lincoln & Guba 1985). There are several techniques used in qualitative research to ensure this, and hence the validity of its findings. These are generally accepted as being member checking, negative case analysis, triangulation and constant comparison analysis.

Respondent or member checking

Has the author used member checking? If so, do they explain how comments from informants were handled?

Member checking refers to the process of feeding back the researcher's interpretations of the data to informants to determine whether they can recognise and agree with them (Bloor 1983). It can also involve feeding back transcripts to informants to ask them to clarify or elucidate certain points. Lincoln & Guba (1985) assert that respondent checking is a powerful tool to check the credibility of the research findings because it allows the researcher to check and correct interpretations, gain additional information, and get the informants' seal of approval, thus confirming that the researcher 'got it right'.

Member checking, however, is not unproblematic (Bloor 1983, Emerson & Pollner 1988). There may be differences or tensions between how the researcher and the informant interpret the informant's world. Consequently, member checking may be limited to asking informants if the researcher's interpretation represents a *reasonable* interpretation of their accounts. There is also the question of how much researchers can reasonably ask of informants. Informants, having already allowed the researcher to explore their world, often do not want additional contact which will take up more of their time and energy. Informant checking also puts informants potentially in the position of being critical of the researcher, something they may not be prepared to do.

Despite these limitations, member checking, especially when combined with other strategies for ensuring the validity or credibility of qualitative research, is a useful strategy for increasing confidence in the validity of the findings. If member checking is used, the researcher should clearly indicate how they did it, as well as how comments were handled.

Negative case analysis

Did the researcher actively seek out disconfirming or inconsistent evidence and report how it was dealt with?

There is a risk in qualitative data analysis of making the data look more 'ordered' or regular than it actually is. In order to prevent this, negative case analysis is used. Negative case analysis refers to the process of actively searching for cases that appear to be inconsistent with the emerging analysis (Glaser & Strauss 1965). By systematically seeking out exceptional cases, the researcher can refine their analysis (Silverman 1989) until they develop constructs that incorporate most of the available data. By demonstrating in their detailed account or audit trail how they sought out negative cases and how they dealt with them, the researcher therefore strengthens the credibility of research findings.

Triangulation

Did the author attempt to search for negative cases or alternative explanations using either different methods or researchers or sources?

Have they illustrated their findings using quotes from several different informants?

Have they used more than one method for collecting data?

During analysis, was more than one point of view used to develop coding structure and final accounts?

Has the researcher attempted to apply multiple theoretical perspectives to interpret the data?

Triangulation is considered one of the most significant strategies for strengthening the credibility of qualitative research (Lincoln & Guba 1985, Miller & Crabtree 1994, Morse 1994). The underlying assumption of triangulation is that if multiple sources, methods, investigators or theories provide similar findings, their credibility is strengthened. Denzin (1970) identifies four different triangulation strategies.

- *Source/data triangulation*: refers to the use of more than one data source to develop an account. This commonly involves including different informants from the same setting and presenting quotes from several different informants to support a finding.

- *Method triangulation*: qualitative findings increase in validity when different and contrasting methods of collection produce very similar results from the same sample set (Bloor 1997). It is not uncommon for findings produced from quantitative methods to be triangulated with qualitative findings but more commonly, a phenomenon is approached using two or more of the qualitative methods outlined in the previous section.

- *Investigator triangulation*: involves multiple investigators studying the same phenomena independently to see if they arrive at the same results. It is most commonly employed during data analysis but it is not uncommon to have two researchers collecting data. It can also involve exposing the data to more than one researcher so that alternative perspectives can be entertained and alternative interpretations explored.

- *Theoretical triangulation*: refers to approaching the data with multiple perspectives and hypotheses in mind so that different theoretical points of view can be compared and contrasted.

Researchers use triangulation in many different ways. Methods and source triangulation are the most commonly used and theoretical triangulation tends to be the least common. The question is, of course, not simply whether triangulation has been used, but how well it has been used and whether in a meaningful manner.

Constant comparative analysis

Did the author use the constant comparison method of analysis and was this clearly reported?

The constant comparative method means that the researcher is always seeking out cases in the dataset during data collection that support or 'shape' the provisional hypothesis (Silverman 2000). This can be done while collecting data, but Glaser & Strauss (1967) assert that it can also involve inspecting and comparing all the different types of data after they have been collected. This can include quantitative data, observations, written accounts – all the different types of data that can arise in a single study. This usually requires a dataset that is fully transcribed. Using a small part of the dataset, the researcher develops a set of categories or themes. These are tested out (and sometimes modified) as the researcher incorporates the remaining dataset. The goal of this strategy is to 'use' the entire dataset instead of just parts of it, in order to avoid the temptation to select only those bits of data that fit with the current analytical argument (ten Have 1998). In this way, the constant comparative method ensures that the dataset is given comprehensive treatment.

Appraising transferability: how well can the findings fit contexts outside the study situation?

Has the researcher provided a detailed account of the research context and informants?

Has the research produced a theoretical inference that can be examined in other settings?

The quantitative notion of generalisability refers to the extent to which findings from research produced in one setting are applicable to other similar settings. However, this perspective downplays or ignores the importance of time and context upon research findings. Within the qualitative paradigm, it is accepted that findings are highly contextualised, partial and temporal. Consequently, direct comparability between research settings is almost impossible. Qualitative researchers have opted for the concept of transferability instead of seeking to be able to generalise from their findings. In utilising the concept of transferability (Lincoln & Guba 1985) qualitative researchers recognise that, while direct comparisons between research settings cannot be made, some similarities will exist and it is possible to develop working hypotheses that can potentially transfer between different settings. Transferability requires providing sufficient descriptive detail for another researcher to be able to make an informed judgement about whether this is likely to be the case (Kennedy 1979). Being able to evaluate the possibility of transferability depends heavily upon the provision of a 'thick description' (Geertz 1973) or a very detailed account of the methodological and interpretive strategy in the form of fieldnotes.

Thick description

Was the researcher explicit about every step of the research process?

This should include detailed descriptions of:

Research context(s)

- Site selection and sampling strategy
- How informants were accessed
- How data were collected and recorded
- How analysis was conducted.

Transferability greatly depends on other researchers being able to determine how research findings are produced. This is achieved through the provision of 'thick descriptions'. These provide a thorough and detailed account of: the contexts or settings where the research took place; sampling strategies; how informants or settings were accessed; and the process of data collection and analysis. Also referred to as 'audit trails' by Guba & Lincoln (1989) and 'auditability' by Beck (1993), thick descriptions allow others to examine the processes by which the researchers have arrived at their conclusions. Consequently, transferability is assessed by the extent to which the researchers have made transparent the decision trail that led them to their conclusions.

It must be noted that the provision of a thick description of the research process is often unseen in published qualitative research. When reading qualitative journal papers, it cannot be inferred that the lack of a detailed audit trail means that one was not done. In many cases, the authors of such papers have written a detailed account of their audit trail, often in the form of fieldnotes, which is available for exploration and inspection upon request.

Appraising dependability: given the instability of the social world, how has the researcher been able to produce plausible accounts?

The quantitative notion of internal reliability refers to the extent to which, given a set of previously generated concepts, new researchers would match these concepts with the data in a similar way. Within qualitative research, this poses difficulty for a research paradigm committed to naturalistic inquiry, where the researcher is the research instrument (LeCompte & Goetz 1982) and the social world is constantly changing. Guba & Lincoln (1989) suggest that another way of approaching the issue of internal reliability is to determine how plausible or dependable the accounts produced are, *given* the instability of the social world. Therefore, the concept of dependability refers to the degree to which it is possible to deal with instability/idiosyncrasy and design-induced change and produce plausible accounts (Kirk & Miller 1986).

As qualitative researchers do not believe that accepting the inevitability of changes in reality produces unreliable findings, the emphasis is upon design/researcher-induced changes. The techniques used in qualitative research to improve the dependability of the research include: flexible research design;

use of mechanically recorded data; and verbatim transcription. Researcher triangulation and member checking are also used to ensure the dependability of the accounts.

Flexibility in research design

Did the researcher encounter anything unexpected when entering the field?

Did the researcher report how they adapted to any unexpected changes?

Given that the social world is constantly changing and often unpredictable, qualitative inquiry cannot be completely specified in advance of fieldwork. Whilst a study design will have an initial question and plans for exploring this question, the naturalistic and inductive nature of the inquiry makes it both impossible and inappropriate to specify operational variables, state hypotheses or finalise a research instrument or sampling strategy (Patton 1990). Consequently much of qualitative research design unfolds as the study progresses.

Due to the requirements of funding agencies or dissertation committees, qualitative researchers tend to develop a strategy for exploring a particular phenomenon before entering the field. When in the field, the researcher will need to demonstrate a high level of tolerance for ambiguity or uncertainty, and attempt to deal with it in a pragmatic and flexible manner. For example, if the researcher finds during the course of a study that their original idea about how to gain access to informants is not working, they will need to re-evaluate their approach and decide upon a more appropriate strategy or strategies. The researcher is required to demonstrate what happened during fieldwork, why it happened, and how it might impact on the research findings in the thick description of data collection.

Use of mechanical recording devices and transcripts

Has the researcher used mechanical recording devices?

Did they obtain permission to use these devices from the informant(s)?

How were the tapes handled?

What rules were followed for transcription?

How were any identifying features handled?

The dependability of qualitative research is closely related to the quality of the data (Silverman 1993). Using mechanical devices for recording data is a common strategy to ensure the quality and accuracy of qualitative data, thus increasing its dependability. Mechanical devices produce highly reliable accounts, as they are not dependent on the researcher's ability to recall what took place. Mechanical recordings are usually done with a video camera or a tape recording machine. Researchers are required to report what type of device was used and if permission was given by the informant to use it. Researchers who do not gain the informant's permission prior to recording an interaction are considered to be ethically questionable.

Tapes are transcribed verbatim, often according to a specific set of rules (see Poland 1995), to create the raw materials that researchers work from. At this point in the process, identifying features are often removed in order to protect the anonymity of the informants. If anonymisation of the data has taken place, it is essential that it be reported. In addition, the researcher should explain how tapes were stored to protect the identities of informants.

The result of this process is a highly detailed and publicly accessible representation of the interactions under investigation. This allows other researchers to examine the data and assess their credibility and dependability.

Assessing confirmability: has the study explained how the researcher might have affected the research findings?

The concept of confirmability focuses attention on both the investigator and interpretations. What is known by quantitative researchers as 'external reliability' poses many problems for qualitative researchers. External reliability refers to the extent to which independent researchers would discover the same phenomena or generate the same findings in the same or similar settings. This requires neutrality or objectivity on the part of the researcher. Confirmability is suggested as a qualitative parallel for the quantitative notion of external reliability. Confirmability refers to the degree to which findings are determined by the respondents and condition of the inquiry, and not by the biases of the inquirer (Lincoln & Guba 1985). Thus, qualitative researchers are expected to account for their interests and motivations by showing how they have affected the interpretations. One strategy, described previously, is to provide a thick description of how decisions were made during every stage of the research process. Another is the technique called reflexivity.

Reflexivity

Has the researcher(s) attempted to be reflexive about their impact on the research process either in the form of an autobiographical account or in their analysis?

Within quantitative research, the goal is always to limit the influence of the researcher on the research findings through standardisation of procedures. However, in qualitative research, the commitment is to a naturalistic setting and this partly requires asking questions in a way that is appropriate to the person you are speaking with. There is also a recognition that in order to study the social world, one must enter it (Hammersley & Atkinson 1995). While objectivity or distance is not possible, reflexivity allows for researchers to limit the impact they have on what is produced.

Reflexivity refers to sensitivity to the ways in which a researcher's presence affects data collection, or how their own assumptions have shaped the data analysis. This requires a certain degree of self-conscious reflection upon the way in which the research outputs have been shaped by the person who has conducted it. It requires being explicit, often in the form of an autobiographical account (see Litva 1997), about the personal and theoretical assumptions the researcher brings to the research. It also requires recognition of how such things as the researcher's social position, appearance, voice, age, gender and other characteristics will influence the research process (Silverman 1993). The use of the technique of reflexivity is most common in the analysis of data, where the author may reflect on how they have shaped or influenced what has been found.

It must be noted here that editorial limits on the length of journal papers mean that authors cannot always provide a detailed account of how they addressed the issue of confirmability. Thus it may often appear to be poorly handled in qualitative papers. An example of this is illustrated in Table 6.1 where we provide a worked example of a paper by Hanratty et al (2002). In this study, doctors' views of palliative care for patients with heart failure were explored, with the aim of identifying any barriers to improving the care of this patient group. Seven groups of doctors, chosen to reflect the specialties that most frequently provide care for patients with heart failure, were recruited to participate in focus group meetings. The published report is particularly strong in the areas of credibility and dependability. It is less strong in the area of transferability, and weak in the area of confirmability. In brief, the people who were involved in the study are likely to recognise the researchers' account of their ideas and experiences, as these are plausible and the researchers have taken into account the nature of the social

TABLE 6.1 WORKED EXAMPLE OF PAPER BY HANRATTY ET AL

Evaluation criteria	Techniques used	Criteria being met
Design	1. Focus groups were used to explore doctors' views on terminal care for patients with heart failure.	**Dependability**: i) Given the need to respond to the nature of the doctor's world (lack of time, busy), focus groups provide a reasonable way to collect information about doctors' views. The research is responsive to the nature of the doctors' social world. The study design works *with* their constraints and realities. ii) By using focus groups, the informants can clarify their own ideas around the topic. In this way, the researcher has responded to the possible needs of the informants to discuss the issues, rather than imposing a research tool upon them.
Site/location	Not reported.	**Transferability**: Whilst details of the informants' professions and usual place of work are given, the authors failed to provide the thick description of: i) how informants were obtained, ii) where they were obtained from (the geography of their sample), and iii) where the focus groups took place. This lack of detail means that the reader is unable to make an informed judgement about the transferability of any working hypotheses to other patients and settings.
Sample	Purposive and maximum variation sample.	**Credibility**: The researchers appear to have implemented source triangulation by using multiple sources to gain access to informants, thus ensuring that

(Continued)

TABLE 6.1 (CONTINUED)

Evaluation criteria	Techniques used	Criteria being met
		informants do not all come from one social network. It would have been helpful if this had been made explicit in the paper, thus reducing uncertainty around the issue. Although the rationale for using this sampling strategy is not clearly stated, the strategy is appropriate for an 'exploratory' study. Use of this 'pragmatic' approach to recruitment suggests a highly responsive approach to getting informants, using multiple sources.
Data collection	1. Tape recording. 2. Verbatim transcripts with transcript check. The focus groups were tape recorded, transcribed verbatim and the written and recorded accounts were then compared to establish accuracy. 3. Investigator triangulation: at each focus group there were two researchers: one facilitating and one observing.	**Dependability**: Use of a mechanical recording device can ensure that the quality and accuracy of the data are high. Checking the transcripts against the tape recording can improve the quality of the final dataset. The use of two researchers to collect the data aims to reduce the impact of one researcher on the data and thus improve its dependability. **Credibility**: How the observations were combined with the transcripts of the focus groups is not clear, thus reducing the credibility of the findings. **Transferability**: The researchers failed to provide the details of how permission was obtained from the informants or how the tapes were handled. This lack of 'thick description' affects other researchers' ability to repeat this study in another location.

(Continued)

TABLE 6.1 (CONTINUED)

Evaluation criteria	Techniques used	Criteria being met
Data analysis	1. Constant comparison method. 2. Use of qualitative software. 3. Investigator triangulation. 4. Theoretical triangulation.	**Credibility**: Researchers report using the constant comparative method, whereby emerging themes are constantly checked to see if they confirm what has been previously found or if a negative case arises. No further details are provided. A qualitative software package (Nvivo) was used to manage the data. The use of the constant comparative method in analysis improves the plausibility of the final account. Computerised software can make the job of analysing all the data easier. Under-reporting of this method raises questions as to how well it was applied. **Dependability**: Several researchers were involved in the analysis, thus ensuring that the interpretations are not the result of one person's view of the data. The coding framework was developed out of several researchers' examination of the data. These researchers came from a variety of backgrounds, thus allowing many possible interpretations of the data. **Transferability**: Use of multiple researchers for analysis is also a form of theory triangulation as everybody involved came from a different academic background, thus bringing multiple interpretations of the data from which the most plausible was agreed and is presented in the paper.

world being explored. It is also reasonable to expect that, should this project be repeated in a different location or for a different aspect of care of patients with terminal heart failure, similar findings would be shown. Reporting of the study is weakest with regard to the issue of confirmability, leaving the reader wondering about the extent to which the researchers thought about their impact on the research process. This is problematic as it does not assist future researchers in doing the research *better* should they wish to conduct similar studies.

How can qualitative research inform clinical practice?

Finally, we turn to the question of how qualitative research can inform clinical practice. Evidence-based medicine is the 'conscientious, explicit, and judicious use of current best evidence in making decisions about the care of individual patients' (Sackett et al 1996). It is now recognised that the *practice* of evidence-based medicine requires a strategy that combines the best available evidence with individual clinical expertise and patient preferences, in order to devise a strategy that is most appropriate for the patient (Muir Gray 1997). The advantage that qualitative methods bring to the practice of evidence-based medicine is that they can systematically examine the kinds of questions that cannot usually be answered by experimental methods (Green & Britten 1998). Some examples of questions that qualitative methods can address are presented in Box 6.5.

Qualitative methods can be used to explore the impact of patient attitudes and beliefs on their care. For example, clinical evidence indicates that giving thrombolytic therapy early in a heart attack episode maximises its benefit and prevents premature death and disability (Weston et al 1994). However Rushton et al (1998), in a qualitative study undertaken to explore reasons for delays in the delivery of thrombolytic therapy for patients having heart attacks, found that patients often delay seeking treatment because they fail to recognise their symptoms as cardiac in origin. As a result, the window of opportunity during which thrombolytic therapy can be given and have the best outcome is inadvertently reduced.

A study using in-depth interviews with parents living in the south east of England explored the process by which they decided whether or not to call the doctor out (Houston & Pickering 2000). The study findings showed that parents employed reasonable strategies, such as waiting to see if their child improved or using over-the-counter drugs such as paracetamol, when attempting to manage their child's illness. The authors of the study

BOX 6.5 Examples of clinical evidence questions that lend themselves to qualitative research methods

- Why do patients seek or delay medical care/treatment?
- Where else do patients seek help?
- What are the factors that facilitate or limit help-seeking behaviour?
- What are patients' perceptions of causes of their illnesses and how do these differ from those of health-care professionals?
- What is the impact of the doctor–patient relationship upon treatment decisions?
- What concerns do health-care professionals have about treatments?
- Why do health-care professionals make particular decisions about patient management?
- What factors contribute to or inhibit patient adherence to treatment?
- What do patients perceive their treatment needs to be?
- What are the factors that inhibit or facilitate practitioners or health-care teams in following particular clinical guidelines?

concluded by stating that health professionals needed to rethink the 'problem' of out-of-hours calls. Parents were struggling not so much with a lack of knowledge on how to treat minor illness as with the problems of coping with uncertainty and so may need help in developing strategies for doing so.

A qualitative study by Howitt & Armstrong (1999) demonstrates how patient attitudes to the risks and benefits of treatment can impact upon clinical decision making. These authors explored uptake of antithrombotic treatment for atrial fibrillation. They identified patients who were at increased risk of thromboembolism and educated them on the relevance of aspirin and warfarin as preventive treatment. The study revealed that giving patients an active role in deciding whether to take warfarin tended to result in a low uptake. One of the conclusions of the study was that a barrier to the implementation of evidence-based medicine is that patients must consent to treatment. In deciding whether to give consent, patients draw on their own understandings of the risk of having a stroke against the costs of taking the treatment. Howitt & Armstrong (1999) suggest that while patients have most to benefit from the implementation of effective treatment, without their support evidence-based medicine is limited in its applicability.

Qualitative methods are also effective for comparing patients' and/or practitioners' perceptions about service provision. We have previously mentioned the study by Hanratty et al (2002) which used focus groups to identify doctors' perceptions of the need for palliative care for heart failure and the barriers to using palliative services for these patients. This study identified that different types of doctors were in agreement in terms of supporting the development of a more holistic palliative care service, with the general practitioner acting as a central figure. However, they felt that the nature of the present health-care system worked against the provision of such care and this was compounded by territoriality between different medical factions. A study conducted by Murray et al (2002) that used interviews with patients dying from lung cancer and cardiac failure supports the findings from Hanratty et al's study by demonstrating that dying patients perceived a need for the provision of both health and social care service that would meet their unique needs.

Qualitative methods can be a very effective way to explore health issues of a sensitive nature. Tomlinson & Wright (2004) used semi-structured interviews with men who suffered from erectile dysfunction. This approach was flexible enough to allow the men to discuss the serious distress and effects such a problem had on their self-esteem and relationships.

The above examples are all studies where qualitative methods were used as a single strategy. In conjunction with quantitative methods, qualitative approaches may also be better at identifying the appropriate variables to be measured or questions to be asked. Insights from qualitative data can help to develop quantitative instruments that are more sensitive to respondents' meanings and interpretations (Coyle & Williams 2000). One question on which qualitative methods have been extremely useful is why some randomised controlled trials have such difficulty recruiting subjects. For example, Donovan et al (2002) audiotaped the consultations with men who were being recruited to participate in a RCT of treatments for prostate cancer. They found that recruiters had difficulty discussing the concept of equipoise and presenting the treatment options equally, and they often used terminology that led to misinterpretation. The findings from this qualitative part of the RCT informed the content and presentation of information to potential participants, resulting in it being more acceptable to them and increasing the efficiency of the recruitment process.

It is because of their ability to answer questions which cannot be addressed by experimental methods that qualitative approaches have a place alongside RCTs and meta-analysis in producing applicable clinical evidence, thus contributing to the effective practice of evidence-based medicine. This will require qualitative research that explores questions relevant to practice (Barbour 2000).

Conclusions

In this chapter we have explored the value of qualitative methods for the practice of evidence-based medicine. We began the chapter by asserting that qualitative methods have a very active role to play in the development of applicable and appropriate approaches to health-care research. There are many qualitative strategies that can be used to explore questions that are relevant to the practice of evidence-based medicine. When selecting which, careful thought must be given to which is the most appropriate strategy to answer the question being asked. Only when used appropriately can qualitative methods become a powerful research tool for addressing questions about clinical practice.

It is essential that if qualitative research methods are to be incorporated into the process of production of clinical evidence, they are used in a systematic and careful way to formulate findings that are of the highest quality. In the latter part of this chapter, we define four criteria that can be used to assess the quality or 'goodness' of qualitative research and the techniques used to address each criterion. The application of qualitative methods to evidence-based medicine will undoubtedly produce some very challenging and exciting results. It will contribute to the production not only of clinically and cost-effective treatment, but also of clinical practice that is appropriate for everyone.

Summary

- The purpose of the qualitative approach is to produce insights on the social world that are developed within the contexts in which it exists. It focuses upon the meanings, experiences and practices of those who are being investigated. It is inductive research that seeks to understand social phenomena within their own context, incorporating many different perspectives in order to provide a holistic perspective.

- Qualitative data collection is driven by the question of what is the most appropriate strategy to explore the social phenomena under investigation. It can involve the use of interviews, focus groups, observations or investigation of texts.

- Because of the many traditions within qualitative research, it is necessary to avoid a 'checklist' approach to evaluating qualitative research. Instead, evaluation should be considered in terms of critically assessing how different techniques have been used to increase the credibility, transferability, dependability and confirmability of the research.

- Qualitative research can inform clinical practice by examining the kinds of question that cannot be answered using experimental methods alone. By combining qualitative methods with quantitative approaches, the ability to produce applicable clinical evidence is greatly increased.

References

Atkinson P, Coffey A 1997 Analysing documentary realities. In: Silverman D (ed) Qualitative research: theory, methods, and practice. Sage, London

Barbour R S 2000 Checklists for improving rigour in qualitative research: a case of the tail wagging the dog? British Medical Journal 322:1115–1117

Beck C T 1993 Qualitative research: the evaluation of its credibility, fittingness and auditability. Western Journal of Nursing Research 15:263–266

Black N 1994 Why we need qualitative research. Journal of Epidemiology and Community Health 48:425–426

Bloor M 1976 Bishop Berkeley and the adenotonsillectomy enigma: an exploration of the social construction of medical disposals. Sociology 10:43–61

Bloor M 1983 Notes on member validation. In: Emerson R M (ed) Contemporary field research: a collection of readings. Little, Boston

Bloor M 1994 On the conceptualization of routine medical decision-making: death certification as a habitual activity. In: Bloor M, Taraborrelli P (eds) Qualitative studies in health and medicine. Avebury, Aldershot

Bloor M 1997 Techniques of validation in qualitative research: a critical commentary. In: Miller G, Dingwall R (eds) Context and method in qualitative research. Sage, London

Bogdewic S P 1992 Participant observation. In: Crabtree B F, Miller W L (eds) Doing qualitative research. Sage, London

Britten N 1995 Qualitative interviews in medical research. British Medical Journal 311:251–253

Bryman A 1988 Quantity and quality in social research. Unwin Hyman, London

Chapple A, Rogers A 1998 Explicit guidelines for qualitative research: a step in the right direction, a defence of the 'soft' option or a form of sociological imperialism? Family Practice 15:556–561

Coenen S, Van Royen P, Vermeire E, Hermann I, Denekens J 2000 Antibiotics for coughing in general practice: a qualitative decision analysis. Family Practice 17(5):380–385

Coyle J, Williams B 2000 An exploration of the epistemological intricacies of using qualitative data to develop a quantitative measure for user views of health care. Journal of Advanced Nursing 31(5):1235–1243

Davies E, Clarke C, Hopkins A 1996 Malignant cerebral glioma II: Perspectives of patients and relatives on the value of radiotherapy. British Medical Journal 313:1512–1516

Denzin N 1970 The research act. Prentice Hall, Englewood Cliffs, NJ

Denzin N, Lincoln Y 1994 Entering the field of qualitative research. In: Denzin N, Lincoln Y (eds) Handbook of qualitative research. Sage, Thousand Oaks, CA

Dingwall R, Murphy E, Watson P, Greatbach D, Parker S 1998 Catching goldfish: quality in qualitative research. Journal of Health Services Research and Policy 3(3):167–172

Donovan J, Mills N, Smith M et al 2002 Improving design and conduct of randomized trials by embedding them in qualitative research: Protec T (prostate testing for cancer and treatment) study. British Medical Journal 325:766–770

Emerson R M, Pollner M 1988 On members' responses to researchers' accounts. Human Organisation 47:189–198

Farooqi A, Nagra D, Edgar T, Khunti K 2000 Attitudes to lifestyle risk factors for coronary heart disease amongst South Asians in Leicester: a focus group study. Family Practice 17(4):293–297

Geertz C 1973 The interpretation of culture. Basic Books, New York

Glaser B G, Strauss A 1965 The discovery of substantive theory: a basic strategy underlying qualitative research. American Behavioral Scientist 8:5–12

Glaser B G, Strauss A 1967 The discovery of grounded theory. Aldine, Chicago

Gold R L 1958 Roles in sociological field observations. Social Forces 36:217–223

Green J, Britten N 1998 Qualitative research and evidence based medicine. British Medical Journal 316:1230–1232

Guba E G 1981 Criteria for assessing the trustworthiness of naturalistic inquiries. Educational Communication and Technology Journal 29:75–92

Guba E G, Lincoln Y 1981 Effective evaluation. Jossey-Bass, San Francisco, CA

Guba E G, Lincoln Y 1989 Fourth generation evaluation. Sage, Newbury Park, CA

Hammersley M 1990 Reading ethnographic research. Longman, New York

Hammersley M 1992 What is wrong with ethnography? Routledge, London

Hammersley M, Atkinson P 1995 Ethnography: principles in practice. Routledge, London

Hanratty B, Hibbert D, Mair F et al 2002 Doctors' perceptions of palliative care for heart failure: focus group study. British Medical Journal 325: 581–585

Hassell K, Noyce P R, Rogers A, Harris J, Wilkinson J 1997 A pathway to the GP: the pharmaceutical 'consultation' as a first port of call in primary care. Family Practice 14(6):498–502

Houston A M, Pickering A J 2000 'Do I don't I call the doctor': a qualitative study of parental perceptions of calling the GP out-of-hours. Health Expectations 3:234–242

Howitt A, Armstrong D 1999 Implementing evidence based medicine in general practice: audit and qualitative study of antithrombotic treatment for atrial fibrillation. British Medical Journal 318:1324–1327

Junker B H 1960 Field work: an introduction to the social science. University of Chicago Press, Chicago

Kennedy M 1979 Generalising from single case studies. Evaluation Quarterly 3:661–678

Kirk J, Miller M 1986 Reliability and validity in qualitative research. Sage, Newbury Park, CA

Kitzinger J 1995 Introducing focus groups. British Medical Journal 311: 299–302

LeCompte M, Goetz J P 1982 Problems of reliability and validity in ethnographic research. Reviews of Educational Research 52:31–60

Lincoln Y 1992 Sympathetic connections between qualitative methods and health research. Qualitative Health Research 2(4):375–391

Lincoln Y, Guba E G 1985 Naturalistic inquiry. Sage, Newbury Park, CA

Litva A 1997 'Placing' lay perceptions of health and illness. PhD dissertation, McMaster University, Canada

Malinowski B 1922 Argonauts of the Western Pacific. George Routledge, London

Marshall C, Rossman G 1989 Designing qualitative research. Sage, London

Mays N, Pope C 1995 Observational methods in health care settings. British Medical Journal 311:182–184

Miller B F, Crabtree B 1994 Clinical research. In: Denzin N, Lincoln Y (eds) Handbook of qualitative research. Sage, Thousand Oaks, CA

Miller J, Pinnington M A, Stanley I M 1999 The early stages of low back pain: a pilot study of patient diaries as a source of data. Family Practice 16(4):395–401

Morse J 1994 Designing funded qualitative research. In: Denzin N, Lincoln Y (eds) Handbook of qualitative research. Sage, Thousand Oaks, CA

Muir Gray J A 1997 Evidence based health care: how to make health policy and management decisions. Churchill Livingstone, New York

Murphy E, Dingwall R, Greatbatch D, Parker S, Watson P 1998 Qualitative research methods in health technology assessment: a review of the literature. Health Technology Assessment Report 2(16):1–274

Murray S A, Boyd K, Kendall M, Worth A, Benton F T, Clausen H 2002 Dying of lung cancer or cardiac failure: prospective qualitative interview study of patients and their carers in the community. British Medical Journal 325:929

Patton M Q 1990 Qualitative evaluation and research methods. Sage, London

Poland B 1995 Transcription quality as an aspect of rigor in qualitative research. Qualitative Inquiry 1(3):290–310

Popay J, Williams G 1998 Qualitative research and evidence-based health care. Journal of Royal Society of Medicine 91(35):32–37

Pope C, Mays N 1995 Reaching the parts other methods cannot reach: an introduction to qualitative methods in health and health services research. British Medical Journal 311:42–45

Rier D A 2000 The missing voice of the critically ill: a medical sociologist's first-person account. Sociology of Health and Illness 22(1):68–93

Rushton A, Claton J, Calnan M 1998 Patients' action during their cardiac event: qualitative study exploring differences and modifiable factors. British Medical Journal 316:1060–1065

Sackett D L, Rosenberg W M C, Muir Gray J A, Haynes R B, Richardson W S 1996 Evidence-based medicine: what it is and what it isn't. British Medical Journal 312:71–72

Sandelowski M 1986 The problem of rigor in qualitative research. Annals of Advances in Nursing Science 8:27–37

Seale C G, Silverman D 1997 Ensuring rigour in qualitative research. European Journal of Public Health 7:379–384

Silverman D 1989 Telling convincing stories: a plea for a cautious positivism in case studies. In: Glassner B, Moreno J D (eds) The qualitative-quantitative distinction in the social sciences. Kluwer Academic, Dordrecht

Silverman D 1993 Interpreting qualitative data: methods for analysing talk, text and interaction. Sage, London

Silverman D 2000 Doing qualitative research: a practical handbook. Sage, London

Smith J 1984 The problem of criteria for judging interpretive inquiry. Educational Evaluation and Policy Analysis 6:379–391

ten Have P 1998 Doing conversation analysis: a practical guide. Sage, London

Tomlinson J, Wright D 2004 Impact of erectile dysfunction and its subsequent treatment with sildenafil: qualitative study. British Medical Journal 328:1037

Weston C F M, Penny W J, Julian D G 1994 Guidelines for the early management of patients with myocardial infarction. British Medical Journal 308:767–777

Further reading

Bloor M 1997 Techniques of validation in qualitative research: a critical commentary. In: Miller G, Dingwall R (eds) Context and method in qualitative research. Sage, London

Denzin N, Lincoln Y (eds) 1994 Handbook of qualitative research. Sage, Thousand Oaks, CA

Hammersley M 1990 Reading ethnographic research. Longman, New York

Kirk J, Miller M 1986 Reliability and validity in qualitative research. Sage, Newbury Park, CA

Systematic reviews: what are they and how can they be used?

Rosalind L Smyth

KEY POINTS

- Systematic reviews use rigorous methods to reduce bias and can provide reliable summaries of relevant research evidence.
- Because systematic reviews include a comprehensive search strategy, appraisal and synthesis of research evidence, they can be used as shortcuts in the evidence-based process.
- The Cochrane Library, which is updated every 3 months, electronically, includes a database of up-to-date systematic reviews across the whole of health care.
- Critical appraisal of systematic reviews is necessary to ensure that they have been conducted to rigorous standards.

- Meta-analysis is a statistical technique used in systematic reviews. It can answer the questions 'does this intervention have a beneficial effect?' and if so, 'what is the size of that effect?'.

What are systematic reviews?

Reviews for health-care professionals take many shapes and forms, depending on the type and expertise of the audience to which they are addressed. They may include chapters in textbooks, reports to expert committees and 'state of the art' reviews for clinical journals. The main purpose of these reviews is to bring their audience rapidly up to speed with the current information in specific clinical areas.

It is partly because of the explosion in information technology that we have come to rely increasingly on reviews. Indeed, evidence-based health care has been described as having 'the potential to rescue us from sinking in a sea of papers' (Bradley & Field 1995). It is because health professionals are bombarded by so many publications that may be relevant to their area of clinical practice on a weekly or monthly basis, and it is impossible to sift through all of these, that they have come to rely on summaries of the evidence in the form of reviews. Many of these review articles are well researched, beautifully illustrated and highly entertaining and informative. However, as 'bottom line' summaries of which treatments, diagnostic tests, etc., are effective, they may be misleading. One reason for this is that reviews are often written by acknowledged experts, who are likely to have already formed an opinion about what works, and who may not review the evidence in an unbiased manner. Another reason is that writing reviews is not always regarded as the most important academic activity and less time is devoted to it than, for example, writing up original scientific research. So those writing the reviews may cut corners and rehash something they have written previously, rather than undertaking an exhaustive search and critical appraisal of all the evidence.

Let us take the example quoted by Professor Paul Knipschild in the book *Systematic Reviews* (Knipschild 1995). He describes how the distinguished biochemist Linus Pauling, writing in his book *How to Live Long and Feel Better* (Pauling 1986), quoted more than 30 trials that supported his contention that vitamin C could prevent the common cold. Knipschild and colleagues then went on to do their own 'systematic review' which showed that even large doses of vitamin C cannot prevent a cold although they may slightly decrease its duration and severity. A critical review of what

Pauling had written showed that he had omitted a number of important studies which did not support the contention that he so enthusiastically proposed. There are now many examples that have shown that unsystematic or narrative reviews do not routinely incorporate all relevant up-to-date scientific evidence.

This shortcoming has led to the notion that reviews need to be performed systematically. This means that the same rigour which we expect of people undertaking primary research should be demanded of reviewers undertaking this very important task of 'research synthesis' or 'secondary research'. You will have seen from Chapters 4 and 5 that in studies such as randomised controlled trials and diagnostic tests, the study can be designed so that bias is reduced or eliminated. Strategies such as blinding (or masking) investigators and participants in clinical trials to whether they are in the experimental or the control group may be introduced to prevent the human element of bias.

In the same way, strategies can be introduced to the reviewing process to eliminate the human element of bias caused, for example, by the reviewer having a strong opinion about whether the treatment under review works. The methodology of a systematic review is outlined in Box 7.1. The research needs to start with a protocol which first of all states clearly the hypothesis or question which the investigator is addressing. In Chapter 2 we have already discussed the importance of formulating an appropriate question. A systematic reviewer needs to define their question very precisely as everything else in the methodology will flow from this.

The search itself should be comprehensive, including not only electronic databases (e.g. MEDLINE) but also, where possible, accessing unpublished studies. This may seem odd, but there is a phenomenon known as 'publication bias'. For any intervention, there may be studies which do not show a clear benefit of the intervention compared with the control group and the evidence indicates that these are less likely to be published (Easterbrook et al 1991). Excluding unpublished studies from systematic reviews may bias the results of the review towards studies in which a benefit of the intervention was observed. Unpublished studies can be retrieved in a number of ways, none of which is perfect. One way of doing this is to search for abstracts of studies presented at conferences. These are available in the abstract books of relevant international conferences. Another common feature of systematic reviews, which may impair their quality, is that they may exclude study reports which are not published in English. Important information may be contained in such studies. For example, in the field of complementary medicine, many studies of acupuncture are

---

BOX 7.1 How to conduct a systematic review

1. State objectives and hypotheses.
2. Outline eligibility criteria, stating types of study, types of participants, types of interventions and outcomes to be examined.
3. Perform a comprehensive search of all relevant sources for potentially eligible studies.
4. Examine the studies to decide eligibility (if possible with two independent reviewers).
5. Construct a table describing the characteristics of the included studies.
6. Assess methodological quality of included studies (if possible with two independent reviewers).
7. Extract data (with a second investigator if possible) with involvement of investigators if necessary.
8. Analyse results of included studies, using statistical synthesis of data (meta-analysis), if appropriate.
9. Prepare a report of review, stating aims, materials and methods and describing results and conclusions.

---

published in non-English language journals, particularly those from China (Linde et al 2001).

The next step in the review is to decide what studies should be included. This should be done according to rigorous inclusion and exclusion criteria so that systematic bias can be avoided. These criteria should be stated in the review. The studies should be defined according to their design, the types of participants, the types of interventions and types of outcomes. For example, Poustie et al (1999) have published a review on the Cochrane Library entitled 'Oral protein calorie supplementation for children with chronic disease'. The review states that the types of participants were children aged 1–16 years with any defined chronic disease. Trials undertaken in children suffering from malnutrition who did not have an associated disease were not included.

The clear description of eligibility criteria can then be applied to all the studies retrieved from the search. Again, to reduce bias it is best if more than one reviewer can do this, working on their own. Two reviewers can then compare which studies they have independently included. They should have previously worked out a mechanism for deciding what to do if there are differences between their lists of included studies. This may mean involving a third reviewer. In the review of oral protein calorie supplementation, the search identified a very large number of studies conducted in children suffering from the effects of famine. The question of whether this intervention is effective in children with severe undernutrition in this setting is a very important one, but was not the question addressed in Poustie and colleagues' review and thus these studies were excluded.

Having decided which studies are eligible for inclusion, the reviewers need to tabulate their characteristics. This description should include the study methods, details of the participants, the precise nature of the interventions and the outcomes measured. You will notice that, in tabulating the study characteristics, the reviewers are describing the studies under the headings by which they have determined whether or not the study is eligible for inclusion in the review. For this reason, it may be helpful if steps 4 and 5 (Box 7.1) are done together. When reviewers are trying to determine whether a study is eligible for inclusion in a review, in many cases it is very obvious whether this is the case or not. However, by tabulating the characteristics of all studies where one or more reviewers think the study may be included, it will soon become apparent whether the inclusion criteria have been fulfilled. The final table of included studies, which all reviewers have agreed, will appear in the review and the readers can judge if the reviewers got it right. For each study excluded, the reviewers need to state, in the review, the reason for this exclusion, and again the reader can judge whether this is valid.

For example, Table 7.1 provides details of a study by Kalnins et al (2005) which was included in the review of oral protein calorie supplementation. This study included children and adults with cystic fibrosis over the age of 10, but the review addressed children only. However, the reviewers were able to obtain summary data on the children included in the trial by contacting the investigators in the original study. All the outcomes evaluated in the trial are listed and those which are evaluated in the review are asterisked. When reading a review, examination of the 'Characteristics of included studies' can help the reader to decide whether the review is applicable to their question. The reader may have in mind a particular age of patient or a specific type of intervention. If none of the studies has included this age of patient or type of intervention, then it is less likely that the review will be relevant.

The protocol should describe how the quality of the included studies will be assessed and how the data will be extracted and analysed. Again, it is best if these steps are performed by more than one person. The quality of the studies should be assessed using a checklist or scoring system. There are many of these now available for the assessment of randomised controlled

TABLE 7.1 CHARACTERISTICS OF INCLUDED STUDY (COPYRIGHT COCHRANE LIBRARY, WITH PERMISSION)

Study	Methods	Participants	Interventions	Outcomes
Kalnins et al 2005	Quasi-randomised, parallel design	Cystic fibrosis patients aged > 10 years, <90% ideal weight for height, or greater than 5% reduction in ideal weight for height over previous 3 months	High-calorie drinks to increase energy intake by 20% of predicted energy needs. Control group received nutritional counselling to increase energy intake by 20% of predicted energy needs by normal diet. Study period: 3 months	Z scores for weight and height;[a] percentage ideal weight for height;[a] anthropometric measures;[a] pulmonary function;[a] energy and nutrient intake;[a] faecal balance studies

[a] Protocol-defined outcome measures.
Data from Kalnins et al (2005).

trials and other tools are being developed for other study designs. Generally, studies are graded according to whether they are of high, medium or low quality. It may be possible to separately analyse the high-quality studies. If the results of this analysis are the same as those obtained when studies of all standards of quality are analysed, this would reassure the reader that the results had not been biased by including low-quality studies. This is known as a 'sensitivity analysis'. In Knipschild's systematic review of vitamin C and the common cold, he identified 61 trials (Knipschild 1995). By applying a rigorous quality scoring, he found that only 15 were of high quality. When the trials which Knipschild included in his review were compared to the ones which Pauling considered, five of Knipschild's top 15 trials were not included by Pauling. Pauling did mention two preventive trials, which did not show any effect of vitamin C, but said that they were 'flawed'. Methodological quality of included studies is very important in a review, but it needs to be judged in an unbiased way.

The next steps in the review process are to extract the data and analyse them. When the reviewers stated their outcomes, they would have provided some indication of what measures they expected to find. The measures used in individual studies will be further described in the table of study characteristics. For example, in Table 7.1 it will be seen that in the trial by Kalnins et al (2005), there were various measures of nutritional status, pulmonary function and energy intake. In extracting the data, the reviewers need to examine exactly what these measures are, for each trial, for the outcomes in which they are interested. They should draw up their own data extraction form, listing the measures made in each trial. In some situations statistical analysis of the results may not be possible. For example, slightly different measurements of outcomes may have been made in each of the included trials and because of this, they cannot be combined as one summary outcome measure. In this situation, reviewers should summarise the results of the individual studies, in narrative or tabular form, in the review. If a meta-analysis has not been possible, the results of the review (which should be the best possible summary of the evidence) are still robust.

Meta-analysis will be explained in detail later in this chapter. Essentially, in the analysis, sensible comparisons should be made and the results should be expressed in a way that is easy to understand. It is an often stated truism that 'no evidence of effect' is not the same as 'evidence of no effect' (Altman & Bland 1995). A review may conclude that there is no evidence to show that a treatment works, but this does not mean that the treatment does not work. Results from analysis of specific groups of patients (known as 'subgroups') should be interpreted with caution. The conclusions should be supported by the results and extravagant claims avoided.

By writing a protocol before they start the review, the reviewers are ensuring that their methods will not be influenced by prior knowledge of the studies that they are going to encounter. The methodology is made clear and if there are any potential sources of bias, it is available for people to examine externally. It is this methodology that largely distinguishes a systematic review from a narrative or literature review.

Cochrane Systematic Reviews

In most descriptions of evidence-based practice, a four-step approach is proposed (Box 7.2). It will be apparent from the previous discussion that if you are able to directly access a systematic review which addresses the question posed, the systematic review would have already performed steps 2 and 3. Systematic reviews are therefore a 'shortcut' which the evidence-based practitioner can use to answer specific questions relating to clinical management. The very laborious tasks of searching and critical appraisal will already have been done by the reviewer. However, to be confident of this process, one would need to be reassured that the systematic reviews being accessed were of high quality. In the end, rather than accessing databases of primary research studies such as CINAHL or MEDLINE, would it not be much more convenient to access the database of systematic reviews? This is, in effect, what the Cochrane Database of Systematic Reviews, which is contained in the Cochrane Library, provides. The Cochrane Library has been referred to previously but here I shall discuss its merits as a source of systematic reviews.

There are two main problems with systematic reviews published in paper journals. The first is that in reviewing the evidence, one wishes to be assured that the systematic review is up to date. In a paper journal, a systematic review can only be current up to the date of publication. This means that studies published subsequently will not have been included and these may change the results and conclusions of the systematic review. Secondly, systematic reviews require a lot of work, particularly in the meticulous searching for appropriate studies and their critical appraisal. It would be very

---

BOX 7.2 Four steps in an evidence-based approach

1. Ask a clinically relevant question.
2. Search for the best available external evidence.
3. Critically appraise that evidence for its validity and relevance.
4. Apply the evidence in clinical practice.

disheartening indeed to discover just before you were due to submit a manuscript of a systematic review for publication that you had been 'pipped to the post' by somebody doing the same systematic review.

Both of these problems have been addressed by the Cochrane Collaboration. This is an international body of researchers who have responded to the challenge of the British epidemiologist Archie Cochrane. It was he who observed that 'it is surely a great criticism of our profession that we have not organised a critical summary by specialty or subspecialty adapted periodically of all relevant randomised controlled trials' (Cochrane 1979). Systematic reviews published on the Cochrane Library are regularly updated. Later in the chapter, two systematic reviews from the Cochrane Library are used as examples. The version that has been used is Disk Issue 4, 2005. As you may be reading this some time later, these reviews are likely to have been updated and may contain new information. Duplication of effort is avoided as individual review groups within the Collaboration publish the titles of all systematic reviews as soon as the review process has started. The other important advantage of Cochrane Systematic Reviews is that they are of high quality. For example, Jadad et al (2000) have published an evaluation of reviews and meta-analyses of treatments used in asthma. Of the 50 reviews they included, 40 were found to have serious or extensive methodological flaws. They found that Cochrane Reviews had higher overall quality scores than those published in peer review journals.

The methodology for Cochrane Reviews has been developed by the Cochrane Collaboration and follows the same steps outlined in Box 7.1. Before the review is published, the protocol of the review is published first of all on the Cochrane Library so that readers of the Library can examine the methodology before the results of the review are available. The coverage of the Cochrane Library does not extend to the whole of health care as yet. However, Disk Issue 4, 2005 contained 2524 completed systematic reviews. I searched the Cochrane Library using the free text term nurs* and achieved hits on 1005 of these 2524 reviews, so many of them are relevant to nursing practice. Clearly, if one is able to identify a systematic review on the Cochrane Library that addresses the question of interest, this is a much quicker process than starting with other electronic databases. One can also be confident that all the relevant clinical studies will have been included.

Critical appraisal of systematic reviews

Box 7.3 shows a checklist adapted from Oxman (1994) for assessment of review articles. This checklist should clearly enable the reader to distinguish

BOX 7.3 Checklist for appraising systematic reviews

1. Was the purpose of the review clearly stated?
2. Did the reviewers report a systematic and comprehensive search strategy to identify relevant studies?
3. Were inclusion and exclusion criteria for studies reported and were they appropriate (i.e. was selection bias avoided)?
4. Was the quality of included studies assessed appropriately?
5. Were the results of the included studies combined systematically and appropriately?
6. Were the conclusions supported by the data?

between narrative and systematic reviews, but should also enable the reader to assess the quality of systematic reviews and the rigour of the methodology. The latter point is particularly important as there is now evidence of considerable variation in quality of systematic reviews. The term 'systematic review' may have been applied to something inferior, in order to give it legitimacy.

Bias may be introduced as a result of the affiliations of the review authors. For example, a study by Barnes & Bero (1998) evaluated the quality of review articles on the health effects of passive smoking. They found that in these reviews, a conclusion that passive smoking was not harmful was associated with authors who were affiliated with the tobacco industry. In Jadad's review of reviews on asthma (Jadad et al 2000), all six reviews funded by the pharmaceutical industry were among the 40/50 with serious or extensive methodological flaws. All but one of these six studies had results and conclusions that favoured the intervention related to the companies sponsoring the review. These and other studies should make us aware that the heading 'systematic review' is not a guarantee that the results are reliable.

Understanding meta-analysis

Like all quantitative studies, systematic reviews often include a statistical analysis. This involves combining the data from the included studies in a process referred to as 'meta-analysis'. This analysis may be very powerful. The individual studies that make up a review are often small and unable, on their own, to detect whether or not a treatment is effective, but when the data from a number of similar small studies are combined, valid conclusions may be drawn. Often the terms 'meta-analysis' and 'systematic review' are

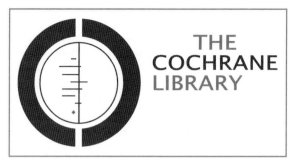

Figure 7.1 The Cochrane Library logo indicating a meta-analysis of seven randomised controlled trials comparing corticosteroids versus no corticosteroids in pregnant women about to deliver prematurely. (From the Cochrane Library, Disk Issue 3, 2001. Update Software, Oxford, with permission.)

used interchangeably. This is inappropriate because, as can be seen from Box 7.1, meta-analysis is simply one of the final steps in what must be a rigorous process. Statistical aggregation of the data in a meta-analysis does not mean that the individual studies included in the meta-analysis were reviewed systematically or appropriately. The most important part of the process is the one that I have already described, which refers to all the elements in the review process set up to prevent bias.

The Cochrane logo (Figure 7.1) is a stylised diagram of a meta-analysis from a systematic review. This systematic review included data from seven randomised controlled trials, which investigated the effect of corticosteroids administered to pregnant women who were about to deliver prematurely. The outcome examined was the survival of their infant. The vertical line is where these results would be expected to cluster if this treatment had a similar effect to the control group (placebo or no treatment) and each horizontal line represents the results of one trial. The shorter the line, the more certain the result, because the 95% confidence intervals are narrow. If the horizontal line lies entirely to the left of the vertical line, the treatment has shown significant benefit. If it touches or crosses the vertical line then clear benefit was not demonstrated in that trial. If the horizontal line were to lie entirely to the right of the vertical line, then more babies would have died in the treatment group than in the control group, i.e. the treatment would have been harmful. The trial at the top of the diagram was performed in 1972 and did show benefit, but the four subsequent trials did not. The sixth trial did show benefit and the seventh did not. On a simple 'vote count' (five of the trials showed no benefit) one might be persuaded not to use this intervention. However, when a systematic review was performed with meta-analysis

TABLE 7.2 A 2 × 2 TABLE SHOWING HOW RESULTS OF A PROSPECTIVE
STUDY ARE REPRESENTED

		Group 1	Group 2	Total
Outcome present	Yes	a	b	a + b
	No	c	d	c + d
	Total	a + c	b + d	n

and first reported in 1989 (Crowley 1996), this showed that corticosteroids administered to pregnant women reduced the odds of their babies dying by between 30% and 50%. This meta-analysis is indicated by the solid diamond at the bottom of the diagram.

Meta-analysis can answer two main questions about a treatment: 'Does this intervention have a beneficial (or harmful) effect?' and if so 'What is the size of that effect?'. I will consider this with reference to specific examples. First, there are some terms used in expressing results that need to be explained. The first is known as the 'relative risk'. The risk (or proportion, probability or rate) is the ratio of people with an event in a group compared with the total in that group. In Table 7.2, the risk of the outcome being present in group 1 is:

$$\frac{a}{a + c}$$

In 1992, a clinical trial published by Northeast et al (1990) compared two types of bandaging for the treatment of venous ulcers. One was elastic, high-compression bandaging, which is widely used in the UK, and the other was low-compression bandaging, used in standard practice in mainland Europe and Australia. The outcome that we will consider is complete healing of the ulcer within the trial period. There were 49 patients in the high-compression bandaging group and 52 in the low-compression group. Table 7.3 shows the numbers in each group which had complete healing. So the risk of complete ulcer healing in the high-compression group is 31/49 and the risk of complete healing in the low-pressure group is 26/52.

In a clinical trial, the relative risk is the ratio of the risk in the intervention group to the risk in the control group. For this trial, the relative risk is:

$$\frac{31/49}{26/52} = \frac{0.63}{0.5} = 1.26$$

TABLE 7.3 RELATION BETWEEN COMPLETE ULCER HEALING AND HIGH-COMPRESSION OR LOW-COMPRESSION BANDAGING

		High compression		Low compression		Total
Complete healing	Yes	31	a	b	26	57
	No	18	c	d	26	44
	Total	49			52	101

Data from Northeast et al 1990.

If the risk in the treatment group is the same as that in the comparison group, the ratio will be 1. This means that there is no difference between the treatment and the comparison group.

The 'odds ratio' is the ratio of the odds of an event in the treatment group compared to the odds of an event in the comparison group. The odds are the ratio of the number of people in a group with an event compared to the number without an event. So, looking again at Table 7.2, the odds of a patient in group 1 having the outcome present are:

a/c

In the Northeast trial, the odds of complete ulcer healing in the high-compression group are:

31/18 = 1.72

In the low-compression group, the odds of complete ulcer healing are:

26/26 = 1.0

The odds ratio of complete ulcer healing in the two groups is:

1.72/1 = 1.72

If the odds of the event in the treatment group are the same as those in the comparison group then the odds ratio is again 1. That is, there is no difference between the treatment and comparison groups.

Where the outcome of interest is rare, in Table 7.2, a will be very small and a/(a + c) will be approximately equal to a/c. Similarly b/(b + d) will approximately equal b/d. Thus, when the outcome is rare, the risks of the outcomes in the two groups will be very similar to the odds of the outcomes in the two groups and the relative risks will be very similar to the odds ratios.

Ninety-five percent confidence intervals are an expression of how precise the estimate of the odds ratio or relative risk is. This gives an estimate of the range to 95% certainty that the true result for odds ratio or relative risk lies within the range stated.

Let us consider now a systematic review by Cullum et al (2001), which assessed the effectiveness of compression bandaging and stockings in treatment of venous leg ulcers. Included in this review was the comparison between high-compression and low-compression bandaging, which we have referred to previously. Three trials that made this comparison were found, including the study by Northeast et al (1990) described previously. This meta-analysis is illustrated in Table 7.4. The ratios shown in the column labelled 'Expt' indicate the number of patients in the experimental group (elastic high compression) with complete healing compared with the total number of patients in that group. These risks are shown both for each individual study and, at the bottom, for the three studies combined. The term 'risk', as used here, is misleading, because the effect of ulcer healing is beneficial, but I have retained it for consistency. The combined result gives a relative risk of 1.54. This represents the relative benefit increase for healing for the high-compression bandaging. You will recall that if the two treatments were equally effective, this ratio should be 1. Because instead it is 1.54, this means there is a 54% relative benefit increase for healing in the high-compression bandaging group. Cullum et al (2001) calculated the 95% confidence intervals for the relative risks. For this relative benefit increase of 54%, the 95% confidence intervals were 19% to 99%. This is a very wide range, within which the true benefit increase is estimated to lie, 95% of the time. However, even the lowest estimate of 19% indicates clear benefit of the high-compression bandaging over the low-compression bandaging, and this is a statistically significant result.

In the text of their review, Cullum et al (2001) chose to express their results as relative risk, rather than odds ratios. However, in Table 7.5, the right-hand column demonstrates the odds ratio with 95% confidence interval:

2.26 [1.40, 3.65]

Now look at the fourth column. You will see a number of 'blobs' through which go horizontal lines. Reading the figures along the bottom axis, the point where the blob is represents the odds ratio for each individual trial.

TABLE 7.4 COMPRESSION FOR VENOUS LEG ULCERS. THE COMPARISON SHOWN IS FOR ELASTIC HIGH-COMPRESSION VERSUS INELASTIC COMPRESSION (MULTILAYER) (RR AND 95% CONFIDENCE INTERVAL). THE OUTCOME IS COMPLETE HEALING IN TRIAL PERIOD (VARYING LENGTHS) (COPYRIGHT COCHRANE LIBRARY, WITH PERMISSION)

Review: Compression for venous leg ulcers
Comparison: 02 Elastic high compression vs inelastic compression (multilayer) (RR and 95% Confidence Interval)
Outcome: 01 Complete healing in trial period (varying lengths)

Study	Elastic multilayer n/N	Inelastic multilayer n/N	Relative risk (fixed) 95% CI	Weight (%)	Relative risk (fixed) 95% CI
Callam	35/65	19/67		36.7	1.90 [1.22,2.95]
Gould	11/20	7/20		13.7	1.57 [0.77,3.22]
Northeast	31/49	26/52		49.5	1.27 [0.90,1.79]
Total (95% CI)	134	139		100.0	1.54 [1.19,1.99]

Total events: 77 (Elastic multilayer), 52 (inelastic multilayer)
Test for heterogeneity chi-square = 2.11
df = 2 p = 0.35 I² = 5.1%
Test for overall effect Z = 3.28 p = 0.001

0.1   0.2   0.5   1   2   5   10
Inelastic better   Elastic better

TABLE 7.5 COMPRESSION FOR VENOUS LEG ULCERS. THE COMPARISON SHOWN IS FOR ELASTIC HIGH-COMPRESSION VERSUS INELASTIC COMPRESSION (MULTILAYER) (OR AND 95% CONFIDENCE INTERVAL). THE OUTCOME IS COMPLETE HEALING IN TRIAL PERIOD (VARYING LENGTHS) (COPYRIGHT COCHRANE LIBRARY, WITH PERMISSION)

Study	Expt n/N	Ctrl n/N	Peto OR 95% CI	Weight (%)	Peto OR 95% CI
Callam	35/65	19/67 +		47.7	2.85 [1.43,5.68]
Gould	11/20	7/20		15.1	2.20 [0.64,7.52]
Northeast	31/49	26/52		37.2	1.71 [0.78,3.73]
Total (95% CI)	134	139		100.0	2.26 [1.40,3.65]
Total events	77	52			

Chi-square 0.93
(df = 2) p = 0.63
Z = 3.35 p = 0.0008

.10   .20   1   2   5   10

Inelastic better   Elastic better

Data from Cullum et al (2001).

The horizontal line represents the 95% confidence interval of the individual trial. In this situation if both the odds ratio and the 95% confidence interval lie entirely to the right of the vertical line at 1, this means that there is a statistically significant benefit, in this case of elastic, high-compression stockings compared to inelastic, low-compression stockings, for the outcome being examined (complete healing of the ulcer in the trial period). If one looks at the three individual trials, it will be seen that this applies to only one trial (Callam). In the other two trials (Gould and Northeast) the horizontal line crosses the vertical line of 1. This means that, although the odds ratio lies to the right of the line, the 95% confidence intervals include the line, so it is possible that the true result is 1 or even slightly less than 1 which means that there is no significant benefit. However, if the results from all three trials are combined, the total result shown by the diamond at the bottom, where the 'blob' lies to the right of 1, indicates that the combined result is significant. The odds ratio of 2.26 suggests a large benefit of high-compression bandaging over low-compression bandaging. Cullum et al (2001) chose to express their results as relative risks rather than odds ratios, because their outcome of interest (complete ulcer healing) was not rare in either group. You will recall from the previous discussion that relative risks and odds ratios are only similar if the outcome is rare. The authors felt that to quote odds ratios would give an inflated impression of the magnitude of the effect.

In a meta-analysis, each study does not make an equal contribution to the pooled estimate. Rather, studies are given a 'weight', specified as a percentage, to reflect the amount of information that they contain. The more informative the study, the more weight it is given and the greater its contribution to the pooled estimate. The contribution to the pooled estimate of each of the three studies is shown in the column labelled Weight %.

How can systematic reviews inform practice?

Let us suppose that you are a practice nurse working in a busy inner-city practice. There are high rates of unemployment and social deprivation within your practice population. You are concerned to find that three men, all in their early 40s, have recently died from acute myocardial infarction. All three men were on your GP's list but none had attended the surgery for the last 5 years. All were smokers.

These tragedies have prompted you to consider setting up a 'well man' clinic. The aim of the clinic would be to identify men with risk factors for cardiovascular disease, and try to implement lifestyle changes which may reduce these risks. You plan to review all men on the practice list aged 40–60 in the first instance. Because of the large number of people that this will involve, you will have a limited time for detailed discussions with each individual. You are in a dilemma about whether it would be appropriate to include specific counselling on smoking cessation for smokers who attend the clinic. You are not sure if they would take much notice of what you said anyway. You decide to look at the evidence for the effectiveness of advice from nurses on smoking cessation in this primary care setting.

You start by searching on the Cochrane Library. An advanced search on NURS* AND (SMOKING AND CESSATION), restricted to the abstract, yields two systematic reviews in the Cochrane Database of Systematic Reviews. One of these, entitled 'Nursing interventions for smoking cessation' (Rice & Stead 2001), seems relevant to your question. A review of the 'criteria for considering studies' found that studies included were randomised trials in which adult smokers of either gender were recruited in any type of health-care setting. The types of intervention included the provision of advice and/or other content and strategies to help patients quit smoking. The main outcome assessed was smoking cessation. The review group divided the interventions into low and high intensity for comparison. A low-intensity intervention was defined as trials where advice was provided (with or without a leaflet) during a single consultation lasting up to 10 minutes with up to one follow-up visit. High-intensity intervention was defined as trials where the initial contact lasted more than 10 minutes, there were additional materials (e.g. a manual) and/or strategies other than simple leaflets and the participants had more than one follow-up session. You were interested to look at the low-intensity comparison separately from the high-intensity comparison. This was because you knew your time would be limited and it would be feasible to spend up to 10 minutes with each man, provide a leaflet and see them for one follow-up visit, but you would not have the resources to do more than this.

The review included 29 trials. Six of these evaluated the 'low-intensity' intervention. These results are illustrated in Table 7.6. The pooled odds ratio for this group was, as you can see, 1.76 (95% CI 1.23–2.53). This was similar to the pooled odds ratio for the 14 trials of high-intensity interventions, which was 1.43 (95% CI 1.24–1.64). The results for these 14 trials are not shown here, but can be viewed on the Cochrane Library. You were concerned that a number of trials had evaluated nursing interventions for smoking cessation in hospitalised patients and you felt that the results might be better in that setting than in the clinic you were planning to set up. The analysis of all the studies which looked at non-hospitalised patients is shown in Table 7.7. This again showed an odds of success of well over 50%

TABLE 7.6 NURSING INTERVENTIONS FOR SMOKING CESSATION. THE COMPARISON SHOWN IS FOR LOW-INTENSITY INTERVENTION VERSUS CONTROL. THE OUTCOME IS SMOKING CESSATION AT LONGEST FOLLOW-UP (COPYRIGHT COCHRANE LIBRARY, WITH PERMISSION)

Study	Expt n/N	Ctrl n/N	Peto OR 95% CI	Weight (%)	Peto OR 95% CI
Low-intensity intervention					
Aveyard 2003	9/413	3/418		1.3	2.79 [0.89,8.71]
Davies 1992	2/153	4/154		0.7	0.51 [0.10,2.57]
Janz 1987	26/144	12/106		3.5	1.68 [0.84,3.38]
Nebot 1992	5/81	7/175		1.1	1.62 [0.47,5.63]
Tonnesen 1996	8/254	3/253		1.2	2.52 [0.76,8.31]
Vetter 1990	34/237	20/234		5.3	1.77 [1.00,3.12]
Subtotal (95% CI)	1282	1340		13.0	1.76 [1.23,2.53]
Total events	84	49			

Chi-square 3.26
(df = 5) $p = 0.66$
$Z = 3.07$ $p = 0.002$

.10   .20   1   5   10

Favours control   Favours treatment

Data from Cochrane Library (2005).

TABLE 7.7 NURSING INTERVENTIONS FOR SMOKING CESSATION. THE COMPARISON SHOWN IS FOR SMOKING INTERVENTION ALONE VERSUS CONTROL IN NON-HOSPITALISED PATIENTS. THE OUTCOME IS SMOKING CESSATION AT LONGEST FOLLOW-UP (COPYRIGHT COCHRANE LIBRARY, WITH PERMISSION)

Study	Expt n/N	Ctrl n/N	Peto OR 95% CI	Weight (%)	Peto OR 95% CI
Smoking intervention alone in other non-hospitalised smokers					
Aveyard 2003	9/413	3/418		4.8	2.79 [0.89–8.71]
Canga 2000	25/147	3/133		10.2	5.12 [2.35,11.17]
Curry 2003	4/156	3/147		2.8	1.26 [0.28,5.63]
Davies 1992	2/153	4/154		2.4	0.51 [0.10,2.57]
Hollis 1993	79/1997	15/710		28.5	1.73 [1.09,2.77]
Janz 1987	26/144	12/106		12.8	1.68 [0.84,3.38]
Lancaster 1999	8/249	10/248		7.1	0.79 [0.31,2.03]
Nebot 1992	5/81	7/175		4.0	1.62 [0.47,5.63]

Terazawa 2001	8/117	1/111	3.5	4.75 [1.26,17.99]
Tonnesen 1996	8/254	3/253	4.9	2.52 [0.76,8.31]
Vetter 1990	34/237	20/234	19.4	1.77 [1.00,3.12]
Subtotal (95% CI)	3948	2689	100.0	1.90 [1.48,2.43]
Total events	208	81		

Chi-square 15.23
(df = 10) p = 0.10
Z = 5.02
p = <0.00001

.10 .20   1   5   10

Favours control   Favours treatment

Data from Cochrane Library (2005).

in the nursing intervention group compared with the control group (OR 1.90, 95% CI 1.48–2.43).

The quality of the review is appraised as described in Box 7.3. The objectives of the review clearly lay out the research question. A detailed search strategy has been prepared within the collaborative review group responsible for the review and this is comprehensive. Specific inclusion and exclusion criteria are reported and the quality of the included studies is clearly described. The meta-analysis addressed appropriate comparisons and was easy to understand. The conclusions of the review, which were that 'the results indicate potential benefits of smoking cessation advice counselling given by nurses to their patients, with reasonable evidence that intervention can be effective', appear appropriate and supported by the evidence obtained in the review. You now feel very confident that introducing a smoking cessation strategy into your follow-up clinic for patients with risk factors for cardiovascular and respiratory disease will be effective and you are able to go ahead and plan the clinic.

It will be clear by now that systematic reviews are an important element of evidence-based practice. They are considered the 'gold standard' for assessing the effectiveness of a treatment or intervention. As a research activity, they are important and need to be performed thoroughly. This chapter has described their basic methodology. All practitioners will need to use systematic reviews, so it is important to understand these methods and how the results are presented. They also need to be able to judge the quality of reviews to assess whether their results are valid.

References

Altman D G, Bland J M 1995 Absence of evidence is not evidence of absence. British Medical Journal 311:485

Barnes D, Bero L 1998 Why review articles on the health effects of passive smoking reach different conclusions. Journal of the American Medical Association 279:1566–1570

Bradley F, Field J 1995 Evidence-based medicine. Lancet 346:838–839

Cochrane A L 1979 A critical review, with particular reference to the medical profession. In: Teeling-Smith G (ed) Medicines for the year 2000. Office of Health Economics, London, pp.1931–1971

Cochrane Library 2005 The Cochrane Library, Disk Issue 4, 2005. John Wiley, Chichester*

Crowley P 1996 Prophylactic corticosteroids for preterm birth (Cochrane Review). Cochrane Database of Systematic Reviews, Issue 1. Art. No.: CD000065. DOI: 10.1002/14651858.CD000065*

Cullum N, Nelson E, Fletcher A, Sheldon T 2001 Compression for venous leg ulcers (Cochrane Review). Cochrane Database of Systematic Reviews, Issue 2. Art. No.: CD000265. DOI: 10/1002/14651858.CD000265

Easterbrook P J, Berlin J A, Gopalan R, Matthews D R 1991 Publication bias in clinical research. Lancet 337:867–872

Jadad A R, Moher M, Browman G, Sigouin C, Fuentes M, Stevens R 2000 Systematic reviews and meta-analyses on treatment of asthma: critical evaluation. British Medical Journal 320:537–540

Kalnins D, Corey M, Ellis L et al 2005 Failure of conventional strategies to improve nutritional status in malnourished adolescents and adults with cystic fibrosis. Journal of Pediatrics 147:399–401

Knipschild P 1995 Some examples of systematic reviews. In: Chalmers I, Altman D G (eds) Systematic reviews. BMJ Publishing, London, pp.9–16

Linde K, Jobst K, Panton J 2001 Acupuncture for chronic asthma (Cochrane Review). In: The Cochrane Library, Disk Issue 3, 2001. Update Software, Oxford*

Northeast A, Layer G, Wilson N, Browse N, Burnand K 1990 Increased compression expedites venous ulcer healing. Royal Society of Medicine Venous Forum

Oxman A D 1994 Checklists for review articles. British Medical Journal 309:648–651

Pauling L 1986 How to live long and feel better. Freeman, New York

Poustie V, Watling R, Smyth R L 1999 Oral protein calorie supplementation for children with chronic disease (Cochrane Review). Cochrane Database of Systematic Reviews, Issue 3. Art. No.: CD001914. DOI: 10.1002/14651858.CD001914*

Rice V, Stead L 2001 Nursing interventions for smoking cessation (Cochrane Review). In: The Cochrane Library, Disk Issue 3, 2001. Update Software, Oxford*

* Cochrane Reviews are regularly updated as new information becomes available and in response to comments and criticisms. The reader should consult The Cochrane Library for the latest version of a Cochrane Review. Information on The Cochrane Library can be found at http://www.cochrane.org/reviews/clibintro.htm

8

CHAPTER

Integrating research evidence into clinical decisions

Joan Livesley and Michelle Howarth

KEY POINTS

- Research evidence is, on its own, insufficient to ensure the robust clinical decisions necessary for clinically effective health care.
- Good clinical decisions require the sophisticated application of research findings in the context of clinical expertise, patient preferences and values, and the individual situation.
- Patient preferences, beliefs and experiences shape and inform evidence-based decisions.
- The availability of resources influences how research evidence is interpreted and applied.

Introduction

Having worked through previous chapters, you will understand the role of high-quality, scientific research evidence in informing health-care practice but should also appreciate that research evidence alone is insufficient to make robust judgements and clinical decisions. Indeed, for many clinical situations, research evidence may be unavailable, of poor quality or not applicable. Clinical decision making is a complex process that necessitates the integration of professional expertise and client/patient preferences, values and beliefs alongside available best research evidence. Resource availability is another important consideration. This chapter explores these 'non-research' aspects of evidence-based practice and considers how they impact on clinical decision making.

Whilst a detailed explication of decision making is beyond the scope of this chapter, it is useful to consider the concept in its broadest sense. Thompson & Dowding (2002) draw on Dowie's (1993) work in which it is suggested that a judgement is defined as 'the assessment of alternatives' and a decision defined as 'choosing between them'. Previous chapters have already explored how evidence-based practice requires practitioners to ask questions about their practice, locate evidence through systematic searching, and appraise the evidence to ascertain its trustworthiness, findings and usefulness prior to implementation. Applying the findings, in other words, assessing alternatives before choosing between them, is the next step and one which requires close collaboration with the patient.

At this stage of the process, the practitioner and patient are required to 'step back' and consider the basis for, and the potential implications of, their proposed interventions and actions. Seen in this way, professional expertise and patient preference can be used to challenge research findings, just as research findings can be used to challenge our professional expertise and patients' preferences.

More than research is needed

For some, the drive for evidence-based practice is seen to be dominated by research evidence alone but, as Sackett et al (2000) took care to acknowledge, research evidence is on its own insufficient to make robust clinical decisions, as for them, evidence-based practice is: '. . . the integration of *best research evidence* with *clinical expertise* and *patient values* . . .' (emphasis added). It is these three elements of evidence-based practice operating together that allow health-care practitioners and patients to work in partnership to optimise clinical outcomes that are acceptable to patients and their families (Sackett et al 2000). Kitson et al (1998) highlight the need to also consider the situational context in which the care episode or consultation is taking place.

If research evidence were applied without due regard for clinical expertise, the patient's or the family's wants or needs, and the situational context, the likelihood of achieving an outcome acceptable to the patient and family would be compromised. Consider the terminally ill patient who, after months of exhausting treatments, has reached the decision to receive palliative care only. On developing a bacterial chest infection, for which there is good evidence that antibiotics reduce morbidity and mortality, the decision to administer antibiotics must surely take account of the patient's wishes. The health-care practitioner must draw on his or her clinical expertise to ascertain the patient's wishes and to determine the most appropriate way to assist the patient with reaching clinical decisions that are right for him/her.

A 'cook-book' approach to health care, in which a recipe of research evidence is mindlessly applied regardless of context, is clearly not compatible with evidence-based practice, as highlighted by Sackett et al (1996):

'External evidence can inform, but can never replace, individual clinical expertise, and it is this expertise that decides whether the external evidence applies to the individual patient at all, and if so, how it should be integrated into a clinical decision. Similarly, any external guideline must be integrated with individual clinical expertise in deciding whether and how it matches the patient's clinical state, predicament and preferences, and thus whether it should be applied.'

Clinical effectiveness and evidence-based practice

Clinical effectiveness is one way of thinking about how, as nurses, we must work towards finding out what our patients' preferences are and how our own values, beliefs and experiences may prejudice and bias clinical decision making. Most simply expressed by the Royal College of Nursing (1996) as seven rights (see Box 8.1), clinical effectiveness can only be achieved by working in partnership with clients. Partnership working requires us to take account of any differences that exist between the patient and our

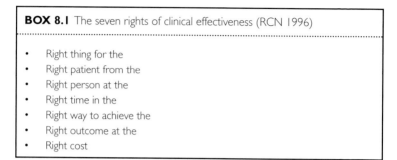

BOX 8.1 The seven rights of clinical effectiveness (RCN 1996)

- Right thing for the
- Right patient from the
- Right person at the
- Right time in the
- Right way to achieve the
- Right outcome at the
- Right cost

own professional understanding of the problem, suggested interventions and intended outcomes. As Guyatt et al (2004) note: '. . . because clinicians' values differ from those of patients even those who are aware of the [research] evidence risk making the wrong recommendations if they do not involve patients in the decision making process . . .' (p.329).

Clinical expertise

Clinical expertise has been described as:

- the professional artistry and practice wisdom inherent in professional practice (Manley et al 2005)
- the proficiency and judgement that individual clinicians acquire through clinical experience and clinical practice (Sackett et al 1996)
- the ability to use our clinical skills and past experience to rapidly identify each patient's unique health state and diagnosis, their individual risks and benefits of potential interventions, and their personal values and expectations (Sackett et al 2000).

Some of the key elements of clinical expertise are teased out by Miles et al (2000) when they note that competent practice relies not only on the findings derived from scientific research, such as large population studies or qualitative research, but also on the practitioner's intuition, common sense and a clear understanding and knowledge of the meaning that the situation has for the patient and their family. Exploring the unique elements of clinical expertise will help us gain insight into this important aspect of evidence-based practice, and to understand more fully how it can be integrated with the other components that influence clinical decisions.

Different forms of knowing

Different typologies of knowledge have been described. Hek et al (2002) identify tradition and rituals, intuition, common sense, trial and error, authority and scientific evidence as sources of knowledge for practice, whilst Parahoo (1997) incorporates tradition, intuition, experience and research under this umbrella term. In her seminal work on fundamental patterns of knowing in nursing, Carper (1978) discusses the following.

- *Empirical* knowing is that derived from factual, scientific evidence. This form of knowing is usually systematically organised into laws and often equated with research-based evidence.

- *Ethical* knowing is that derived from ethical principles of what is right and wrong and what should inform decision making.

- *Aesthetic* knowing is that knowledge that rests on the art of nursing, derived from an understanding of the meaning the situation has for others who are involved.

- Finally, *personal* knowing is that knowledge derived from self-conscious, personal awareness of prejudices and how these may interfere with the interaction and decision-making processes, especially when the nurse's views of an intervention differ significantly from those of the person with whom he/she is working.

Two other elements can be considered here.

- *Sociopolitical* knowing, added by White (1995) to capture the importance of the context, time and space in which the interaction between the nurse and patient is taking place.

- Benner (1984) highlighted that the core of nursing rests on relationships and cannot therefore be adequately described without articulation of the *context and situation*.

Carper's thesis on ways of knowing has been criticised for oversimplifying what is in essence a very complex concept (Edwards 2001). Nonetheless, it provides some insight into the complexities of decision making and has helped to develop our understanding of how different forms and different types of knowledge are blended by expert nurse practitioners into evidence-based decision making. Box 8.2 illustrates the impact of different types of knowledge on clinical decisions using a case study. As shown, the information or knowledge available to the nurse (and the patient) is complex and requires sophisticated partnership working and expert blending of all the issues to ensure that the patient's preferences remain central to the final decision.

> **BOX 8.2** Case study illustrating the impact of types of knowledge on clinical decisions
>
> Mrs Lovely is a 70-year-old woman with hypertension. She is otherwise healthy, has had no previous vascular events, is a non-smoker and, whilst overweight, is not obese. Her blood pressure has consistently been recorded at 160/100.
>
> While there is good research evidence to support the use of antihypertensive medication to reduce her risk of stroke (Mulrow et al 1998), Mrs Lovely explicitly states that she will not take any medication, being a firm believer in 'self-healing' through lifestyle changes.
>
> The nurse is aware from current research evidence that antihypertensive medication significantly reduces the risk of stroke and cardiovascular disease in patients with raised blood pressure (SIGN 2001) (empiric knowing). The nurse's desire to uphold Mrs Lovely's autonomy to decline medication (ethical knowing) might be tempered not only by his/her knowledge of empiric evidence, but also by his/her views on pharmacological interventions as a treatment modality (personal knowing), knowledge of national targets to reduce the incidence of stroke (sociopolitical knowing) and by recent experiences of clients' successes or failures at managing hypertension through lifestyle changes only (aesthetic knowing). Knowledge of Mrs Lovely's apparent motivation and physical and mental ability to make the required changes in diet and levels of physical activity (aesthetic knowing) must be countered with the empiric knowledge that lifestyle changes alone are likely to result in only modest reductions to diastolic and systolic blood pressure (NICE 2004).

Accumulating expertise

Benner (1984) is credited with developing the theoretical understandings of expertise in nursing practice. In her influential work *From Novice to Expert*, Benner (1984) details how a beginner moves through the stages of novice to advanced beginner, competent practitioner, and proficient practitioner before becoming expert. Central to this work is the notion that clinical expertise develops over a period of time through exposure to practice in the clinical area. For Benner (1984) expertise develops through: '. . . A process of comparing whole similar and dissimilar clinical situations with one another, so the expert has deep background understanding of the clinical situations based upon many past paradigm cases . . .' (p.294).

Drawing on the work of educationalists seeking to examine the development of clinical expertise, Greenhalgh (2002) concludes that novices start off by learning and rigidly applying 'rules' about how to diagnose and manage each condition. Discretionary judgement is not used. Over time, and

as they develop expertise, they build up a bank of clini/
as stories, which they can draw on to 'break the rules'
is unique about each patient/care episode. Their act
a deep, tacit understanding, and analytic approach…
unfamiliar or problematic situations.

Reflective practice

Reflective practice provides the opportunity to look back at a clinical situation, analyse it and learn from it. How effective was the intervention? Did it achieve its intended outcome? If not, why not? Is there a better alternative? What types of knowledge impacted on the decisions made and did these have a positive or negative effect in terms of patient outcome? What aspects of my behaviour were helpful/obstructive? What could I do to ensure a better outcome next time?

'Reflective practice' is one way of overcoming the contradictions that lie within our personal and professional experiences and those of the patients and carers with whom we work. Indeed, Johns' (1995) popular model of reflection is based on Carper's (1978) early work on fundamental ways of knowing. As such, it prompts us to think about the different sources and types of knowledge used in a particular situation so that we can become reflexively aware of the need to question all aspects of our practice – in other words, 'to think, and think about that thinking' (Manley et al 2005).

Intuitive practice

Inextricably linked to clinical expertise, and its development, is intuition. Although the contribution of intuition to evidence-based practice is not well researched, it has long been accepted as playing a pivotal role in decision making (Benner 1984) and, subsequently, quality of patient care (McCutcheon & Pincombe 2001). The term 'intuition' defies precise definition but attempts have been made to describe it. For Parahoo (1997), intuition is a way in which we know and behave about a situation that is not based on conscious reasoning or rational thought processes. Benner (1984) asserts that 'intuitive grasp' is impossible without sufficient clinical experience in similar and dissimilar situations; it rests on personal experiences and tacit knowledge that is difficult to articulate. Greenhalgh (2002) describes intuition as a rapid unconscious process that cannot be explained through cause and effect rules (in other words, that Y will happen because of X); rather, intuitive practice builds on repeated practice situations, it is context specific and it enables the integration of complex pieces of data to derive a decision that is difficult to articulate through linear rules.

If, as Schon (1991) suggests, reflective practice is the bedrock on which learning from experience helps to develop practice-based theory then systematic, critical reflection with colleagues is a necessary pre-requisite for the use of clinical expertise in the formulation of decisions. It becomes an essential component in person-centred evidence-based practice.

What is clear from all these authors is that intuition and clinical expertise/experience are interdependent.

Expert opinion in clinical decision making

Much of the literature on expert opinion in decision making focuses on evidence-based guidelines. Indeed, in instances where there is no good-quality research evidence to underpin practice, expert opinion becomes the source of evidence on which clinical recommendations/guidelines are based. To illustrate, the Scottish Intercollegiate Guideline Network (SIGN) (2003) guidance on the management of obesity in children and young adults advocates an increase in activity and a reduction in both energy intake and sedentary behaviour. The evidence for this recommendation is based on the 'clinical experience of the guideline development group'. Similarly, despite research evidence that 'most' people with sore throats will not need antibiotics (Little et al 1997), it is acknowledged that the final decision on whether or not to prescribe antibiotics rests with the practitioner; 'where the practitioner is concerned about the clinical condition, antibiotics should not be withheld' (SIGN 1999). Again the basis of this recommendation is expert opinion.

However, experts' opinions of what constitutes an effective or harmful intervention might not always be correct. Their beliefs may be based on misconceptions or on recollections of a situation that was not representative of the norm, and their opinion might not represent the view of other experts. Despite this, the benefits that experienced practitioners bring to the clinical decision-making arena, in terms of both interpreting evidence in light of the unique clinical situation and their observations of what has worked, are immense.

Reaching consensus

Thompson & Dowding (2002) observe that, as nurses, we rarely make decisions on our own, having a preference for gleaning 'oral' evidence from colleagues when formulating decisions. They describe decision making as a 'social activity'. Indeed, clinical decisions are often the result of multidisciplinary team meetings. Reaching consensus of opinion on health-care interventions, especially where a number of practitioners or professions are involved or where there is no relevant research evidence to support the decision, can be problematic and there will be occasions when all those present do not agree on what is proposed for a patient. The nominal group technique is one method of dealing with such difficulties. Similarly, the Delphi research method can facilitate the development of consensus amongst practitioners. These techniques are described more fully in Chapter 9.

Consensus may not necessarily mean unanimous support for a particular decision. Simply translated, consensus usually denotes agreement, harmony or compromise. This invariably means that those involved in the decision making, the patient or professional, need to reach agreement through discussion and negotiation. Even when using this 'tolerant' definition, consensus is not always possible, as illustrated in the paper by Fass et al (2001). In the absence of good-quality research evidence on which to develop diagnostic tests for irritable bowel syndrome, Fass et al (2001) relied on consensus derived from expert opinion. Despite using the Delphi method, not all experts could agree or reach consensus for some diagnostic procedures. In view of this, the resulting diagnostic algorithm incorporated coding to show which recommendations comprised 'expert consensus disagreement'.

Integrating the components of clinical expertise

What do these insights into ways of knowing, clinical expertise, reflection, intuition and consensus tell us, and how can we make use of them? Perhaps their most important contribution is to prompt us to recognise that in situations which are relatively novel to us, we become novices and as such, our ability to successfully help patients reach the right decision for them is reduced; the case for consulting with an expert in such situations is a strong one. Moreover, we must recognise that our personal prejudices and beliefs that we bring to any patient consultation can influence the eventual outcome, so it is worth examining these critically to ensure they do not override other important considerations.

Patient preferences, values and beliefs

Sackett et al (2000) describe patient values as: 'the unique preferences, concerns and expectations each patient brings to a clinical encounter and which must be integrated into clinical decisions if they are to serve the patient' (p.1).

Patients' clinical and personal circumstances and outlooks *are* unique. Kitson (2002) notes that even patients with the same diagnosis or similar needs do not form a homogeneous group; each person has significant individual differences and acknowledgement of these differences is fundamental in working towards clinical effectiveness. Kitson reminds us that it is often necessary to implement different interventions with different patients even when the presenting problem is similar.

An illustration of differences between people in terms of their preferences is given by Devereaux et al (2001), who investigated patients' and physicians' thresholds for commencing antithrombotic treatment in people with atrial fibrillation. In this study, patients varied widely on the risk of haemorrhage they would accept in return for a reduction in risk of stroke. Whilst at least half of the patients in the study were willing to accept as many as 22 extra episodes of bleeding per 100 warfarinised patients over a 2-year period to prevent eight strokes in these 100 patients, more than 10% of the patients would accept only five, or less than five extra episodes of bleeding for this benefit. These data demonstrate marked differences between patients in their attitudes to the risks and benefits of taking warfarin. This same study showed a striking difference between clinicians and patients in how many bleeding episodes were acceptable. In contrast to the patients, only a small proportion of clinicians (fewer than 10%) were prepared to accept as many as 22 extra episodes of bleeding per 100 patients over 2 years to prevent eight strokes in the 100 patients. Moreover, thresholds for the risk of bleeding varied markedly between clinicians. The authors of this study conclude their report with the following statement:

'. . . *Patients' preferences should be incorporated into decisions about antithrombotic treatment in atrial fibrillation. If physicians make decisions about management without such input, then they risk finding themselves out of step with the people whose care they strive to optimise* . . .'

Incorporating patient values into clinical decisions

Stevenson et al (2000) draw on the work of Charles et al (1999) to demonstrate the four conditions necessary for shared decision making to take place:

- both practitioner and patient are involved
- both share information

- both build a consensus on preferred treatment options
- both agree on which treatment to implement.

Central to this model is the need for effective communication and partnership working. Working in partnership to reach health-care decisions is a laudable aim and one that demonstrates respect for patients' autonomy; indeed, Rogers (2002) states that actions which disregard the choices of others could be viewed as coercive or manipulative. However, it is not easy to get the balance right: each patient and patient encounter is unique. Patients form a broad spectrum in terms of age, social, ethnic, cultural and educational backgrounds, personal circumstances, etc. In addition, their health status and experiences of the health-care system all vary. Each of these factors ultimately influences their approach to clinical dialogue. To make matters more complex, there is often a considerable range of options available to patients, although their immediate clinical situation will dictate the options available and the extent to which they can be involved in decision making (Rogers 2002). An additional consideration is the potential for patients to try to make the 'right' choice in order to please the health-care practitioner, thus becoming reluctant collaborators (Waterworth & Luker 1990).

Barry et al (2000) remind us of the importance of understanding the patient's perspective in their study examining patients' unvoiced agendas in the context of general practitioner consultations. They discovered that most patients seemed comfortable to talk about symptoms and request a diagnosis or prescription but often did not disclose information relating to their social context or their understanding of the problem. Follow-up case studies revealed that the outcomes of these consultations were often major misunderstandings, non-adherence to prescribed treatment and unwanted prescriptions. The message that can be taken from this study is that failure to ascertain patients' preferences for particular interventions can potentially jeopardise the opportunity to probe any concerns that the patient may have, to allay any ill-founded fears and to present alternative options.

Non-adherence with drug, exercise and other health intervention programmes is a potential cause for continued ill health in patients, and one that can increase risks for morbidity and mortality and lead to wasted resources. Knowing what factors impact on non-adherence is part of the tacit knowledge that nurses and patients bring to each care episode. This tacit knowledge can be complemented by research evidence as illustrated in the case study presented in Box 8.3. Clearly, it is important to ascertain patients' understanding and values regarding a proposed intervention before prescribing it. Whitstock (2003) goes even further, suggesting that adherence

---

BOX 8.3 Case study illustrating use of research evidence in overcoming non-adherence

Consider Mr Patel, discharged from hospital 3 months ago following surgical intervention for osteoarthritis in his left knee. It emerges that he has not continued with the prescribed exercise regimen as he understood the surgical intervention would 'cure' his problem and he says he has had difficulty in finding the time to fit the exercises into his daily routine. Research tells us that non-compliance is associated with difficulty in incorporating prescribed exercises into daily routines, the severity of the illness and the patient's experience (Campbell et al 2001). As Barry et al (2000) remind us, patients may have many unvoiced agendas and misunderstandings of what is proposed that may remain unheard during consultations.

---

to some interventions might be improved if patients were involved in their development:

'. . . Patients are the final consumers of research. . . . if patients find a proposed therapeutic intervention unacceptable, then it is important to know why and to consider whether the reason for this could have been more usefully addressed as part of the process of developing the intervention . . .' (Whitstock 2003, p.217)

You're the nurse, you tell me

Of key importance in clinical effectiveness is recognition of the extent to which the patient is able or willing to be involved in decision making, and appreciation that this level of willingness is unlikely to remain static during the course of the patient's disease trajectory/health-care episode. Caress et al (2005) undertook a cross-sectional survey of 230 adult patients with asthma and established that only 23.9% of these wanted to be actively involved in treatment decisions, 35.7% wanted to collaborate and 40.4% wished to take a passive role.

In qualitative interviews to explore preferences for involvement in decision making in patients with asthma (Caress et al 2002), possession of sufficient information, the practitioner's ability to listen, effective practitioner/patient relationship, continuity of care, the longer the time with the condition and patient assertiveness appeared to facilitate patient involvement in decision making. Conversely, lack of knowledge about treatments, poor interpersonal skills, lack of time, the personality characteristics of the patient, lack of willingness by the practitioner to accept patient expertise and life-threatening situations were perceived to inhibit patient involvement.

Translating research evidence

If the information needed to make a decision is inaccessible or obscure, there is far less chance of patients being able to make informed choices. Given this, how can we translate the findings from quantitative studies into 'lay-friendly' terminology so that patients can actively participate in health-care decisions? A good example is provided by Haynes et al (2002), who interpret the findings from the warfarin study conducted by Devereaux et al (2001) (discussed earlier) as follows:

'. . . if you take 1 warfarin tablet a day with weekly blood checks to guide the dose, your risk for stroke in the first year would decrease from 6% (6 in 100) to 2.3% (about 2 in 100). Half of strokes resulting from atrial fibrillation will be major, resulting in permanent disability, and half will be minor, allowing the person to function independently . . .'

This interpretation is far more user friendly than an equally accurate format incorporating more complicated statistics. For example, compare the above quote with '. . . the relative risk reduction of stroke for patients receiving warfarin is 62% . . .'.

Figure 8.1 shows how risk data can be displayed graphically to help patients who may have difficulty in interpreting numbers to make sense of numerical data.

A popular way of expressing research data about interventions (provided the data are dichotomous) is in terms of 'number needed to treat' (NNT). NNT is defined as 'the number of patients you need to treat to prevent one additional bad outcome (e.g. death, stroke, etc.). For example, if a drug has an NNT of 5, it means you have to treat five people with the drug to prevent one additional bad outcome' (Centre for Evidence-Based Medicine: www.cebm.net/nnts.asp). The Knowledge Library section of the *Bandolier* website (www.jr2.ox.ac.uk/bandolier/index.html) provides some examples of NNTs:

- the NNT for antibiotic prophylaxis following dog bites is 16 (95% confidence interval (CI) 9–92). On average, one patient out of 16 receiving prophylactic antibiotics avoids infection as a result of this prophylaxis (Cummings 1994)

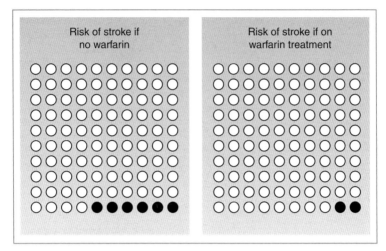

Figure 8.1 Graphical representation of percentage risk

- the NNT for a programme of interventions delivered to patients with chronic pain, within an inpatient setting, is 2.8 (95% CI 1.8–6.1). On average, for every three patients treated as inpatients rather than outpatients, one patient fewer was taking analgesic or psychotropic drugs at 1 year after the end of treatment (de C Williams 1995).

An NNT of 1 is the perfect result. It means that every patient in the intervention group had a favourable outcome, and that no patients in the comparison group had a favourable outcome. NNTs are much easier to comprehend than many other statistical terms and allow straightforward comparisons between different interventions – hence their use by practitioners when helping patients to reach decisions about a particular intervention. NNTs should be expressed with 95% confidence intervals. These tell you that you can be 95% certain that the true NNT lies somewhere inside these intervals.

As well as accurately translating often complicated research findings, health-care practitioners are also charged with ensuring that patients understand how applicable the findings are to them. This concept of applicability is discussed in more detail in Chapter 5.

Decision aids

One way of helping patients to access high-quality information on the options available to them is through the use of decision aids. These are educational resources designed to help people understand the range and type of options available, and consider the personal importance of the possible advantages and disadvantages of each option (O'Connor et al 2003). A systematic review undertaken to examine the benefits of decision aids found that they can improve knowledge, improve realistic expectations, enhance active participation, lower decisional conflict and decrease the proportion of those undecided. Furthermore, decision aids do not appear to increase patients' anxiety levels (O'Connor et al 2003).

Decision aids are increasingly popular as a way of helping patients and health-care professionals make informed, reliable decisions but their effectiveness remains unknown. In the UK the NHS Connecting for Health has developed a Service Level Agreement with the National Institute for Health and Clinical Excellence (NICE) 'to appraise the effectiveness of computer-based clinical decision support systems'. In addition, work has recently commenced with NHS Direct Online to 'appraise and, if appropriate, introduce patient decision aids'.

Decision aids can take many forms. For example, some use simple sets of questions to enable patients to determine what matters most to them in the context of their daily lives in order to make a decision about a proposed intervention. MSdecisions, an interactive web-based resource funded by the Department of Health, aims to enable people diagnosed with multiple sclerosis to decide if they should start disease-modifying drugs and which, from the four available, would most suit their needs (see www.msdecision.org.uk). Similarly, NHS Direct (the official website for the NHS and 24-hour helpline (www.nhsdirect.nhs.uk)) has a number of interactive decision aids to help people decide what action/intervention they should pursue in relation to presenting symptoms and whether they can safely self-care or need to seek urgent professional help (see www.nhsdirect.nhs.uk/SelfHelpGuide/).

Kim et al (2005) developed an interactive computer package aimed at helping patients decide whether to undergo screening for colorectal cancer and helping them to select the screening test most appropriate/acceptable to them. To ensure patients were provided with a balanced view of the potential benefits and harms of screening, the package included a range of health-care professionals' and patients' perspectives in the form of short video clips. Less 'high-tech' resources, such as pamphlets and simple flow charts, are also used. A variety of decision aids developed by the Ottawa Health Research Institute can be viewed at decisionaid.ohri.ca/decaids.html. Because these particular aids are designed to be used outside doctor/nurse consultations, fairly detailed information is provided and this is presented in a clear, unambiguous way. Not all decision aids are suitable for use in this way; most require interpretation by health-care practitioners and are simply prompts for further discussions.

The expert patient

Patients are well placed to know what works for them in the context of their lives. Regardless of the extent of their clinical knowledge, they are the ones who live with the condition and who are experts in terms of their social circumstances, preferences, values and attitudes to risk (Department of Health 2001). In contrast, health-care practitioners' expertise lies in establishing diagnoses, prognoses, treatment options and outcome probabilities (Department of Health 2001). By working together, patients and health-care practitioners can pool their separate areas of expertise.

Patients are also being encouraged to participate at the research stage: INVOLVE is a UK advisory group which was established to promote public involvement in research. Funded by the Department of Health, INVOLVE aims to promote and maintain active public involvement in public health, NHS and social care research. It is able to achieve this through involving members of the public in research that is 'more relevant to people's needs and concerns, more reliable and more likely to be used'. INVOLVE suggests that 'research which reflects the needs and views of the public, is more likely to produce results that can be used to improve practice in health and social care'. More information about INVOLVE can be found on their website at www.invo.org.uk/.

In the UK, expert patients are actively contributing to national initiatives such as the National Service Frameworks (NSFs). NSFs seek to improve specific areas of care by setting measurable goals, within set timeframes, to raise the quality of services and decrease variance in quality. During the development phase of the NSF for long-term conditions, extensive consultations were held with patients to harness their expert opinions. The NSF reflects these opinions in its recommendations: the opinions are coded to differentiate them from professional expert opinion (Department of Health 2005), as shown in Box 8.4.

Currently, there is a move towards further developing patients' expertise. The UK expert patient initiative (Department of Health 2001) offers user-led self-management courses that give patients with chronic conditions (such as asthma, multiple sclerosis, arthritis) the opportunity to develop the confidence, skills and knowledge to effectively manage their conditions,

---

BOX 8.4 Types of evidence cited in the NSF for long-term conditions (adapted from Department of Health 2005, with permission. Reproduced under the terms of the Click-Use Licence)

Each piece of evidence cited in the NSF is given either an 'E' or an 'R' rating.

R reflects research-based evidence.

E reflects expert (user/carer/professional) evidence. This is evidence expressed through consultation or consensus processes rather than research.

E1 reflects the expert opinion of users and/or carers or other stakeholders.

E2 reflects the expert opinion of professionals.

---

and thereby gain greater control over their lives. The evidence supporting such initiatives is accumulating, and shows that patients' severity of symptoms and quality of life can improve with increased self-management (Department of Health 2001).

As health-care practitioners, we need to bring about a fundamental shift in the way in which we care for patients such that they are enabled and encouraged to actively manage their own care – to be 'experts'. It is not enough to simply educate patients about their condition or instruct them on what to do. A more holistic approach must be taken to develop their confidence and motivation to become active in self-management of their condition. Perhaps Jones' (2003) definition of expert patients outlines the attitudes, skills and knowledge to be encouraged in our patients:

> *'Expert patients are people who understand that the quality of their lives is primarily up to them; believe they can exert significant control over their own lives; are determined to live a healthy life despite their chronic condition; are realistic about the impact of their disease; and have worked out what services exist and how they can be accessed.'*

In this era of easily accessible information, there are excellent opportunities for patients to develop expertise in terms of clinical knowledge. For instance, Jadad & Haynes (1998) describe how the Cochrane Collaboration Consumer Network was developed to facilitate the dissemination of research findings to patients, their families and advocates by notifying the lay press of significant developments and sharing information amongst network members. The National Library for Health (www.library.nhs.uk) is also working to produce a comprehensive digital library for patients and the public, while the DIPEX website (www.dipex.org) enables patients to share their experiences by making available personal experiences of health and illness. The DIPEX website aims to cover the 100 main illnesses and conditions and make contemporaneous evidence-based information accessible to aid people in decision making. More examples of such initiatives can be seen on the UK professional nursing body website (www.rcn.org.uk) and the Nursing and Midwifery Council website (www.nmc-uk.org). Both give free online access to information for patients and the public.

The influence of the media on patient expertise

The mass media play a pivotal role in the way new evidence is projected to the public. To help the patient and clinician rapidly ascertain the reliability of the reports, the National Library for Health (NLH) has incorporated a Hitting the Headlines section on its webpage. It features appraisals of 'the reliability of both the journalists' reporting of health stories, and the research on which they are based', as provided by the Centre for Reviews and Dissemination (CRD) at the University of York.

At the time of writing, UK daily newspapers had published the interim findings from the Herceptin Adjuvant Trial (Piccart-Gebhart et al 2005), a study which investigated the efficacy of herceptin in patients with HER2-positive breast cancer. The NLH commentary states that the 'newspapers reported the results of the trial accurately, though the front page headline, 'Wonderdrug is "cure" for breast cancer, say doctors', is overly enthusiastic' (Hitting the Headlines 2005). The commentary went on to describe how one of the newspapers did not accurately state that the results applied only to those women with HER2-positive breast cancer (an estimated 15–25% of breast cancers; Piccart-Gebhart et al 2005). As evidence-based practitioners, we should point patients in the direction of resources that provide high-quality information, and should be ready to correct any misinterpretation of research findings (Thomas 2005).

Integrating the components of patient preference

As this section illustrates, the patient's unique experiences should play a pivotal role in the decision-making process. Patient preferences, values and beliefs should be integrated into clinical decisions and acknowledged as a key attribute of evidence-based practice. For shared decisions to occur, effective communication and partnership working need to be evident to avoid the 'unvoiced agendas' highlighted in Barry et al's (2000) study. Thus we are reminded that patient preferences may lay claim to be a legitimate form of evidence and as such should be accepted within the evidence-based decision-making process.

Limited resources for health care

While research evidence and clinical guidelines form the basis for legally defensible interventions, it is for practitioners to make the final decision on how to proceed, having taken account of all data that impinge on what should happen in any given situation (Kitson 2002). After all, it is practitioners, not guidelines, who make decisions. Hurwitz (1999, p.662) underlines this in his discussion of the legal implications of guidelines:

'. . . *Expert testimony helps the courts to ascertain what is accepted and proper practice in specific cases, ensuring that professionally generated standards from real clinical situations are generally applied rather than standards enunciated in the rhetoric of clinical guidelines . . .*'

While research evidence, clinical expertise and patient preference might all point towards a particular intervention, shortfalls in resources might not allow for that intervention to be implemented. Health-care providers are faced with difficult decisions about health-care rationing and approaches will differ. To illustrate, in the USA, the 'flu vaccine' is available to those aged 55 and over, while in Ontario, it is available to everyone (Watkins 2005).

Conclusion

Evidence-based practice is the bedrock on which clinical effectiveness (the seven rights) stands. Clinical decisions, reached through an evidence-based practice approach, take account not only of research findings but also of the patient's and nurse's expertise, preferences, values and beliefs and the unique clinical situation. Each of these elements of decision making is influenced by numerous factors, some of which are described in this chapter (displayed graphically in Figure 8.2). The challenge for us as aspiring evidence-based practitioners is to tap into and understand the workings of these elements, and to truly integrate them into the decision-making process.

Individual nurses will undoubtedly bring their unique perspective to any problem. The interpretation of research findings and how they are applied

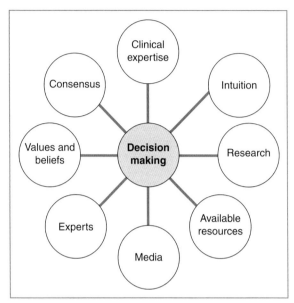

Figure 8.2 Influences on clinical decision making

will always be different according to the level of knowledge, expertise and experiences of both the nurse and patient involved, and the available resources. In essence, the reality of evidence-based practice is that it puts the needs of the patient at the centre of decision making; the final decision of how to apply the research findings or clinical guidelines is left to the nurse and patient. Research evidence is indeed an essential component of evidence-based practice, but this must be contextualised through clinical expertise, patient preferences and the situation.

References

Barry C, Bradley C, Britten N, Stevenson F, Baker N 2000 Patients' unvoiced agendas in General Practice consultations: a qualitative study. British Journal of Medicine 320:1246–1250

Benner P 1984 From novice to expert: excellence and power in clinical nursing practice. Addison-Wesley, Menlo Park, CA

Campbell R, Evans M, Tucker M, Quilty B, Dieppe P, Donovan J 2001 Why don't patients do their exercises? Understanding non-compliance with physiotherapy in patients with osteoarthritis of the knee. Journal of Epidemiology and Community Health 55:132–138

Caress A, Luker K, Woodcock A, Beaver K 2002 A qualitative exploration of treatment decision making role preference in adult asthma patients. Health Expectations 5:223–235

Caress A, Beaver K, Luker K, Campbell M, Woodcock A 2005 Involvement in treatment decisions: what do adults with asthma want and what do they get? Results of a cross-sectional survey. Thorax 60:199–205

Carper B 1978 Fundamental of patterns of knowing in nursing. Advances in Nursing Science 1:13–23

Cummings P 1994 Antibiotics to prevent infection in patients with dog bite wounds: a meta-analysis of randomised trials. Annals of Emergency Medicine 23:535–540

de C Williams A C 1995 NNTs used in decision making in chronic pain management. Available online at: www.jr2.ox.ac.uk/bandolier/band22/b22-2.html May 2006

Department of Health 2001 The expert patient: a new approach to chronic disease management for the 21st century. Product code 25216. Stationery Office. Available online at: www.dh.gov.uk 28 December 2005

Department of Health 2005 National Service Framework for long term conditions. Product code 265109. Stationery Office. Available online at: www.dh.gov.uk 20 January 2006

Devereaux P, Anderson D, Gardner M et al 2001 Differences between perspectives of physicians and patients on anticoagulation in patients with atrial fibrillation: an observational study. British Medical Journal 323:1–7

Edwards S 2001 Philosophy of nursing: an introduction. Palgrave, Basingstoke

Fass R, Longstreth G, Pimentel M et al 2001 Evidence and consensus based practice guidelines for the diagnosis of irritable bowel syndrome. Archives of Internal Medicine 161:2081–2088

Greenhalgh T 2002 Uneasy bedfellows? Reconciling intuition and evidence based practice. Young Minds Magazine 59. Available online at: www.youngminds.org.uk/magazine/59/greenhalgh.php 28 December 2005

Guyatt G, Cook D, Haynes B 2004 Evidence based medicine has come a long way (editorial). British Medical Journal 329:990–991

Haynes B, Devereaux P, Guyatt G 2002 Clinical expertise in the era of evidence-based medicine and patient choice. Evidence Based Medicine 7:36–38

Hek G, Judd M, Moule P 2002 Making sense of research: an introduction for health and social care practitioners, 2nd edn. Continuum, London

Hitting the Headlines 2005 Herceptin for treating HER-2 positive breast cancer. Available online at: www.nelh.nhs.uk/hth/herceptin.asp

Hurwitz B 1999 Clinical guidelines: legal and political considerations of clinical practice guidelines. British Medical Journal 318:661–664

Jadad A, Haynes B 1998 The Cochrane Collaboration – advances and challenges in improving evidence-based decision making. Medical Decision Making 18:2–9

Johns C 1995 Framing learning through reflection within Carper's fundamental ways of knowing in nursing. Journal of Advanced Nursing 22:226–234

Jones F R 2003 Can expert patients be created? Expert Patient Conference. Available online at: www.rpsgb.org.uk/pdfs/exptpatsem6.pdf

Kim J, Whitney A, Hayter S et al 2005 Development and initial testing of a computer-based patient decision aid to promote colorectal cancer screening for primary care practice. Biomed Central Informatics and Decision Making 5:36. Available online at: www.biomedcentral.com/content/5/1/36

Kitson A 2002 Recognising relationships: reflections on evidence-based practice. Nursing Inquiry 9:179–186

Kitson A, Harvey G, McCormack B 1998 Enabling the implementation of evidence based practice: a conceptual framework. Quality in Health Care 7:149–158

Little P, Williamson I, Warner G, Gould C, Kinnmouth A 1997 Open randomised trial of prescribing strategies in managing sore throat. British Medical Journal 314:722–727

Manley K, Hardy S, Titchen A, Garbett R, McCormack B 2005 Changing patients' worlds through nursing expertise. Royal College of Nursing, London

McCutcheon H, Pincombe I 2001 Intuition: an important tool in the practice of nursing. Journal of Advanced Nursing 35:342–348

Miles A, Charlton B, Bentley P, Polychronis A, Grey J 2000 New perspectives in the evidence-based healthcare debate. Journal of Evaluation in Clinical Practice 6:77–84

Mulrow C, Lau J, Cornell, Brand M 1998 Pharmacotherapy for hypertension in the elderly. Cochrane Database of Systematic Reviews, Issue 2. Art. No. CD 00028

National Institute for Health and Clinical Excellence (NICE) 2004 CG18 Hypertension (persistently high blood pressure) in adults: full guideline. Available online at: www.nice.org.uk/page.aspx?o5CG018fullguideline January 2006

O'Connor A, Stacey D, Entwistle V et al 2003 Decision aids for people facing health treatment or screening decisions. Cochrane Database of Systematic Reviews. Issue 1. Available online at:mrw.interscience.wiley.com/cochrane/clsysrev/articles/ CD001431/frame.html

Parahoo K 1997 Nursing research: principles, process and issues. Macmillan, Basingstoke

Piccart-Gebhart M, Proctor M, Leyland-Jones B et al (The Herceptin Adjuvant Trial Study Team) 2005 Trastuzamab after adjuvant chemotherapy in HER2-positive breast cancer. New England Journal of Medicine 353(16):1659–1672

Rogers W 2002 Evidence-based medicine in practice: limiting or facilitating patient choice? Health Expectations 5:95–103

Royal College of Nursing 1996 Clinical effectiveness. Royal College of Nursing, London

Sackett D, Richardson W, Rosenberg W, Haynes R 1996 Evidence based medicine: how to practice and teach EBM. Churchill Livingstone, New York

Sackett D, Strauss S, Richardson W, Rosenberg W, Haynes R 2000 Evidence based medicine: how to practise and teach EBM, 2nd edn. Churchill Livingstone, London

Schon D 1991 The reflective practitioner, 2nd edn. Jossey Bass, San Francisco, CA

Scottish Intercollegiate Guideline Network (SIGN) 1999 Management of sore throat and indications for tonsillectomy. SIGN Guideline No 34. Scottish Intercollegiate Guideline Network, Edinburgh. Available online at: www.sign.ac.uk/guidelines/fulltext/34/index.html 28 December 2005

Scottish Intercollegiate Guideline Network (SIGN) 2001 Hypertension in older people. SIGN Guideline No 49. Scottish Intercollegiate Guideline Network, Edinburgh. Available online at: www.sign.ac.uk/guidelines/fulltext/49/index.html 28 December 2005

Scottish Intercollegiate Guideline Network (SIGN) 2003 Management of obesity in children and young people. SIGN Guideline No 69. Scottish Intercollegiate Guideline Network, Edinburgh. Available online at: www.sign.ac.uk/guidelines/fulltext/69/index.html 28 December 2005

Stevenson F, Barry C, Britten N, Bradley C 2000 Doctor–patient communication about drugs: shared decision making. Social Science and Medicine 50:829–840

Thomas M 2005 Public communication, risk perception and the viability of preventive communicable diseases. Bioethics 19:407–421

Thompson C, Dowding D 2002 Clinical decision making and judgement in nursing. Churchill Livingstone, London

Waterworth S, Luker K 1990 Reluctant collaborators. Do patients want to be included in decisions concerning care? Journal of Advanced Nursing 15:971–976

Watkins J 2005 The UK flu vaccine shortage: who is at fault? British Medical Journal 331:1413

White J 1995 Patterns of knowing: review, critique and update. Advances in Nursing Science 17:73–86

Whitstock M 2003 Seeking evidence from medical research consumers as part of the medical research process could improve the uptake of research evidence. Journal of Evaluation in Clinical Practice 9:213–224

APPENDIX

Useful websites

National Electronic Library for Health: www.nelh.nhs.uk/

Cochrane Library: www.nelh.nhs.uk/cochrane.asp

DIPEX: www.dipex.org

Nursing and Midwifery Council: www.nmc-uk.org

Royal College of Nursing: www.rcn.org.uk/

Scottish Intercollegiate Guideline Network (SIGN): www.sign.ac.uk/

Bandolier: www.jr2.ox.ac.uk/bandolier/index.html

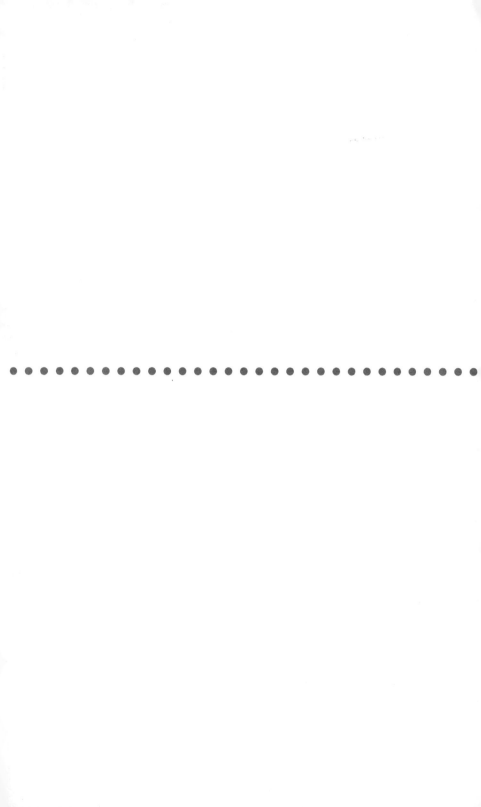

3
SECTION

The process of changing practice

9

CHAPTER

Evidence-based guidelines

Lois Thomas

KEY POINTS

- During the last decade there has been an unprecedented increase in guideline development activity in response to professional, public and political calls for evidence-based treatment delivered to comparable standards across the country.

- A potentially unlimited number of clinical topics may be amenable to guideline development. Criteria for topic selection have therefore had to be agreed.

- Rigorous methods are recommended for guideline development, which is a time-consuming and often costly process.

- Guidelines incorporate varying grades of recommendation depending on the strength of the evidence they are based on.

- Instruments are available to appraise guidelines. These should be applied and the quality of the guideline judged before it is accepted for use.

- Strategies for the implementation of guidelines at local and individual clinician level must incorporate methods that have been demonstrated to be effective.

Introduction

Clinical guidelines are 'systematically developed statements to assist practitioner decisions about appropriate health care for specific clinical circumstances' (Field & Lohr 1990). The topic of a clinical guideline may be a condition (such as asthma or angina; North of England Evidence-Based Guideline Development Project 1999a, b), a symptom (such as pain; Royal College of Nursing 2000) or a clinical procedure (such as urinary catheter care; Seto et al 1991). Guidelines can be used to reduce inappropriate variations in practice and to promote the delivery of high-quality, evidence-based health care. They may also provide a mechanism by which health-care professionals can be made accountable for clinical activities (Royal College of General Practitioners Clinical Guidelines Working Group 1995).

Traditionally, guidelines were based on consensus, individual opinion and/ or current practice (and this remains the case in topics where there is little valid research evidence) but it is now recognised that guidelines should be explicitly evidence-based. To date, most of the development and evaluation of clinical guidelines have been in medicine, but there is increasing interest in the use of guidelines in nursing (McClarey 1997, Royal College of Nursing 1995, Von Degenburg & Deighan 1995).

Guideline characteristics

If guidelines are to be effective, it is recommended that they have most, if not all, of the eleven characteristics listed in Box 9.1 (NHS CRD 1994). Ensuring that guidelines meet these criteria is a resource-intensive task in terms of cost and the time and skills required for both developing evidence-based guidelines and ensuring they remain up to date. The process from start of guideline development to publication has been estimated by the Scottish Intercollegiate Guidelines Network (SIGN 2004) to take up to 30 months, depending on the volume of relevant literature on the topic, the amount of feedback received during the consultation phase and the time constraints of the guideline development group. The National Institute for Health and Clinical Excellence (NICE 2004) estimates that the production of a draft guideline takes 12–18 months. The development of evidence-based guidelines may therefore be beyond the scope of practising health professionals, who may prefer to adopt or adapt guidelines developed nationally.

BOX 9.1 Desirable attributes of clinical guidelines (reproduced from NHS CRD 1994, with permission)

Attribute	Explanation
Validity	Evidence should be interpreted correctly so that if a guideline is followed, it leads to the predicted improvements in health
Cost-effectiveness	Improvements in health care should be at acceptable costs. If guidelines ignore issues of costs and concentrate only on benefits, there is the possibility that practices might be recommended with major implications for resource use which are not reflected in correspondingly large improvements in patient outcome
Reproducibility	Given the same evidence, another guideline development group would produce similar recommendations
Reliability	Given the same clinical circumstances, another health professional would apply the recommendations in a similar fashion
Representative development	All key disciplines and interests contribute to guideline development
Clinical applicability	The target population is defined in accordance with the evidence.
Clinical flexibility	Guidelines identify exceptions and indicate how patient preferences are to be incorporated into decision making
Clarity	Guidelines use precise definitions, unambiguous language and user-friendly formats
Meticulous documentation	Guidelines record participants, assumptions and methods and link recommendations to the available evidence
Scheduled review	Guidelines state when and how they are to be reviewed
Utilisation review	Guidelines indicate ways in which adherence to recommendations can be sensibly monitored

National or local guideline development

While locally developed ('internal') guidelines may need fewer resources and may be more likely to be adopted into clinical practice because of local ownership (Putnam & Curry 1985, Williamson 1978), local groups may not have the extensive skills and resources required for guideline development (Grol 1990a, North of England Study of Standards and Performances in

General Practice 1991). An alternative is the development of guidelines at regional/national level and subsequent modification to suit local circumstances (Grol 1990a, b, 1992).

Prioritising topic areas for guideline development

Nationally funded organisations use various criteria to identify topics that most warrant the significant investments required to develop rigorous evidence-based guidelines. For example, the National Institute for Health and Clinical Excellence, in England, endeavours to develop guidance that 'promotes the best possible improvement in patient care given the available resources' (NICE 2004) and selects topics that satisfy one or more of the following questions.

Does the proposed guidance:

- relate to one of the clinical areas identified as a priority for improvement within the NHS or to other government health-related priorities, such as reducing health inequalities?
- address a condition associated with significant disability, morbidity or mortality in the population as a whole or in particular subgroups?
- relate to one or more interventions that could significantly improve patients' or carers' quality of life and/or reduce avoidable morbidity or premature mortality, if used more extensively or appropriately relative to current standard practice?
- relate to one or more interventions that, if used more extensively, would impact significantly on the resources (financial or other) available to the NHS or to society in general?
- relate to one or more interventions that could, without detriment to patient care, be used more selectively, thus freeing up resources for use elsewhere in the NHS?

NICE (2004) also considers the robustness of the evidence base and whether there is likely to be either inappropriate practice and/or significant variation in clinical practice or access to treatment in the absence of the proposed guideline.

The Scottish Intercollegiate Guidelines Network (SIGN 2004, Section 3.1) states that guidelines should 'address a specific health care need and there should be an expectation that change is possible and desirable and that, if the guidelines are followed, there is potential to improve the quality of care and/or patient outcomes' (SIGN 2004, Section 3.1). SIGN also stipulates that there should be a strong research base providing evidence of effective practice to underpin guideline recommendations (SIGN 2004). In addition, SIGN (2004) criteria for guideline development include:

- areas of clinical uncertainty as evidenced by wide variation in practice or outcomes
- conditions where effective treatment is proven and can reduce mortality or morbidity
- iatrogenic diseases/interventions carrying significant risk
- clinical priority areas for the NHS in Scotland
- the perceived need for the guideline, as indicated by a network of relevant stakeholders.

The idea that guidelines aim to improve quality of care has, at times, been met with scepticism. Some of the earliest criticisms of or misgivings about guideline development arose because of cynicism around their purpose; that is, the suspicion that they could be an exercise in cost containment. Klein (1996) suggests that values, as opposed to research evidence, can determine the judgements made within 'guidelines', citing the example of the accessibility, or limits to the accessibility, of in vitro fertilisation treatment (IVF), where value-judgements are made about the ethics of individuals' situations.

In a recent exercise designed to examine the priorities of nurses in Scotland for the development of 'Best Practice Statements' (www.nmpdu.org.uk), which will use scientific evidence, where it exists, combined with expert nursing opinion and consensus, topics that topped the poll were nutrition, continence, pressure ulcer prevention and others that many would consider 'basic' nursing care. Paradoxically, given the importance of these topics and the resources which their treatment costs the NHS, they have not been tackled by groups specifically resourced to develop national guidelines, such as SIGN. This may be because the topics lack sufficient evidence at the level of randomised controlled trial or well-conducted clinical trial. The prioritisation of topics for guideline development where recommendations are not open to wide dispute is understandable; however, the inevitable consequence of this is that matters that most concern nurses may fail to be prioritised.

How are guidelines developed?

Methods for developing evidence-based guidelines have been formalised both nationally (e.g. NICE 2004, SIGN 2004) and locally (e.g. North of

---

BOX 9.2 Stages of guideline development

- Selection of guideline topic
- Composition of the guideline development group
- Defining the scope of the guideline
- Systematic literature review
- Formation of recommendations
- Consultation and peer review
- Presentation and dissemination
- Local implementation
- Audit and review

England Evidence-Based Guideline Development Project 1999a, b). Recommended stages are presented in Box 9.2.

The guideline development group decides on the scope of the guideline, assesses available research evidence, and produces consensus recommendations which will aid practitioners in their health-care decisions. According to SIGN (2004), five main skills are required in guideline development group members (but each member is not expected to have the full range).

1. Clinical expertise (e.g. nursing, physiotherapy, etc.)
2. Other specialist expertise (e.g. health economics, research methods)
3. Practical understanding of the problems faced in the delivery of care
4. Communication and team-working skills
5. Critical appraisal skills

The group should ideally include representatives from all relevant disciplines and interested parties (Lomas 1993a), with representatives seeking the views of their colleagues to ensure that a balanced approach is taken. The optimum size for a group has been put at 8–10 (Scott & Marinker 1990) but groups of between 15 and 25 members have been used successfully (SIGN 2004). A facilitator ensures that all members are free to contribute, that 'decibel level' does not determine priorities (Northern Regional Health Authority 1994), and that guideline recommendations accurately reflect the consensus of the whole group.

Patient involvement in their care is central to current government thinking in the UK (Department of Health 1997) and in many other countries, and patient involvement in guideline development should be no exception.

> **BOX 9.3** Patient roles within guideline development groups
>
> | Title | Role |
> |---|---|
> | Patient | Presents their own views |
> | Member of patient group | Presents the group's views |
> | Patient advocate | Presents knowledge of patients' views |

Indeed, the NICE (2004) now funds a Patient Involvement Unit whose role is to develop and support opportunities for patient and carer involvement in clinical guideline development (as well as other guidance produced by the NICE). Patients' knowledge, understanding and experience of their illness make them ideally placed to contribute, particularly in areas where guideline development is difficult because of lack of evidence. In the medical literature, however, patient involvement in guideline development groups is rare (Van Wersch & Eccles 1999). To illustrate, Eccles et al (1996) invited a patient with asthma and a patient with stable angina to join the development group for the North of England Evidence-Based Guidelines for asthma and angina respectively. However, the patients were described as 'non-participating observers' of technical discussions to which their contribution was minimal. Patients were not included in the guideline update team. The perceived difference in status between health professionals and patients may inhibit any constructive participation by patients, who may feel themselves to be in an uncomfortable minority (Bond & Grimshaw 1995).

Patients involved in guideline development groups have three potential roles (Box 9.3). Using a patient advocate may be one way of increasing the likelihood of incorporating patients' views into guidelines and preventing the problems outlined above. It may be beneficial for the advocate (who is not a patient) to have:

- a broad knowledge of the subject of the guideline
- a knowledge of patients' experiences of coping with this symptom or condition
- an awareness of patients' feelings and problems
- an understanding of patients' needs
- training in communication or counselling skills (Van Wersch & Eccles, personal communication).

Soliciting patients' views outside the guideline development group and feeding these views back into group discussions may also be effective. This approach was used in the development of the guideline on the recognition and assessment of acute pain in children (Royal College of Nursing 2000): a qualitative study sought children's views and a children's conference was also held, where children described their experiences of pain through play, acting, drawing or interview (Doorbar & McClarey 1999). While anecdotal evidence suggests these approaches may be effective, there has been very little research into how best to use the patients' expertise in guideline development.

Once the group has been established, the scope of the guideline is defined. A number of key clinical questions are identified. A broad topic, for example the management of patients receiving chemotherapy, will take longer to develop and be more labour intensive than a topic that focuses on a single aspect of care such as mouth care in children with cancer.

Next, a detailed literature search is conducted to look for evidence from research studies about the appropriateness and effectiveness of different clinical management strategies. Ideally, this will be a systematic review with defined inclusion and exclusion criteria, explicit criteria for assessing study quality, rigorous methods of data abstraction (for example, data abstracted by two reviewers for each paper) and data synthesis. Although this approach demands a considerable amount of time and effort, applying scientific principles such as these to the review process reduces the risk of bias. Further information on systematic reviews is provided in Chapter 7.

Depending on the topic, the search strategy may include only certain study designs; for example, for the North of England Evidence-Based Guidelines for the Management of Asthma (1999b) only randomised controlled trials, case–control and cohort studies were searched for, while the guideline on the recognition and assessment of acute pain in children (Royal College of Nursing 2000), which was not concerned with the effectiveness of treatments, included a wider range of study designs.

A level of evidence is allocated to each paper, according to its methodological quality. Studies that have used an appropriate study design to address the research question, and are methodologically sound (for example, for a RCT whether randomisation, allocation concealment, completeness of follow-up and intention to treat analysis have been adequately performed), are allocated a high level of evidence. The level is linked to the statement of evidence within the guideline, for example: 'the administration of salbutamol using a large volume spacer with metered dose inhaler is as effective as nebulised salbutamol in patients with acute, but not life threatening, asthma. Level 1' (North of England Evidence-Based Guideline Development Project 1999b).

BOX 9.4 Levels of evidence (from SIGN 50, with kind permission of SIGN.
© Scottish Intercollegiate Guidelines Network (SIGN), 2004)

1++	High-quality meta-analyses, systematic reviews of RCTs or RCTs with a very low risk of bias
1+	Well-conducted meta-analyses, systematic reviews of RCTs or RCTs with a low risk of bias
1−	Meta-analyses, systematic reviews of RCTs or RCTs with a high risk of bias
2++	High-quality systematic reviews of case–control or cohort studies High-quality case–control or cohort studies with a very low risk of confounding, bias or chance and a high probability that the relationship is causal
2+	Well-conducted case–control or cohort studies with a low risk of confounding, bias or chance and a moderate probability that the relationship is causal
2−	Case–control or cohort studies with a high risk of confounding, bias or chance and a significant risk that the relationship is not causal
3	Non-analytic studies, e.g. case reports, case series
4	Expert opinion

The assigned level provides an indication of the potential for bias within the statement and is taken into consideration when recommendations are formulated. There are a number of interpretations of levels of evidence. Box 9.4 shows levels of evidence as defined by SIGN (SIGN 2004).

Next, the evidence is considered by the guideline development group and recommendations are formulated. This is a complex part of the process, especially where the evidence can be interpreted in a number of different ways. The guideline development group members are required to consider all the evidence relating to each question, in the light of its methodological quality, and make recommendations that are explicitly based on the most robust evidence. Where recommendations vary, a process for reaching consensus is required. Recommendations are graded according to the level of evidence, thus enabling readers to differentiate between those recommendations for which there is strong evidence and those based on weak evidence. Grading also enables guideline users to assess the predictive validity of each recommendation; recommendations based on strong evidence are more likely to achieve the predicted outcome (SIGN 2004). An example of grades of recommendation is shown in Box 9.5 (SIGN 2004).

BOX 9.5 Grades of recommendation (from SIGN 50, with kind permission of SIGN. © Scottish Intercollegiate Guidelines Network (SIGN), 2004)

A

At least one meta-analysis, systematic review or RCT rated as 1++, and directly applicable to the target population; or

A systematic review of RCTs or a body of evidence consisting principally of studies rated as 1+, directly applicable to the target population and demonstrating overall consistency of results

B

A body of evidence including studies rated as 2++, directly applicable to the target population, and demonstrating overall consistency of results; or

Extrapolated evidence from studies rated as 1++ or 1+

C

A body of evidence including studies rated as 2+, directly applicable to the target population and demonstrating overall consistency of results; or

Extrapolated evidence from studies rated as 2++

D

Evidence level 3 or 4; or

Extrapolated evidence from studies rated as 2+

GOOD PRACTICE POINTS

Recommended best practice based on the clinical experience of the guideline development group

---

Finally, the guideline is tested by asking professionals not involved in guideline development to review it for clarity, internal consistency and acceptability. The guideline can be piloted in selected health-care settings to see whether its use is feasible in routine practice.

All guidelines should be reviewed after a specified time period to make sure they are updated to take into account new knowledge. Frequency of review will depend on the amount of new information in the particular topic area. If there have been significant developments in the evidence base, review may need to take place to incorporate these.

Consensus guidelines

If there is no high-quality research evidence to underpin all or some guideline recommendations, the views of a group of experts may be distilled through a consensus development process (Fink et al 1984). Using this

---

BOX 9.6 Stages in the nominal group technique (modified from Jones & Hunter 1995 British Medical Journal 311:376–380, with permission from the BMJ Publishing Group Ltd.)

- Participants write down their views on topic in question.
- Each participant, in turn, contributes one idea to the facilitator, who records it on a flipchart.
- Similar suggestions are grouped together where appropriate. There is group discussion to clarify and evaluate each idea.
- Each participant privately ranks each idea.
- The ranking is tabulated and presented.
- The overall ranking is discussed and re-ranked.
- Final rankings are tabulated and results fed back to participants.

---

process enables guidelines to cover all the areas where clinicians need to make decisions and ensures guidelines are comprehensive, rather than limiting their scope to recommendations where evidence exists. Murphy et al (1998) conducted a systematic review of consensus development in relation to clinical guidelines. They provide some useful pointers regarding the process, suggesting, for example, that a review of the evidence should be given to all participants at an early stage and that information presented in a synthesised form is more likely to be assimilated.

Achieving consensus is not easy and may be hampered by the most assertive or most authoritative group members having a greater say than others (Thomson et al 1995). There are, however, ways of getting the best out of a group, such as the Delphi technique or the nominal group technique (Jones & Hunter 1995). The Delphi technique does not require group members to meet; instead group members generate topics of discussion. These are sent to all participants, who then comment in writing on their co-participants' views. Responses are analysed and collated and sent back to participants. The process continues until a consensus is reached.

The nominal group technique achieves consensus using highly structured meetings. It comprises two rounds in which participants rate, discuss and then re-rate a series of items or questions. The process is shown in Box 9.6. The method can also be used within a single meeting and, in the context of guideline development, will include a detailed review of the literature as background material for the topic under discussion. A modified version of the nominal group technique was used in the development of the pressure ulcer risk assessment and prevention guideline (Rycroft-Malone & McInness 2000). The process is outlined in Box 9.7.

BOX 9.7 Modified nominal group technique used to develop the pressure ulcer risk assessment and prevention guideline (Rycroft-Malone & McInness 2000, reproduced with permission from the Royal College of Nursing)

Stage	Process
Formation of consensus group	A group of 10, reflecting the full range of people to whom the guideline will apply, was formed using purposive sampling based on the parameters of status, knowledge of the research and intended commitment to the process
Synthesis of pertinent information	Consensus group provided with relevant research and two systematic reviews
Ranking of statements	Before the group meeting, participants asked to consider 200 statements developed from the literature and evidence-linked recommendations
	Each participant was asked to rate agreement with each statement on a scale of 1–9 (1 = least agreement, 9 = most agreement)
	Frequency of response to each statement was calculated
	Pattern of responses for the group is presented alongside each member's response to each statement
Nominal group meeting	Statements discussed in turn, focusing primarily on those where there was most disagreement
	All members given the chance to respond, followed by discussion to clarify, defend or dispute issues
	Participants given the opportunity to privately re-rate statements
Mathematical aggregation	Median (measurement of central tendency or average) and inter-quartile range (measure of distribution) calculated from each statement from ratings of second round
	Statements with a median of 7–9 developed into practice recommendations
Development of recommendations	Recommendations drafted based on panel's level of agreement about the statements

Murphy et al (1998), however, sound a note of caution, suggesting that while using the Delphi or nominal group technique may result in convergence of individual judgements, it is not clear whether the accuracy of the group decision is increased.

> **BOX 9.8** Grades of recommendation used in the guideline for the recognition and assessment of acute pain in children (Royal College of Nursing 2000)
>
> Grade I: Generally consistent finding in a majority of multiple acceptable studies
>
> Grade II: Either based on a single acceptable study, or a weak or inconsistent finding in multiple acceptable studies
>
> Grade III: Limited scientific evidence which does not meet all the criteria of acceptable studies or absence of directly applicable studies of good quality. This includes published and unpublished expert opinion
>
> Reproduced by kind permission of the Royal College of Nursing, from *The Recognition and Assessment of Acute Pain in Children*. Technical Report (2000, due to be updated in late 2006)

Example of an evidence-based guideline

The Royal College of Nursing is developing nurse-led guidelines in a number of areas and is now the base for the NICE National Collaborating Centre for Nursing and Supportive Care. Examples include the management of venous leg ulcers and pressure ulcer risk assessment and prevention. The guideline for the recognition and assessment of acute pain in children was produced in 2000 and is described as 'evidence linked', rather than evidence based, as some recommendations are based on expert consensus opinion. The guideline includes a summary of graded recommendations for practice, as well as the rationale for each recommendation and a justification for each rating score. For this guideline, a simple grading system (Box 9.8) was used. An example showing a range of recommendations is given in Box 9.9.

Appraising published guidelines

Developing new evidence-based guidelines is expensive and time-consuming and it is therefore preferable, in the majority of cases, to use previously published guidelines if these are applicable and of good quality. Some useful websites for finding guidelines are given at the end of this chapter. A validated UK instrument is available for appraising the quality of published guidelines (AGREE 2003). A worked example showing the appraisal of the recognition and assessment of acute pain in children guideline (Royal College of Nursing 2000) is shown in Box 9.10.

BOX 9.9 Example of recommendations for the recognition and assessment of acute pain in children (Royal College of Nursing 2000)

2   Indicators of children's pain

2.1   Note changes in children's behaviour, appearance, activity level and vital signs as these may indicate a change in the pain intensity   Grade I

2.2   Use physiological measures (e.g. heart and respiratory rates) but only in addition to self-report and behavioural measures to determine whether children are in pain   Grade II

3   Individual differences

3.1   Obtain a patient history from each child and his/her parents at the time of admission and learn what word the child uses for pain (e.g. hurt, baddie, etc.)   Grade II

3.2   Recognise the importance of and seek to identify cultural factors which may affect the assessment of pain   Grade III

Reproduced by kind permission of the Royal College of Nursing, from *The Recognition and Assessment of Acute Pain in Children*. Technical Report (2000, due to be updated in late 2006)

BOX 9.10 AGREE tool completed for the clinical guideline *The Recognition And Assessment of Acute Pain in Children* (Royal College of Nursing 2000) (AGREE tool reproduced with permission from AGREE Research Trust)

SCOPE AND PURPOSE

Item 1. The overall objective(s) of the guideline is (are) specifically described.
Strongly Agree (Score: 4 points)
A clear description of the purpose and scope of the guideline is given:
The purpose of this clinical guideline is to present information about methods that can be used to improve the recognition and assessment of pain in children.
The guideline was developed with the following aims:
- To identify the best method for recognising pain in children
- To identify reliable and valid measures of pain appropriate for use with children of differing age groups and levels of development.

Item 2. The clinical question(s) covered by the guideline are specifically described.
Strongly Agree (Score: 4 points)

There is a clear statement of key areas covered by the guideline, for example:
- When pain should be assessed
  - Indicators of pain
  - Individual differences
- Who should assess pain in children
  - Role of parents/carers and other family members
  - Role of nurses and other practitioners
  - Role of self-report by children.

Item 3. The patients to whom the guideline is meant to apply are specifically described.
Strongly Agree (Score: 4 points)
A clear definition of 'child' is provided.

STAKEHOLDER INVOLVEMENT

Item 4. The guideline development group includes individuals from all relevant professional groups.
Agree (Score: 3 points)
The group responsible for reviewing evidence was made up of representatives from nursing, medicine and anaesthesia, therapies (including play therapy) and parents. We are not told the names and professions of the guideline development group.

Item 5. The patients' views and preferences have been sought.
Strongly Agree (Score: 4 points)
Parents had a role in reviewing evidence and in determining the 'Philosophy for Care'. The guidelines were also informed by a qualitative study of children's views and a children's conference where children described their experiences of pain through play, acting and drawing.

Item 6. The target users of the guideline are clearly defined.
Strongly Agree (Score: 4 points)
There is a clear statement regarding target users:
Although developed by the Royal College of Nursing, this guideline has been written for everyone involved in managing children's pain.

Item 7. The guideline has been piloted among target users.
Strongly Agree (Score: 4 points)
The clinical guidelines were piloted for applicability, user-friendliness and comprehensiveness amongst a wide range of experts and users.

(Continued)

RIGOUR OF DEVELOPMENT

Item 8. Systematic methods were used to search for the evidence.
Strongly Agree (Score: 4 points)
The guideline provides clear information about the search strategy, including databases used (MEDLINE, CINAHL, sociofile, Psychlit and SIGLE) and search terms. These appear comprehensive.

Item 9. The criteria for selecting the evidence are clearly described.
Strongly Agree (Score: 4 points)
A detailed list of inclusion and exclusion criteria for selecting the evidence is provided.
Examples of inclusion criteria are:

* Studies related to the recognition and assessment of acute pain amongst a paediatric population
* Studies written in English.

Examples of exclusion criteria are:

* Studies dealing solely with the management of pain
* Studies dealing solely with chronic pain.

Item 10. The methods used for formulating the recommendations are clearly described.
Agree (Score: 3 points)
Information is provided about assessment of weak evidence by expert groups who were asked to assess *'whether the recommendations were clinically relevant and correct on the basis of their clinical expertise'*. The authors state that no-one disagreed with recommendations made. However, the process of formulating recommendations from the evidence is not described.

Item 11. The health benefits, side effects and risks have been considered in formulating the recommendations.
Strongly Agree (Score: 4 points)
The benefits and harms of applying most of the recommendations are discussed. For example the recommendation suggesting the use of behavioural measures to indicate that infants are experiencing pain ends with the following statement:
Johnston et al (1995), however, caution against relying solely on behavioural responses with neonates because they may be physically incapable of crying or body movement and their stillness may not indicate that they are pain free.

Item 12. There is an explicit link between the recommendations and the supporting evidence.
Strongly Agree (Score: 4 points)
Evidence is provided for each recommendation, as is the strength of the evidence. More detailed information about individual studies is presented in evidence tables, but this is not ordered according to guideline recommendations.

Item 13. The guideline has been externally reviewed by experts prior to its publication.
Agree (Score: 3 points)
The authors state the guideline has been *'piloted for applicability, user-friendliness and comprehensiveness amongst a wide range of experts and users'* but the methodology is not described.

Item 14. A procedure for updating the guideline is provided.
Agree (Score: 3 points)
It is stated that the guideline will be updated every 2 years, but details of the procedure are not given.

CLARITY AND PRESENTATION.

Item 15. The recommendations are specific and unambiguous.
Strongly Agree (Score: 4 points)
Recommendations are clear and unambiguous.

Item 16. The different options for management of the condition are clearly presented.
Strongly Agree (Score: 4 points)
Different options are suggested for some recommendations (e.g. the use of information sheets for parents and a specific measure of postoperative pain are suggested in recommendation 8.3. *Parents need adequate information to be able to contribute to the assessment of children's pain*) but as this guideline is concerned with assessment rather than management this item is less relevant.

Item 18. The guideline is supported with tools for application.
Disagree (Score: 2 points)
At present the guideline is only supported with a summary document. There is a children's version currently in production.

APPLICATION

Item 19. The potential organisational barriers in applying the recommendations have been discussed.
Agree (Score: 3 points)
The guideline contains a section on organisational issues. For example, there is the suggestion that 'care agreed and contract specifications between commissioners

(Continued)

and providers of children's health care services must be explicit and comply with DoH guidance and the recommendations arising from the forthcoming Clinical Services Advisory Group (CSAG) Report'.

Item 20. The possible cost implications of applying the recommendations have been considered.
Strongly Disagree (Score: 1 point)
The guideline does not mention the potential cost implications.

Item 21. The guideline presents key review criteria for monitoring and/or audit purposes.
Strongly Disagree (Score: 1 point)
The guideline states that 'evidence-based audit criteria will be developed based on this guideline'.

EDITORIAL INDEPENDENCE

Item 22. The guideline is editorially independent from the funding body.
Disagree (Score: 2 points)
It is stated that the development of the guideline was funded by the NHS Executive, but it is not clear what its influence was on the formulation of final recommendations.

Item 23. Conflicts of interest of guideline development members have been recorded.
Strongly Disagree (Score: 1 point)
There is no statement about the conflicts of interest of group members.

OVERALL JUDGEMENT

Scope and purpose: 12/12 = 100%
Stakeholder involvement: 15/16 = 94%
Rigour of development: 25/28 = 89%
Clarity and presentation: 10/12 = 83%
Application: 5/12 = 42%
Editorial independence: 3/8 = 38%

As the guideline rates highly (3 or 4) on the majority of items and most domain scores are over 60% (with the exception of *application* and *editorial independence*), it can be strongly recommended. This rating indicates that the guideline has high overall quality and that it could be considered for use in practice without provisos or alterations.

Material in italics reproduced by kind permission of the Royal College of Nursing, from *The Recognition and Assessment of Acute Pain in Children*. Technical Report (2000, due to be updated in late 2006)

While using this tool will give a good indication of guideline quality, it is likely that many will not score highly on all sections of the instrument because of lack of documentation on the process of guideline development (Thomson et al 1995).

Adapting nationally developed guidelines for local use

The translation of nationally developed or other guidelines developed 'externally' into protocols for local use is both permissible and, in the opinion of many commentators, desirable. Feder et al (1999) suggest that, just as topics for guideline development need to be prioritised against a set of accepted criteria, so local organisations must develop a system for prioritising the implementation of guidelines locally. The sheer volume of recommendations contained within all of the clinical guidelines that might be applicable to the work of a general practitioner, for example, make prioritising according to local need a necessity. To illustrate, the SIGN organisation has now produced in excess of 20 guidelines whose recommendations have implications for general practice, with NICE producing many more.

Local adaptation of guidelines also has the potential for mitigating some of the objections to their use detailed below; for example, that they may lack local relevance. Asking local clinical teams to appraise 'external' guidelines and prioritise their implementation may also bring a sense of ownership that can be difficult to achieve otherwise.

Issues of resource availability and potential returns in terms of health gain also need to be considered. This, though, raises the issue of when local adaptation becomes unacceptable, potentially recreating the situation guidelines are designed to address. NICE has recently issued guidance on the use of beta-interferon for people with multiple sclerosis and has made a judgement against its use. Had NICE decided for its use, it may have had little effect on the budgets of some health authorities/boards in areas of low incidence, whilst in other areas where there is a higher than average incidence of multiple sclerosis (as in the south west of Scotland), the costs would have been high and would arguably have meant that other services could have suffered as a result. Interestingly, Hurwitz (1999) suggests that 'users of guidelines are expected to behave as learned intermediaries,

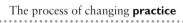

exercising customary clinical discretion and consulting other sources of relevant information'.

Patient versions of guidelines

Versions of guidelines which patients can understand and which are written in their own language are considered essential by NICE. While there are patient versions available, for example of the Intercollegiate National Clinical Guidelines on Stroke (Intercollegiate Working Party for Stroke 2000) and the recognition and assessment of acute pain in children (Royal College of Nursing 2000), there has been little research into the effectiveness of these and what their role is in providing information or helping patients to manage their condition.

Introducing the guideline into practice

Once a clinical guideline is ready for use, there are two stages which facilitate its introduction into practice: dissemination and implementation. Dissemination is generally taken to refer to the method by which the guidelines are made available to potential users. Strategies include publication in professional journals and sending the guideline to targeted individuals, as well as strategies involving an educational intervention. Several studies have assessed the effectiveness of different strategies: dissemination by publication or direct mailing has been found to be the least successful (Freemantle et al 2001, Grol 1992, Lomas et al 1989) but has the advantage of being cheap and reproducible. Strategies involving an educational component, especially where this is specifically targeted rather than in the form of continuing education, are more likely to result in behaviour change (Lomas et al 1991). However, dissemination alone without an appropriate implementation strategy is unlikely to influence behaviour significantly (Grimshaw et al 1995).

Implementation is a means of ensuring that users subsequently act upon the recommendations. 'Implementation is a more active process, involving tailoring the message to the needs of the target audience, and actively working to overcome barriers to behaviour change' (Lomas 1993b). Implementation strategies try to ensure that users adopt and apply guidelines to which they have access. Grol (1992) suggests that in designing an implementation strategy, it is necessary to be aware of barriers to behaviour change; these may include both structural and attitudinal factors and appropriate interventions might be targeted at both the structure and the process of care. Some implementation strategies supply accessible reminders of the guideline. For example, patient-specific prompts at the time of consultation are thought to be a powerful strategy (Emslie et al 1993, Grimshaw & Russell 1993, Lilford et al 1992). Audit and feedback have also been shown to be capable of affecting doctors' behaviour: a systematic review of randomised controlled trials found effects to be small, but potentially worthwhile (Thomson-O'Brien et al 2001).

A recent systematic review of the effectiveness and efficiency of guideline dissemination and implementation strategies targeting medically qualified health-care professionals (Grimshaw et al 2004) found that all interventions achieved improvements in care. A median absolute improvement in performance of 14.1% was found in cluster randomised comparisons of reminders, 8.1% in cluster randomised comparisons of dissemination of educational materials, 7.0% in cluster randomised comparisons of audit and feedback, and 6.0% in cluster randomised comparisons of multifaceted interventions involving educational outreach. Only a quarter of studies included economic data on the costs of developing guidelines and introducing them into practice. Health-care organisations therefore have little evidence to inform decisions on whether the costs involved in guideline development and introduction outweigh potential benefits.

There are few studies evaluating dissemination and implementation strategies in nursing (Richens et al 2004). The systematic review by Thomas et al (2001) found three studies evaluating dissemination and implementation strategies; findings appear to suggest that educational interventions (e.g. lectures, teaching sessions) are of more value than passive approaches (e.g. postal distribution) in the dissemination of guidelines but methodological flaws limit the credibility of findings. Further research is needed into the roles nurses and other professions play in guideline dissemination and implementation, as what is effective for doctors may not be for nurses (Puffer & Rashidian 2004, Richens et al 2004).

Evaluating the effectiveness of clinical guidelines in nursing and allied health professions

Most of the literature on clinical guidelines comes from medicine. However, a systematic review for the Cochrane Collaboration (which is currently being updated) examined whether clinical guidelines are effective in

---

BOX 9.11 Key points from systematic review of the effectiveness of clinical guidelines in nursing, midwifery and professions allied to medicine (Thomas et al 1998, 2001)

Significant changes in some processes of care were found in four out of five studies measuring process.

Six out of eight studies measuring outcomes found significant differences favouring the group who received guidelines.

Three studies evaluated dissemination and implementation strategies: findings appear to suggest that educational interventions (e.g. lectures, teaching sessions) are of more value than passive approaches (e.g. postal distribution) in the dissemination of guidelines; however, methodological flaws limit the credibility of findings.

Studies examining the ability of guidelines to enable skill substitution generally support the hypothesis of no difference between nurse protocol-driven and physician care.

---

changing the behaviour of nurses, midwives and health visitors and other allied health professions (Thomas et al 1998, 2001). Key points are summarised in Box 9.11. Eighteen evaluations of guidelines were found; all but one of these studies evaluated the introduction of guidelines targeting nurses. Guidelines evaluated included the management of urinary catheter care (Seto et al 1991), hypertension (Jewell & Hope 1988) and postoperative bleeding after cardiac surgery (Zeler et al 1992).

While this review has provided some evidence that guideline-driven care can be effective in changing the practice of nurses and patient outcomes, there is a long way to go before guidelines meeting the 11 criteria (Box 9.1, p.239) are routinely used by nurses to improve patient care. While all guidelines should be underpinned by evidence of effectiveness, reports of the guideline development process in studies included in the review typically contained scant details of the methods used for identifying and assessing relevant evidence. Although many of the guidelines identified were based on a literature review, the extent to which these reviews were systematic was not described, nor were the quality criteria by which any evidence was assessed. This calls into question the validity of the guidelines and their consequent potential for patient benefit. Guidelines produced by the Royal College of Nursing (1998, 2000) have been rigorously developed but need to be evaluated to see if they are effective in changing professional behaviour and patient outcomes.

Benefits and disbenefits of clinical guidelines

Clinical guidelines, integrated care pathways, protocols of care and any other externally imposed directives pertaining to treatment and intervention with patients (i.e. any directive about a clinician's action which individual clinicians may not have been involved in devising) will arguably all face the same objections, misconceptions and concerns about their use and, importantly, their legal standing. Hurwitz (1999) points out that:

> 'Courts are unlikely to adopt standards of care advocated in clinical guidelines as legal "gold standards" because the mere fact that the guideline exists does not of itself establish that compliance with it is reasonable in the circumstances, or that non-compliance is negligent.'

He also states that guidelines should not be viewed as 'thought-proof' but that they require interpretation and the use of discretion. SIGN (2004) and NICE (2004), however, suggest that significant deviations from the guideline, together with reasons for these, are documented in patients' case notes at the time the decision is taken.

Objections to, and support for, the use of guidelines are based on differing perceptions of the problems they are designed to address and of the related benefits or disbenefits they bring. The use of guidelines has been criticised on the grounds that they can:

- stifle individual clinical judgement
- de-skill professionals by reducing their capacity to think for themselves
- limit quality of care by restricting care/treatment options
- introduce practice which could be ineffective or dangerous
- encourage the illusion that there is a clear-cut direction to be taken in every clinical situation
- be very resource intensive in relation to their development and implementation
- lack local relevance
- concentrate on 'easy' areas; that is, where there is already a body of evidence about appropriate treatment
- allow powerful and vocal individuals to impose their priorities on particular services

- require clinicians to follow courses of action for which they do not have the requisite skills or knowledge
- raise patient expectations about types and standards of care they might expect to receive.

For each of these criticisms or objections there is an opposing assertion or opinion. It has been suggested that guidelines:

- ensure safe practice
- improve consistency of care in different parts of the country/settings of care
- make it more likely that patients receive correct treatment
- build parity of knowledge amongst staff
- bring the expert opinion to everyday clinical care
- allow for individual patient variation; non-application is not forbidden, it simply has to be justified
- provide more information for patients about what they should expect from the health-care system
- distill the vast array of knowledge relating to individual clinical conditions into a manageable guide for busy clinicians
- allow room for the development of local protocols.

The restriction of individual clinical judgement and the apparent requirement to treat all patients the same, regardless of individual idiosyncrasies or characteristics, seems to be at the heart of most objections to or difficulties with the use of guidelines. Likewise, the heart of the defence case for the use of guidelines seems to be the argument that patients deserve the best possible treatment all the time in definable situations, regardless of the individual expertise of the person dealing with them at the time; if guidelines can expedite that best treatment, the argument goes, then they have a legitimate place in the system.

The acid test for clinical guidelines and the answer to any criticisms would surely proceed from proof of their benefit to patient care. As outlined above, more studies are needed to assess the impact of guidelines, particularly in nursing and allied health professions.

Conclusion

If guidelines are to be underpinned by evidence of effective practice, a prerequisite is high-quality evidence of the benefits and costs of the procedures and practices targeted. Further research into the effectiveness of nursing practice and interventions is required in order to provide this evidence base. For questions about the effectiveness of interventions, particular attention should be given to the provision of high-grade evidence from randomised controlled trials, rather than from weaker quasi-experimental designs.

Nurses whose behaviour is targeted by guidelines need to have an active role in their development or adaptation to local circumstances; this approach will encourage 'ownership' of the guideline and is more likely to lead to more positive attitudes towards it. It will also ensure that profession-specific practices and barriers, and any factors that facilitate behaviour change, are taken into account.

Where possible, the introduction of clinical guidelines should be within an evaluative framework. Nursing requires more evidence that those dissemination and implementation strategies which have proved to be most effective in changing doctors' behaviour are also effective in changing the behaviour of nurses.

Clinical guidelines are a potential means by which evidence can be incorporated into nursing practice. However, more research is clearly required to underpin clinical recommendations and to assess the most effective ways of developing, disseminating and implementing clinical guidelines in nursing. Only then will a decision be possible about their potential for improving nursing practice and patient outcomes.

Acknowledgements

With thanks to Rhona Hotchkiss whose contributions to an earlier version have helped to inform this chapter.

References

AGREE 2003 Appraisal of Guidelines Research and Evaluation Instrument. Health Care Evaluation Unit at St George's Hospital Medical School, London. Available online at: www.agreetrust.org

Bond C M, Grimshaw J M 1995 Multi-disciplinary guideline development: a case study from community pharmacy. Health Bulletin 53:26–33

Department of Health 1997 The new NHS: modern, dependable. Department of Health, London

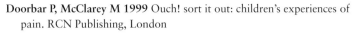

Doorbar P, McClarey M 1999 Ouch! sort it out: children's experiences of pain. RCN Publishing, London

Eccles M P, Clapp Z, Grimshaw J et al 1996 Developing valid guidelines: methodological and procedural issues from the North of England Evidence-Based Guideline Development Project. Quality in Health Care 5:44–50

Emslie C J, Grimshaw J, Templeton A 1993 Do clinical guidelines improve general practice management and referral of infertile couples? British Medical Journal 306:1728–1731

Feder G, Eccles M, Grol R, Griffiths C, Grimshaw J 1999 Using clinical guidelines. British Medical Journal 318(7185):728–730

Field M J, Lohr K N 1990 Clinical practice guidelines: directions for a new program. National Academy Press, Washington DC

Fink A, Kosecoff J, Chassin M, Brook R H 1984 Consensus methods: characteristics and guidelines for use. American Journal of Public Health 74(9):979–983

Freemantle N, Harvey E L, Wolf F, Grimshaw J M, Grilli R, Bero L A 2001 Printed educational materials to improve the behaviour of health-care professionals and patient outcomes (Cochrane Review). Cochrane Library, Issue 3, 2001. Update Software, Oxford

Grimshaw J, Russell I T 1993 Effect of clinical guidelines on medical practice: a systematic review of rigorous evaluations. Lancet 342:1317–1322

Grimshaw J, Freemantle N, Wallace S et al 1995 Developing and implementing clinical practice guidelines. Quality in Health Care 4:55–64

Grimshaw J, Thomas R E, MacLennan G et al 2004 Effectiveness and efficiency of guideline dissemination and implementation strategies. Health Technology Assessment 8(6):1–84

Grol R 1990a National standard setting for quality of care in general practice: attitudes of general practitioners and response to a set of standards. British Journal of General Practice 40:361–364

Grol R 1990b Quality assurance: approaches to standard setting, assessment and change. Atencion Primaria (Barcelona) 7:737–741

Grol R 1992 Implementing guidelines in general practice care. Quality in Health Care 1:184–191

Hurwitz B 1999 Legal and political considerations of clinical practice guidelines. British Medical Journal 318(7184):661–664

Intercollegiate Working Party for Stroke 2000 Care after stroke: information for patients and their carers. Royal College of Physicians, London

Jewell D, Hope J 1988 Evaluation of a nurse-run hypertension clinic in general practice. Practitioner 232:484–487

Jones J, Hunter D 1995 Consensus methods for medical and health services research. British Medical Journal 311:376–380

Klein R 1996 The NHS and the new scientism: solution or delusion? Quarterly Journal of Medicine 89:85–87

Lilford R J, Kelly M, Baines A et al 1992 Effect of using protocols on medical care: randomised trial of three methods of taking an antenatal history. British Medical Journal 305:1181–1184

Lomas J 1993a Making clinical policy explicit. Legislative policy making and lessons for developing practice guidelines. International Journal of Technology Assessment in Health Care 9:11–25

Lomas J 1993b Teaching old (and not so old) docs new tricks: effective ways to implement research findings. Working paper 93–4. McMaster University Centre for Health Economics and Policy Analysis, Toronto, Canada

Lomas J, Anderson G, Pierre K, Vayda E, Enkin M, Hannah W 1989 Do practice guidelines guide practice? The effect of a consensus statement on the practice of physicians. New England Journal of Medicine 321: 1306–1311

Lomas J, Enkin M, Anderson G, Hannah W, Vayda E, Singer J 1991 Opinion leaders vs audit and feedback to implement practice guidelines. Delivery after previous cesarean section. Journal of the American Medical Association 265(17):2202–2207

McClarey M 1997 Identifying priorities for guideline development as a result of nursing needs. DQI Network News 6:4–5

Murphy M K, Black N A, Lamping D L et al 1998 Consensus development methods and their use in clinical guideline development. Health Technology Assessment 2(3):1–88

National Institute for Clinical Excellence (NICE) 2004 The guideline development process. An overview for stakeholders, the public and the NHS. National Institute for Clinical Excellence, London

NHS Centre for Reviews and Dissemination (NHS CRD) 1994 Implementing clinical practice guidelines. University of Leeds, Leeds

North of England Evidence-Based Guideline Development Project 1999a The primary care management of stable angina. Centre for Health Services Research, Newcastle upon Tyne

North of England Evidence-Based Guideline Development Project 1999b The primary care management of asthma in adults. Centre for Health Services Research, Newcastle upon Tyne

North of England Study of Standards and Performances in General Practice 1991 Overview of the study. Centre for Health Services Research, Newcastle upon Tyne

Northern Regional Health Authority 1994 Guidelines – a resource pack. Northern Regional Health Authority, Newcastle upon Tyne, pp.1–40

Puffer S, Rashidian A 2004 Practice nurses' intentions to use clinical guidelines. Journal of Advanced Nursing 47(5):500–509

Putnam R W, Curry L 1985 Impact of patient care appraisal on physician behaviour in the office setting. Canadian Medical Association Journal 132:1025–1029

Richens Y, Anderson E G, Rycroft-Malone J, Morrell C 2004 Getting guidelines into practice: a literature review. Nursing Standard 18:33–40

Royal College of General Practitioners Clinical Guidelines Working Group 1995 The development and implementation of clinical guidelines. Royal College of General Practitioners, London

Royal College of Nursing 1995 Clinical guidelines: what you need to know. Royal College of Nursing, London

Royal College of Nursing 1998 The management of patients with venous leg ulcers. RCN Publishing, London

Royal College of Nursing 2000 The recognition and assessment of acute pain in children. Royal College of Nursing, London

Rycroft-Malone J, McInness E 2000 Pressure ulcer risk assessment and prevention. Technical Report. Royal College of Nursing, London

Scott M, Marinker M L 1990 Medical audit and general practice. British Medical Journal, London

Scottish Intercollegiate Guidelines Network (SIGN) 2004 SIGN 50: a guideline developers' handbook. Scottish Intercollegiate Guidelines Network, Edinburgh. Available online at: www.sign.ac.uk/guidelines/fulltext/50/index. html

Seto W H, Ching T Y, Yuen K Y, Chu Y B, Seto W L 1991 The enhancement of infection control in-service education by ward opinion leaders. American Journal of Infection Control 19:86–91

Thomas L H, McColl E, Cullum N, Rousseau N, Soutter J, Steen N 1998 Effect of clinical guidelines in nursing, midwifery and the therapies: a systematic review of evaluations. Quality in Health Care 7:183–191

Thomas L H, McColl E, Cullum N, Rousseau N, Soutter J, Steen N 2001 Systematic review of the effectiveness of clinical guidelines in nursing, midwifery and professions allied to medicine (Cochrane Review). Cochrane Library, Issue 1. Update Software, Oxford

Thomson R, Lavender M, Madhok R 1995 How to ensure that guidelines are effective. British Medical Journal 311:237–242

Thomson-O'Brien M A, Oxman A D, Davis D A, Haynes R B, Freemantle N, Harvey E L 2001 Audit and feedback to improve health professional practice and health care outcomes (Cochrane Review). Cochrane Library, Issue 1. Update Software, Oxford

Van Wersch A, Eccles M 1999 Patient involvement in evidence-based health in relation to clinical guidelines. In: Gabbay M (ed) The evidence-based primary care handbook. Royal Society of Medicine Press, London, pp.91–103

Von Degenberg K, Deighan M 1995 Guideline development: a model of multi-professional collaboration. In: Deighan M, Hitch S (eds) Clinical effectiveness: from guidelines to cost-effective practice. Department of Health, London, pp.93–97

Williamson J W 1978 Formulating priorities for quality assurance activity. Description of a method and its application. Journal of the American Medical Association 239:631–637

Zeler K M, McPharlane T J, Salamonsen R F 1992 Effectiveness of nursing involvement in bedside monitoring and control of coagulation status after cardiac surgery. American Journal of Critical Care 1:70–75

Further reading

Thomas L H, McColl E, Cullum N, Rousseau N, Soutter J, Steen N 2001 Systematic review of the effectiveness of clinical guidelines in nursing, midwifery and professions allied to medicine (Cochrane Review). Cochrane Library, Issue 1. Update Software, Oxford

This Cochrane Review examines the effectiveness of clinical guidelines in changing professional behaviour and patient outcomes in nursing, midwifery and professions allied to medicine.

Thomas L H, McColl E, Cullum N, Rousseau N, Soutter J 1999 Clinical guidelines in nursing, midwifery and the therapies: a systematic review. Journal of Advanced Nursing 30(1):40–50

This paper describes the characteristics of guidelines evaluated and the effectiveness of different dissemination and implementation strategies used.

APPENDIX

Useful websites

Agency for Healthcare Research and Quality: www.ahrq.gov

AGREE Research Trust: www.agreetrust.org

Canadian Medical Association: www.gacguidelines.ca/

eGUIDELINES: www.eguidelines.co.uk/

Guidelines International Network: www.g-i-n.net/

National Electronic Library for Health guidelines database:
www.nelh.nhs.uk/guidelines_database.asp

National Guideline Clearinghouse: www.guideline.gov/

New Zealand Guidelines Group: www.nzgg.org.nz/index.cfm

National Health and Medical Research Council:
www7.health.gov.au/nhmrc/publications/index.htm

National Institute for Health and Clinical Excellence: www.nice.org.uk/

Royal College of Nursing (RCN clinical guidelines can be accessed from this
site): www.rcn.org.uk/services/promote/clinical/clinical_guidelines.htm/

Scottish Intercollegiate Guidelines Network:
www.show.scot.nhs.uk/sign/guidelines/

10

CHAPTER

Implementing best evidence in clinical practice

Lin Perry

KEY POINTS
....

- Where to start?
  - Identifying appropriate topics to address
  - Choosing a project manager
  - Diagnosing the situation.
- What changes are needed?
  - Ensuring change is based on best available evidence
  - Turning evidence into recommendations
  - Establishing key objectives.
- How to implement the changes
  - Developing a dissemination and implementation strategy
  - General approaches to managing change
  - Specific approaches to managing change.
- Evaluating the progress and effects of the changes.

Introduction

The aim of this chapter is to help nurses understand how best evidence can be applied in everyday practice. It draws on ground covered in previous chapters and presents information in the context of real clinical settings: examples are taken from work focused on development of clinical services in a variety of settings and locations, primarily the multi-site South Thames Evidence-based Practice (STEP) project. This project aimed to implement and evaluate evidence-based guidance for specific areas of health care, across a number of hospital trusts in the UK. Eight clinical topics were identified, representing areas of practice supported by relatively better developed evidence bases. Topics included, for example, acute hospital care, discharge planning, community management of leg ulcers, breastfeeding initiatives, nutrition in stroke and psychotherapeutic intervention. The message to be taken from this is that implementation of evidence-based practice (EBP) is not restricted to any specific area of practice, clinical or professional group. Most topics have varied evidence bases, and each clinical setting presents its own challenges. Despite this, lessons of success and good practice are available across the board, as highlighted within this chapter.

Within the STEP project, a common framework was established incorporating the development and implementation of evidence-based guidelines, preceded and followed by audit of clinical practice and patient outcomes. Hospital trusts within the region were invited to participate. A total of nine were chosen and collaborative partnerships were set up with four university departments. Project managers/leaders/co-ordinators were jointly appointed with eight out of the nine coming from outside the host trusts. Although not a specific requirement, six were nursing appointments. The individual projects were accomplished within 3 years, including the external evaluation of processes and outcomes across the nine sites.

How is this relevant to me?

The lessons learned from each of the hospital trusts participating in the STEP project have direct relevance for health-care practitioners and for clinical governance/effectiveness leads charged with implementing evidence-based changes and service developments. The diversity of project topics, settings (including critical care, acute and rehabilitation wards, mental health services, outpatient and day centres, general practice and domiciliary locations), geographical locations and participants has produced a wealth of information about what worked in which contexts.

For those embarking upon or contemplating changing health-care practice, this chapter offers an illustrated 'basic steps' approach. It supplies examples and explanations for what worked and what did not work, allowing readers to make comparisons with their own environments and identify directly relevant information.

Implementing best evidence – where to start?

Identifying appropriate topics to address

Many topics arise directly from nurses' everyday practice as problems in need of solution or questions to be answered. It may be possible for the nurse to ascertain the best evidence to address these information needs, and to enact this evidence without impacting on colleagues' practice or having to recruit resources. However, most clinical developments have wide implications and carry consequences for other practitioners. Even when choosing the most appropriate dressing for a wound, there are wider considerations. If the evidence indicates dressing A, is it available? If not, why not? If it is, but the dressing is later removed and the patient re-presents, will colleagues also apply knowledge of wound care research in choosing a replacement? Hence individual nurses usually need to think more broadly and beyond their own practice in pursuit of best outcomes for their patients, particularly when embarking on a new course of action.

Changing practice requires energy, motivation and support from others and these need to be sustained over a period of time. Careful selection of the topic is therefore important. There are several key considerations. Patient benefit is of first importance. The primary aim of EBP has been defined as identification and application of 'the most efficacious interventions to maximise the quality and quantity of life for individual patients' (Sackett et al 1996, p.4). Benefiting patients is thus an intrinsic feature. However, it is sometimes not enough that the literature identifies benefits for patients; clinicians have to be persuaded that these will accrue for their patients and be worth the time and trouble that changing working practices entails. Furthermore, changes envisaged need to be congruent with the objectives of the organisation, and accepted as a current priority that warrants the required level of expenditure of time and other resources at this particular time. The persuasion and change management process may not be easy and will make considerable demands upon the person driving or responsible for the changes.

Hence, personal involvement, engagement and motivation to pursue the topic are prerequisites when choosing a topic. If change leaders cannot sustain enthusiastic belief in the merits of changing practice, this is unlikely to be engendered in practitioners. Evaluating nine projects, Redfern et al (2000, p.iv) describe the project leaders as requiring 'motivation and energy to persevere when the going gets tough and obstacles seem to be insurmountable'. Doherty et al (2000, p.15) and Miller et al (1999) highlight the considerable time and emotional investment entailed in steering projects to successful completion. From the outset the motivation and energy of those driving the change are essential. Next, it is sensible to think about how this motivation may be recruited from others.

Consider local and national views on the topic

What are the opinions of patients, colleagues, clinicians and managers? It was apparent for one of the STEP projects that patients were dissatisfied with current nutritional practices, reflected in letters of complaint both locally and nationally (ACHCEW 1997). Internal satisfaction surveys or clinical audits may also provide a useful source of information. For example, audit of documentation of community leg ulcer management demonstrated varied practice amongst primary care teams; Marshall et al (2001) reported that poor results motivated practitioners to change practice.

Prior to one stroke nutritional support project, Community Health Council audits had flagged nutrition in hospital as a local issue, enhancing its priority for local managers (Perry et al 2000). Both nutrition and stroke have been targeted nationally and internationally, and continue to be a priority in health care.

- Within the UK, a patient-focused benchmark for food and nutrition (Department of Health 2001a) has been established. This has received considerable attention within the NHS and in the wider media, for example with the Better Hospital Food Programme (see 195.92.246.148/nhsestates/better_hospital_food/bhf_content/introduction/home.asp).

- Stroke management has been incorporated into various clinical service development initiatives such as the National Service Frameworks for Older People and for Long-Term Conditions (Department of Health 2001b, 2005).

- A new stroke research network has been set up to enhance the research infrastructure for stroke within the UK and to increase collaborative working between academics, stroke clinicians, stroke service users and research funders (Department of Health 2000a; see www.uksrn.ac.uk).

- Examples of developments outside the UK include the Australian national and federal strategies for service development (National Heart, Stroke and Vascular Health Strategies Group 2004) and the proposed European service development for nutritional support (Council of Europe 2003).

- Stroke management is addressed via a number of national clinical guidelines, for example in the UK, America and Australia (Adams et al 2005, Duncan et al 2005, Intercollegiate Stroke Working Party (ISWP) 2004, National Stroke Foundation 2003).

Upton & Brooks (1995) employ a 'change equation' (of $f(D, V, S) R$), anticipating success where dissatisfaction (D) with the present situation, a vision (V) of a more desirable future, and knowledge of the first steps (S) required to achieve this, combine to exceed resistance (R) to or cost of change. For example, within the STEP stroke project, there was general dissatisfaction with dysphagia management (D) combined with nursing and therapists' aspirations towards a more streamlined, faster process (V), but with specific concerns expressed by individual clinicians (R). Once the dissatisfaction, vision and resistances were recognised and first steps agreed (i.e. methods for speeding screening and referral without over-riding decision-making processes), changes took place (Perry et al 2000).

Attitudes to using research evidence

Any change in practice requires commitment from practitioners and managers. There may be training, cost and time implications, and there is often a need to reassess current methods of working. It is therefore important to consider how best to present the project so as to gain support. What evidence is there to defend a course of action other than the status quo? How good is it? What is the prevailing attitude towards 'evidence' and how may it influence quality of care for individual patients?

Despite the obvious advantages identified in the commonly applied definition of EBP as 'the conscientious, explicit and judicious use of current best evidence in making decisions about the care of individual patients' (Sackett et al 1996, p.2), it has not received a universally warm welcome. It has been suggested that this definition can equally be applied to traditional decision making combining practitioners' knowledge of the literature and clinical experience/expertise to meet the needs of individuals (clinicians' 'clinical freedom') and hence EBP does not require any change in practice. In a study of implementation of EBP within acute stroke care in Australia, Perry (2006) reported scepticism voiced about the usefulness of current research evidence to guide clinical practice. Issues raised included selective study recruitment; restricted study populations due to inclusion/

exclusion criteria; discrepancies between nursing, clinical and research priorities. EBP has also been condemned as a 'cook-book' approach and a ploy to undermine practitioners' credibility by revealing obsolete practice. It has been regarded as potentially a means to limit choice of clinical interventions and reduce the costs of health care. However, it has also been argued that this is misinterpretation; that explicit use of evidence enforces updating of knowledge, supports practitioners' accountability for resource use and may in fact increase costs where more expensive interventions or products produce better outcomes (Deighan & Boyd 1996, Sackett et al 1996, pp.2–5).

From a nursing perspective, however, a key issue appears to be the failure to access research information. Faced with a range of situations and sources of information to which they could turn to support their decision making, Thompson et al (2001) reported that most nurses relied heavily on clinical experience, their own or that of colleagues, to supply what they perceived to be clinically useful information. Similar findings were reported by Gerrish & Clayton (2004) studying nurses' use of knowledge to guide pressure damage risk assessment. Once again, it was knowledge derived from hands-on experience that was the primary resource. Thompson (2003) has suggested strategies that may help to address this. Nonetheless, nurses introducing a change in practice need to be aware that they are likely to encounter a range of attitudes amongst colleagues towards the use of research evidence.

Another key consideration when setting out to persuade clinicians to alter their behaviours is both the quantity and especially the quality of evidence. Respected international and national institutions conduct systematic reviews of research evidence and/or present guidance for a wide range of topics relevant to nursing. These include, for example, the Cochrane Library, the National Institute for Health and Clinical Excellence (NICE), the NHS Centre for Reviews and Dissemination, the Scottish Intercollegiate Guidelines Network (SIGN) and the Joanna Briggs Institute. A relevant report may be available. However, in many areas evidence is limited. To illustrate, counting the sources identified as underpinning national evidence-based guidelines for acute stroke management revealed that 50 of 95 (53%) Australian guideline recommendations derived from the expert opinion of their authors (National Stroke Foundation 2003). Of the 277 recommendations contained within the comprehensive UK stroke guidelines (ISWP 2004), 80 (29%) are level A (defined as being derived from meta-analysis of randomised controlled trials (RCTs) or at least one RCT); 96 (35%) are level B (based on at least one well-designed controlled, quasi-experimental or descriptive study); 29 (10%) are level C; and 72 (26%) derive from working party opinion. Hence more than half, and over one-third, of Australian and UK stroke guideline recommendations respectively are not supported by evidence other than published or consensus expert clinical opinion.

This is no denigration of clinical expertise; in many instances it represents 'best available evidence'. However, where the opinions of local experts are not in tune with published recommendations of 'respected authorities', the latter may not be sufficient to effect changes in practice in the face of other competing resistance factors and the prevailing norms of peer group behaviour (Clinical Standards Advisory Group 1998). This may not deter practitioners from addressing a topic that has strong local support. However, gaining support for changes underpinned by level C evidence that local 'experts' do not endorse is likely to present considerable challenge. The practicalities of ensuring changes are based on best available evidence are considered in more detail in the chapters on finding and appraising the evidence.

Even for those topics where there is strong evidence of advantage for changes in practice, those involved in putting this into place must be persuaded of its relative advantage for themselves and their patients. As a consequence, the project co-ordinator should allow time for discussion and negotiation, and reframing the evidence to the local context (Greenhalgh et al 2004).

Summary of key factors in topic selection

There are a number of factors to consider when thinking about pursuing EBP development in a given topic.

- Ensure personal engagement with the issue; motivation and energy are crucial.
- Opt for topics that address local priorities and concerns, to maximise local support.
- Identify links with key policy objectives and national strategies to enlist high-level backing.
- Involve/reflect users' views to ensure relevance to their needs.
- Consider the attitudes and experiences of local practitioners in relation to accessing and applying research evidence for the given topic.
- Bear in mind the strength of evidence on the subject; rigorously developed guidance or evidence from well-conducted systematic reviews is likely to be more persuasive than consensus statements.

- Even good-quality evidence may require a period of discussion, negotiation and refinement before it is accepted as relevant and applicable to the local setting.

First steps

Choosing a project manager

A primary consideration is the practice development or project manager/ leader/co-ordinator role – the person who will hold day-to-day responsibility. Having the right person with the right skills located in the right post within the organisation has been repeatedly identified as crucial for clinical effectiveness/practice development work (Miller et al 1999, Redfern et al 2000, p.155). Miller et al (1999) stress matching the actual post with changes planned; ensuring adequate positional and legitimate authority with salary scale reflecting skills and level of responsibility.

Reviewing the range of skills required by the nine STEP project managers, Ross & McLaren (2000, p.25) noted that these spanned communication, research and audit skills, clinical credibility, guideline development and change management experience. Even more essential was the ability to learn fast. The nurse who occupies this position may have worked locally for many years and be well acquainted not just with the workplace teams or surroundings but with the whole institution and local health-care provision. However, practice development initiatives are also feasible and appropriate when initiated by a nurse new to the area; strengths and limitations attach to both positions.

'Insider' status carries obvious immediate advantages; the nurse knows the system and knows who does what and who to persuade to make things happen. Access to data, personnel and clinical areas may be automatic and clinical credibility with staff has already been established. However, because the nurse is well known, making a role transition or presenting themselves in a different light may not be straightforward. Doherty et al (2000, pp.14–15) describe difficulties and workload pressures when staff and managers continued to perceive an individual as a clinical nurse specialist despite a role change to practice development. The situation may be complicated where the project lead post is part-time and the postholder continues to occupy a previous 'insider' role for the remainder of the week. Kilbride et al (2005) commented that this allowed the postholder the opportunity to maintain clinical credibility and kept her in touch with grassroots stakeholders in a position that facilitated her influence on changes from the bottom up. However, this position was not always comfortable and there were periods when this 'role duality' led to conflicts, for example, due to dual responsibilities, workload issues and staff expressing resentment at her reduced visibility and perceived diminished supportive function due to adoption of the research role.

Further, objectivity for organisational analysis and observation of working practices entails extra effort to see past the familiar. This also presents potential for bias where the nurse may be evaluating practice in which they were a key player, and which represents considerable past personal investment. This situation may also pose personal difficulties if colleagues and friends construe evaluation as criticism.

The position of the 'incomer' is the reverse of this. Neither is better; both require awareness of potential problems and ability to capitalise on strengths. Irrespective of postholders' insider/incomer status, they may experience difficulties in adjusting to juggling several roles simultaneously, for example, those of a health-care professional and a researcher. Kilbride et al (2005) reported difficulties focusing on research where patients and/ or carers prioritised the project co-ordinator's clinical role as a physiotherapist. Perry (2003) discussed being torn between nursing accountability for the needs of an individual patient and the requirements of the project. An important means to help address this entails ensuring that the postholder is appointed early enough to contribute to project planning (Redfern et al 2000, pp.141, 166) and allowing time to mentally step out of the immediate situation and establish the broader picture in order to inform project planning. This is referred to as conducting a situation or diagnostic analysis (NHS CRD 1999). Project leaders should resist the desire to start making changes immediately; time invested at this point is repaid with interest later.

Diagnosing the situation

The organisational environment

The current context of the organisation is a key element which will influence the progress of the project. Important considerations include the presence of strong leadership, good managerial relations, an attitude that supports trying new approaches and taking risks, allied with professional networks and effective audit and feedback systems to keep people abreast of progress (Greenhalgh et al 2004). Organisational stability is also important; of the nine trusts involved in the STEP project, three underwent major reorganisation or merger within the life of the project, two within the first 6 months.

One project manager describes a period during which 'everyone senior was either fearful for their jobs, applying for others or settling into new ones . . . a tense and competitive atmosphere for months' (Bignell, personal communication). Redfern et al (2000, p.155) describe this as 'particularly disruptive . . . (especially) when changes occurred during the early stages of the project'. Trust mergers, restructuring and service reconfiguration are not uncommon but a period of organisational change may not be the best time to seek support for changes in practice; at the very least, practice changes must be planned to take other changes into account (Bignell et al 2000, pp.9–10). The situation at ward and unit level is also important. Bowers & McCann (2002, pp.15, 19–20) recount similar experiences when implementing training for cognitive behavioural interventions on acute psychiatric inpatient wards. One of the case study wards experienced disintegration of the programme following changes of people in key posts. This situation can be difficult to predict and requires active management by a strong project team from the outset.

Even where organisations were not currently involved in major restructuring, effects of recent changes were felt by staff in many trusts, e.g. where closure of a neighbouring accident and emergency department led to workload changes, where wards/departments had relocated or therapy teams had been reconfigured. Many staff reported a sense of 'change overload' and expressed low tolerance of more change (Doherty et al 2000, p.14). However, it is worth bearing in mind that perceptions of change may vary according to management and presentation. Examples were given where changes to the same workplace perceived as ordered from above with little consultation resulted in stress and resentment, but where consensual reorganisation was seen as mutually beneficial for staff and patients. This may be particularly pertinent where a nurse is charged with implementing changes required as a result of policy directives, such as in the UK, National Service Frameworks or Healthcare Commission audits or in Australia, the Council on Healthcare Standards' Evaluation and Quality Improvement Program. In every change management project, it is important to develop a change strategy; where change is externally driven, new practices are highly unlikely to be adopted or sustained without comprehensive and systematic consideration of the supports and barriers in place in the individual location.

It is nonetheless important to consider how the change relates to the organisation's priorities, structures and strategic plans, and the change agent must have a good grasp of these. Ways of achieving this include reviewing public reports, human resources information, clinical audits, minutes of key group meetings (e.g. of trust board, departmental heads, charge nurses); observation of meetings; interviews, focus groups, informal discussions with key figures (Ross & McLaren 2000, pp.32–33). If the selected topic fits within an identified priority area, high-level support may be easier to recruit. Explore existing routes of information dissemination, education and training, avenues by which changes may be introduced. The better the 'fit' between the change initiative and existing priorities and structures, the less time and effort required to introduce it and perhaps the greater the likelihood of success (Miller et al 1999).

Stakeholders and practitioner opinion leaders

The next stage involves identifying the key players in the topic and for the project, including service users and stakeholders (those with a vested interest in the change). All groups who may be affected by the proposed changes should be represented by appropriate practitioners and involved in discussions from the outset. A group representative may be the head of department, someone with recognised expertise in a specific area, for example a senior neurophysiotherapist to represent physiotherapy in a stroke project, or a local opinion leader such as the ward sister or an enthusiastic staff nurse. In the stroke project, nomination of a dynamic senior staff nurse resulted in her being one of the first to complete training and incorporate dysphagia screening within her daily practice; subsequently her ward demonstrated fastest and most complete uptake of the new role (Perry et al 2000). However, thought should be given to how supporters of the new ways of working will themselves be supported. Evaluating an implementation programme of ward-based training in cognitive behavioural interventions in acute psychiatry, Bowers & McCann (2002) found that in the absence of supportive middle management, even ward managers with a strong wish to see change happen were ineffectual in seeing this through. A Canadian study of implementation of pressure ulcer guidelines also found consistent and ongoing administrative support for the leaders to be critical for success (Clarke et al 2005). Ward managers and project co-ordinators themselves need to be supported and supervised; hence a project team needs to consider how and where such support may be recruited.

The views of stakeholders and opinion leaders on the envisaged changes should be explored. Relationships between individuals' beliefs, attitudes, intentions and behaviours are seldom direct and straightforward. However, while they are poor predictors of behaviour, attitudes clearly influence actions. In discussion with key individuals in advance of a project focused on nutrition support post stroke, it became clear that the risk of inappropriate treatment was a major concern (Perry et al 2000). Decisions about nutritional support for severely disabled patients who are perceived to have poor prognoses can be ethically difficult. Artificial nutritional support is regarded as treatment; whilst provision of 'normal' food and fluid is a human right, clinicians are not obliged to provide treatment believed to be futile (British Medical Association 1999). However, prognostication in acute stroke is an inexact science and the problems of prediction can be compounded by differences of interpretation where future quality of life is the issue. One method of addressing these uncertainties, preferred by some practitioners, was to 'wait and see'; to maintain hydration but withhold nutrition, sometimes through a protracted period of uncertainty. Exploring the origins of this approach revealed isolated incidents, sometimes decades earlier, the emotional effects of which were still felt by clinicians. In this instance, without appreciation of underpinning attitudes, it might have been difficult to understand behaviour.

A whole raft of issues may need to be considered when making judgements about the focus of project activities. O'Tuathail et al (2000, p.27) implemented standardised multidisciplinary assessment for older people prior to discharge based on a set of assessment measures assembled via professional consensus (Royal College of Physicians/British Geriatrics Society 1992). A key individual expressed reservations about one component of the assessment measures, namely universal screening for depression. Concerns were that the tool for screening might not transfer from a research setting to everyday clinical practice; that it might be oversensitive and identify clinical depression where patients were experiencing distress accompanying ill health and removal from their home environment. Potentially, this could result in unnecessary medication and iatrogenic morbidity. The individual also felt that time requirements for comprehensive screening in hospital were unrealistic, sudden increases in patients discharged with diagnoses of depression would overwhelm community resources and unnecessary additional workload would detract attention from those really in need. Eventually a compromise position was agreed, allowing formal screening by senior nursing staff whenever suspicion of depression was roused.

It is useful to identify a link person with senior trust management. This is usually someone with managerial responsibilities who can communicate and connect trust and project aims and strategies, including resource issues. Redfern et al (2000, p.155) discuss the importance of this post and suggest the optimal choice as someone senior enough to have authority to make decisions and mobilise responses speedily but also junior enough to have time for the project and more intimate knowledge of the clinical environment. Their attitude towards the project is also important. A clinical lead described as anxious and ambivalent was believed to have conveyed mixed messages about the project to staff. On evaluation, this project was 'not effective' in influencing global staff outcomes (attitudes and perceptions) although patients' health status benefited. These findings may indicate insensitivity of measurement tools in this environment (Redfern et al 2000, p.140); they may also reflect the effect of mixed messages from a very influential manager. It is also important to consider whether existing influential decision-making groups may impact upon project progress, and if so, whether and how the project should ensure representation. For their project implementing stroke unit care, Kilbride et al (2005) highlight the importance of achieving access to and later membership of the medical and managerial Stroke Oversight Committee.

Grassroots workers

Similar considerations argue for investigation of the views of grassroots staff. These are the people who will be asked to enact new ways of working, who will be expected to change their work patterns or activities. One of the key areas to explore is the priority that they accord the topic. Redfern et al (2000, p.49) note that practitioners in all projects and disciplines reported staff shortages and heavy workloads; Bowers & McCann (2002) also reported staff shortages as a key factor affecting the response of practitioners. Conversely, low numbers of patients requiring leg ulcer management in individual nurses' caseload restricted ability to practise skills and gain expertise, compounding difficulties in maintaining project activities as a priority (Marshall et al 2001). The low status accorded to some project activities is believed to have hampered guideline implementation, e.g. continence (Bignell et al 2000, pp.20, 27), leg ulcer care (Doherty et al 2000, p.13), nutrition (Love et al 2000, p.28). The perceived high priority of cardiovascular health promotion was a key element for a successful Canadian programme (Greenhalgh et al 2004, p.291). It is important to ensure that all health-care practitioners are informed of the significance and relevance of the topic; project team members may be best placed to address this within their professional groups.

It is also worth exploring the anticipated impact of the practice change upon resourcing and workload patterns. Doherty et al (2000, p.14) describe a vicious cycle in which lack of time to release community staff nurses for training in leg ulcer management had resulted in a habit of referral to the specialist leg ulcer team. Specialist care effectively decreased community team workload, so there was no motivation to release staff for training that would lighten the load on the specialist team but increase it for front-line staff. It may be possible to identify a 'trade-off'. For example, nursing staff expressed concerns at reintroduction of placement of fine-bore feeding tubes with guidewires within their role, exclusively a medical responsibility for some years. Where would they find time to do anything more? However, they also complained about the effort required to persuade medical teams to re-site displaced feeding tubes, viewed by them as low priority, especially when 'on call'. Checking placement via mandatory chest X-ray was labour intensive, for doctors signing requests and returning to view the X-ray films, porters and nurses in transporting the patient to and from the X-ray department, and for radiographers. Gaining responsibility for siting tubes could therefore be portrayed as labour saving, especially when linked with new placement checking procedures based on nurses checking the pH of gastric aspirate. The exploration of these concerns opened avenues to address them.

Users' views

Service users' views are equally important; clients often 'knew jolly well what they wanted from and liked about the service but were not usually asked' (Bignell, personal communication). The priority accorded to the topic by patients themselves is important; healing of leg ulcers was not always a priority for older patients with high levels of co-morbidity and other more pressing problems (Marshall et al 2001). Exploring patients' and carers' views of stroke rehabilitation, Kelson & Ford (1998) identified their overwhelming need for information – about the stroke itself, its effects, about management plans and what would happen or be available after discharge. Asking patients about their meal experiences highlighted problems (e.g. with ethnic diets and limited choice for some dietary requirements at the evening meal) but also strengths. Missing meals due to investigations/procedures, commonly cited as a problem in the literature, did not occur (Perry et al 2000).

Direct involvement in each stage of the process of change may be difficult; for example, in contributing to the development of evidence-based guidelines it may be unrealistic to ask patients or carers to participate in reviewing and critiquing the literature. They could, however, be asked to generate a list of questions that should be asked of the literature, be included in discussions about proposed changes, and asked to evaluate the changes. Methods for involving service users in guideline development are discussed in Chapter 8.

'The way we do things round here'

This entails putting together a picture of organisational culture at team, ward or unit level as well as trust-wide. Most nurses will be familiar with the marked differences in character encountered even between adjacent wards sharing consultants and patient intake. As 'incomers', Perry et al (2000, p.17) used the Assessment of Ward Environment Schedule (Nolan et al 1998) to gauge the climate of different wards; noticeable differences appeared in staff perceptions of their recognition and regard, working relationships, team climate and workload. One ward had high scores for team-working, recognition and regard, and working relationships coinciding with lower dissatisfaction with workload. This was an admissions ward with very high levels of patient and staff activity. It also boasted earliest and highest compliance with the new guidelines, highlighting the significance of local climate for practice development.

Implementation strategies need to be planned to match local culture and expectations. How is change usually introduced? Are staff accustomed to being told what to do or are they used to self-determination? Where does the usual managerial approach lie between the extremes of enforced compliance and self-motivated adherence? Redfern et al (2000, p.157) describe one project with a mismatch between a project leader with a personal preference to encourage and motivate working with staff who waited to be enforced because that was what they expected and was the norm in their environment. In this instance, guideline implementation was slow until the project leader matched her approach to local expectations instead of trying to change the staff to meet her ideals.

Information on previous experiences of change in the organisation will be helpful. How have previous changes been handled? How was this viewed by staff? What worked well and what problems were reported? The answers to these questions explained the cynicism encountered in one area in response to attempts to involve staff in project development. A previous communication failure over ward relocation had left staff perceiving a *fait accompli* where managers believed they had consulted and discussed. Efforts to include staff were redoubled rather than rejection being taken at face value.

Further information should include whether anything similar has been tried before, and with what result. Perry et al (2000, p.38) found that a nutrition risk screening tool had been introduced a year before, with little success. However, the two wards which used it wanted to keep it, so it was decided to capitalise on and top up previous training and relaunch the same tool. Whilst improvements in nutrition risk screening were achieved, compliance remained poor. It was postulated that rather than building on existing knowledge, relaunch may have been tainted by previous failure. Similar findings occurred across other projects, leading Redfern et al (2000, p.92) to suggest that it may be easier to generate enthusiasm for something new than to enhance or resurrect existing procedures.

BOX 10.1 Force field analysis (from Doherty et al 2000, with permission)

Forces for change	**Forces against change**
Open to communication and collaboration.	Previous bad experience of change in this area.
Will accept and cope with small-scale change.	Excessive recent change/low tolerance for change.
Will co-operate if benefit can be seen in the long run.	Increasing workload and high stress levels.
Ground staff eager to gain skills, increase professional development.	Staff shortage and skills shortage (resource constraint).
Enthusiastic teams, young, eager staff, negotiation.	Management style, viewed as low priority.
Senior managerial and trust board support.	Staff not motivated to provide this care; 'not interested' attitude.
Desire to have more control over own practice.	No feedback/incentives; no perceived need for change.
May perceive relative advantage to change/review practice.	New staff not yet fully integrated into trust; may view change as criticism of their standard of care.

By completion of this phase, possible levers, supports and supporters, potential hindrances or barriers to change will have been identified. At this stage it may be worth pulling it together to highlight key points. One method is to construct a force field analysis (Lewin 1951) which entails identifying those factors that are expected to promote and support the endeavour and those that will hinder and resist it. This approach was employed prior to implementing further practice development within an existing leg ulcer service (Box 10.1; Doherty et al 2000).

Another approach, used before implementing standardised multidisciplinary assessment for older adults prior to hospital discharge (O'Tuathail et al 2000), is the SWOT analysis, where potential or actual Strengths, Weaknesses, Opportunities and Threats offered by the project to the local area are identified (Box 10.2).

Both these approaches concentrate on the 'big issues' and can serve to focus activities, and as a memory aid as the project progresses. However, it is also important not to lose sight of detail such as individual features of wards or teams. It may also be useful to itemise supports, drivers and obstacles

---

BOX 10.2 SWOT analysis (from O'Tuathail et al 2000, with permission)

Strengths
Process to develop care focused
on the patient.
Opportunity to develop teamwork.
Generate multidisciplinary
documentation.
Create data for audit purposes.

Develop evidence-based practice.

Weaknesses
Implementation takes time and effort.

May be seen as yet another change.
Yet more paperwork.

Large project involving so many
disciplines.
Large clinical team.

Opportunities
Develop better outcomes for
patients.
Assist trust's contracting process
and image of promoting quality care.
Marketing initiative regionally and
nationally.
Improve communication across
the primary/secondary interface.

Threats
Lack of time for meetings, education
sessions and ever-increasing workload.
Lack of commitment from individuals
or professional groups of staff.
Overlap with other ongoing projects.

Resistance to change.

---

for individual components of the change. For example, implementing a valid and reliable swallow screening tool was one of the components of a project addressing screening, assessment and management of nutritional risk and the wide range of eating difficulties experienced by patients with acute stroke (Table 10.1). Concise notation of key features retains detail and helps to keep track of individual threads.

In addition to Lewin's approach and the SWOT analysis described above, readers may find the work of Rycroft-Malone et al (2004) useful in ascertaining factors that might have a positive or negative impact on the implementation of a change. Choice of approach is a matter for individual nurses; what is important is to ensure that this key phase for any project is not neglected or skimped. Time spent at this point may prevent time wasted later and avoid opposition or distress.

Summary of first steps

Once the topic has been decided, an early priority is to identify the specific requirements for the project manager/leader/co-ordinator post, identify

TABLE 10.1 DRIVERS AND OBSTACLES TO CHANGING THE PROCESS FOR SCREENING STROKE PATIENTS FOR DYSPHAGIA AND REFERRING TO SPEECH AND LANGUAGE DYSPHAGIA SERVICE FOR FULL CLINICAL ASSESSMENT OF SWALLOWING

Features of swallow screening procedure	Drivers/supports for change	Obstacles to change
Current swallow screen = gag as proxy	1. Only performed by doctors 2. Variability of results 3. Speech and language therapists believe dysphagic patients missed 4. Speech and language therapist concern re inappropriate referrals	A. 'Custom and practice' B. Lack of knowledge re valid methods
Screening only undertaken by doctors	1. Often omitted or delayed 2. Nurses have to request/remind; workload 3. Delayed screening impacts patient care 4. Nurses have little first-hand knowledge of patients' swallow function	A. 'Custom and practice' B. Nurses' lack of knowledge and skills C. Concern re lack of nursing skills D. Workload – another duty for nurses E. Medical sanction required for referral to speech and language therapist
Referral for speech and language dysphagia assessment requires written medical referral	1. Written referral often omitted/delayed 2. Nurses have to request/remind; workload 3. Written referral accompanied by nurses contacting speech and language therapist – nurse workload 4. Omitted written referral wastes speech and language therapist time 5. Delayed referral impacts patient care; concern re time spent with nil orally	A. Potential transfer of referral decision making and hence devolution of management decisions B. Transfer of nutrition support decision making C. Concern re inappropriate nutrition support decision making D. Varied level of concern re duration of times fasting

appropriate support for and appoint the individual who will be responsible for driving the project through. 'Diagnostic analysis' will be an essential first step for the postholder, prior to planning change. Information gained may include:

- the current context and culture at the level of the organisation and in the site(s) where change is planned to occur (at ward/unit/team level)
- identifying organisational priorities, structures and strategic plans into which the changes might fit
- identifying the key players and opinion leaders
- establishing their attitudes, experiences and priorities in relation to the subject
- accessing patients'/users' experiences and views of the topic; involving them directly where feasible
- getting a feel for organisational culture and issues at all levels, formal and informal
- clarifying usual management approaches and exploring previous change experiences.

What changes are needed?

Ensuring change is based on best evidence

Implementation of research evidence into practice has been repeatedly explored in nursing and key barriers identified. A common complaint of clinical nurses in all areas is difficulty accessing and making sense of the evidence (Dunn et al 1997, Funk et al 1995, Newman et al 1998, Redfern et al 2000, p.48). Gerrish & Clayton (2004) found that nurses were much more proficient at accessing organisational information, such as policies, procedures and guidelines, than research evidence.

A number of approaches have been developed to process evidence and present it to health-care practitioners in brief, user-friendly formats. Care pathways are one option, allowing incorporation of research evidence into a structured framework (Wigfield & Boon 1996). On a day-by-day basis the anticipated management and progress of typical patients with specific diagnoses are mapped. Another initiative is that of benchmarking, whereby 'best practice' features are identified for local comparison (Pantall 2001). This approach has been incorporated into a national nursing care quality initiative (Department of Health 2001a). Both of these approaches may make use of evidence-based guidelines comprising recommendations for the interventions and care management that have been shown to produce the best outcomes for a specific situation and patient group. Recommendations are identified according to the type and strength of evidence from which they derive, hence retaining a direct link with and enabling practitioners to read the underpinning evidence if they wish.

Evidence-based guidelines encapsulate 'best practice' for the target patient group and criteria against which clinical practice and patient outcomes can be compared. This enables identification of areas of strength and practice development opportunities. For example, multinational clinical guidelines for stroke management recommend that all patients admitted to hospital with acute stroke should have their swallowing ability screened within 24 hours of hospital admission. Further, where dysphagia is suspected, full clinical assessment should take place within 72 hours of admission (ISWP 2004, National Stroke Foundation 2003). In one project, when practice was audited and compared with these recommendations, it was found that 53% of patients had been screened, with 38% of assessments occurring within the specified time period (Perry & McLaren 2000). Dysphagia screening and referral processes were highlighted as practice development topics.

Evidence-based guidelines can therefore provide a user-friendly means to communicate research evidence and guidance on 'best practice'. In addition, they can encompass audit criteria and may indicate practice development topics. The first stage of guideline development (i.e. seeking robust evidence to support a practice development) may start concurrently with the 'diagnostic analysis' previously described.

Finding the evidence

For both the clinical effectiveness lead initiating a project and the individual nurse seeking help with a practice issue, literature searching is a starting point. Chapter 3 addresses this in detail and this section simply reiterates the importance of making full use of all available resources. Chief of these is the local health librarian who may help with accessing relevant databases and setting up and running search strategies. Discussion with a librarian can often overcome the twin stumbling blocks of searches that find either nothing or 30,000 papers. For many topics, recent systematic reviews or evidence-based guidelines from well-known sources of expertise are available. However, these still may not answer every aspect of the question; for example, users' views and patients' perspectives may not have been addressed, patients studied may not be representative of the local population or the nurse's caseload. Further searching for relevant evidence will be required.

Appraising the evidence

Practice recommendations or guidelines are only as good as the evidence on which they rest, and the manner in which this has been handled. Irrespective of the source of the evidence, it is important to appraise and critique the literature. Key questions to ask include:

- whether the design and methodology adopted by a study is an appropriate means to answer the particular question
- whether the methods used by the study match quality criteria required for that particular design
- whether limitations of study design and methods have been acknowledged and taken into account when results are used to produce recommendations.

Chapters 4–7 and 9 deal with this process in detail, and provide information about appropriate appraisal instruments.

Even if, what appear to be, evidence-based guidelines have been identified, it is important to evaluate their merits, not least because some topics have been repeatedly addressed. An American source of critically appraised guidelines, the National Guideline Clearinghouse (found at www.guideline.gov/), accessed in September 2005, yielded four guidelines focusing on pressure damage or ulceration, nine on continence and 10 for acute pain management, all focused on adult care and all published after 2002. Chapter 9 discusses an appraisal instrument that can be used as a checklist or reminder for guideline developers or groups assessing guidelines prior to undertaking local modification. This option, tailoring nationally developed guidelines to suit local circumstances, has been commended by the NHS Executive (1996) and Greenhalgh et al (2004). It may offer the twin benefits of minimising time spent on literature searching and appraisal whilst maximising input of local clinicians to ensure that guidelines address local circumstances and needs.

Turning evidence into recommendations

The process of developing and grading recommendations according to the strength of evidence has been discussed in Chapter 9. Recommendations that are based on evidence with a very low risk of bias are assigned a high grade. There is, however, limited availability of good-quality data in many important areas of care. In addition, the applicability of findings from controlled studies to patients in a specific clinical setting may be questionable, especially where studies have concentrated on specific subgroups. Doherty et al (2000, p.15) discuss working with a heterogeneous patient caseload with multiple risk factors, resulting in only 35% of their ulcers being of purely venous origin. However, the evidence base underpinning leg ulcer management is predominantly focused on venous leg ulcers. In this and many other situations, guidelines and advice may be needed most where evidence is weak or lacking.

Many topic areas are only addressed via anecdote, description, prescription and discussion. These nonetheless frequently represent important areas of patient care that are the subject of everyday treatment and management decisions. In these situations guidance is still required, perhaps to a greater degree than where strong evidence is in the public domain. The option here is to use opinion derived from clinical experience and experts in the field. This may be available in the form of consensus statements from working parties, standing committees and conference meetings; for example, for stroke management, prior to the development of evidence-based guidelines, 'best evidence' was derived from a published consensus statement agreed at an international conference (Aboderin & Venables 1996). Where even this does not exist, consensus agreement can be sought using formal methods such as the nominal group process or Delphi technique (see Chapter 9) or consensus development panels (Bowling 1997, pp.362–365). Modified nominal group process, used to develop guidelines for pressure damage (Rycroft-Malone 2000), entailed participants rating statements derived from the literature on the basis of their expertise and the quality and strength of the evidence. The distribution of responses was presented and discussed and statements re-rated; recommendations were drafted reflecting and indicating extent of agreement. For the guidelines for nutrition support, a consensus development panel was brought together. Representation from all relevant areas of local expertise agreed local guidance for timing of initiation of artificial nutrition support in patients with unsafe swallow post stroke (Perry et al 2000). Whilst a major multicentre trial (the FOOD Trial) was in progress, there was no clear evidence for optimal timing.

Using the full range of evidence (but selecting a lower level of evidence only when there is no valid primary research using an appropriate study design) in the development and presentation of guidelines allows aggregation of data from a variety of sources (from systematic review to expert opinion) in a concise format that acknowledges and identifies its origins. Not only is this transparency a quality criterion in guideline development, it is also important for implementation.

Establishing key objectives

Comparing baseline to guideline-supported practice

As indicated by Cluzeau et al (1999), rigorous guidelines identify clear standards or targets and define measurable outcomes that can be monitored. With this in mind, before proceeding to plan changes in practice, it is useful to carry out a baseline evaluation of current practice for later comparison. Clinical audit staff are a useful resource here and may guide the choice of data and manner of collection. Much information is routinely collected within organisations. Whilst there may be some difficulties about the manner in which it is presented (e.g. data on length of hospital stay may only be recorded as finished consultant episodes), its detail and accuracy (e.g. diagnostic coding; Stegmayr & Asplund 1992), what is required may be available without additional data collection. However, this information may not be routinely collected or it may be that additional effort and resources are warranted to achieve greater accuracy/relevance. Audit and data collection techniques are beyond the scope of this chapter but texts are available in most health libraries.

A baseline audit will also enable identification and prioritisation of areas of guideline-related practice where changes are required. With depiction of baseline practice and outcomes established, there is a means to evaluate the effects of guideline implementation via later repetition of the data collection exercise. This is essential if the organisation is to learn what has been gained from this whole process. Consequences of a change in practice may not only occur in intended and predicted areas; there may also be unintentional and unpredictable outcomes ('knock-on' effects) that the organisation may need to address. Repeat evaluation may also be a useful 'selling' point for the change management strategy; on the basis that as changes will be fully evaluated, it may be possible to win provisional support where it would not otherwise be forthcoming.

With standards and outcomes clarified, the next stage entails identifying guideline components that require active intervention to enable staff to meet the specified standards and outcomes. For example, the objectives that

BOX 10.3 Objectives to be met to enable nurses to screen stroke patients' swallowing ability (from Perry et al 2000, with permission)

- Identification of nurses' education and training requirements
- Development of a package to meet these, including theoretical and practical instruction and assessment
- Nomination of educators and assessors
- Agreement of competence criteria
- Location of the new role within the framework of nursing competencies within the trust
- Location of the new training package within the framework of in-service training within the trust
- Multiprofessional agreement to nurses' performance of a previously exclusively medical role
- Identification and agreement of changes to the referral process to access full clinical assessment by dysphagia-trained speech and language therapists for patients screened by nurses

were identified and addressed to enable nurses to screen stroke patients' swallowing ability on admission to hospital are set out in Box 10.3. The processes that will accomplish identified objectives need to be considered in the light of requirements for guideline dissemination (making sure that all relevant practitioners are aware of the guidelines and their contents) and the change management process (persuading/facilitating/supporting/ensuring practice change).

Summary – what changes are needed?

Identifying practice development objectives and achievable outcomes entails:

- accessing and appraising the evidence in relation to the characteristics of the patient group and the context in which it will be used
- when developing guidelines or modifying national guidelines to meet local requirements, presenting the evidence as practice recommendations appropriate to the strength of supporting information
- where evidence is lacking, consensus expert opinion can be recruited
- identifying and auditing current practice and outcomes
- establishing topics or standards to be addressed via guideline implementation; outcomes that will be monitored

- pinpointing interventions and activities required to support and enable staff to implement guideline recommendations.

How to implement the changes

Developing a dissemination and implementation strategy

By this stage the guidelines will have been developed and the activities required to prepare staff identified. The next stage entails considering how to inform and motivate practitioners for the practice change. The nurse managing such a project needs to bear in mind that every situation and context is unique; no two projects will work the same way and there are no 'off-the-peg', sure-fire strategies. Reviewing implementation studies, Greenhalgh et al (2004, p.292) concluded that many of the factors identified as key to the success and sustainability of changes in practice were highly individual to studies' contexts, and interacted in unique and often unpredictable ways. This group reiterated the importance of being sensitive to the characteristics and needs of the local area, and the importance of close monitoring and feedback to respond to what works well or less well as the project progresses.

If the proposed changes are small and localised, the nurse may not need an elaborate implementation strategy. However, it is always wise to think the process through from all angles before launching into change. It is important to ensure that potential implications for any other areas of practice have been considered. For a large guideline requiring a lot of preparation for implementation (for example, a guideline for nutritional support, involving nursing and medical teams, therapy departments and catering and continuing beyond hospital discharge), it might be beneficial to stage the launch and address components incrementally. If it is to be introduced across a large area, a rolling programme (perhaps one ward or team at a time) may allow focused intensive input. Identifying one area to function as a 'demonstration project', with systematic evaluation disseminated prior to roll-out, has been identified as a contributor to the success of a Canadian cardiovascular health promotion programme (Greenhalgh et al 2004, p.290). Early successes may be achieved and seen to be achieved, thus encouraging practitioners and supporting the implementation process. However, there are time implications; incremental implementation may take longer and although it may achieve better or more sustained compliance, may not be feasible within the time available.

General approaches to managing change

A range of approaches can be taken when planning change (see also Chapter 11 and Greenhalgh et al 2004, pp.70–120). Grol (1997) talks of *educational approaches* which derive from striving for professional competence, clearly demonstrated in the linkage of continuing professional development (CPD) with educational sessions, ranging in style from didactic lectures to workshops and small group discussions. Appealing to clinicians as rational beings, *epidemiological stances* focus on the presentation of the evidence, e.g. in the form of guidelines, and stress the scientific merits of a new course of action. The validity, reliability, credibility and presentation of the evidence are therefore key. Implementation can also be viewed as the *marketing of a product, information or strategies* that will be useful for clinicians; both the presentation of the product and the channels of information will be important. *Behavioural* change may also be utilised, underpinned by classic theories of behaviour conditioning reliant on the influence of specific stimuli before or after the desired actions, for example, audit and feedback or performance review. It may also be possible to incorporate reminders, for example from patients, tagged to notes or built into software, e.g. for clinic review, hospital admission or discharge procedures. *Social interactionism* capitalises on the essential gregariousness of human culture, including workplace society; the influence of fellow practitioners and patients is recognised. Opinion leaders, role models, patient pressure, peer support and group norms are all acknowledged agents or resistors of change. Moving from individual to *organisational approaches*, quality care is seen as dependent upon a cascade of inter-related actions which can be supported or hindered by the structures of the organisation itself. This approach is reflected in attitudes towards adverse incidents in moving away from individual fault-finding towards whole-systems approaches (Department of Health 2000b).

Each of these approaches offers different avenues and strategies for guideline implementation and change management. It is not envisaged that any one will meet all requirements; a combination tailored to individual situations and needs is recommended (Greenhalgh et al 2004, pp.259–260, NHS CRD 1999).

Specific approaches to managing change

At this stage, the project co-ordinator/manager will need to check that:

- realistic goals and time frames have been set
- resources are sufficient. Redfern et al (2000, pp.157, 161) suggest that it may be unreasonable to expect projects to be cost-neutral throughout; it may

be more realistic to anticipate some degree of investment that will be recouped later. For all STEP projects, resourcing was an issue; projects where the patients' health status was eventually shown to have been improved significantly by the intervention all requested and received additional funding. The level was not great (approximately £2500 each; for example, to fund bank nurse and locum speech and language therapists' time; see Box 10.4) and a cost-benefit analysis case study of the stroke nutrition project indicates that the investment has been repaid

- opportunities have been taken to trial or pilot changes where possible

- interim review points have been identified with flexibility built in to enable changes if necessary in light of progress

- the project manager/leader/co-ordinator role is enabled to fulfil required activities

- review dates for guideline implementation and for the guidelines themselves have been set.

Information from the 'diagnostic analysis' will be invaluable in guiding the choice of implementation strategies from those that have been demonstrated to achieve successful results within similar environments. Even where change is on a small scale and no formal analysis is undertaken, it is beneficial to draw on knowledge of the structures, characters, characteristics, promoting and limiting factors within the change area. Irrespective of the scale of change, the key principle of matching specific strategies to achieve individual objectives applies. Relevant information might include:

- existing initiatives which can support the changes (e.g. for a breastfeeding initiative, where the hospital was seeking UNICEF UK Baby Friendly Hospital status)

- existing structures which can accommodate the changes (e.g. nursing and medical in-service training programmes)

- interprofessional interpretation and prioritisation of key activities (e.g. nursing and medical attitudes towards siting of fine-bore feeding tubes)

- the attitudes and beliefs of key figures and groups, to guide the targeting and presentation of information

- the ward, team or organisational climate, guiding choice of appropriate approach to change from encouragement to enforcement, persuasion to compulsion

- supportive forces that can be relied upon; resistance factors that need to be addressed

- anticipated costs; availability of funding.

Interventions should be accommodated within existing structures where possible and strategies tailored to fit individual characteristics and needs within the culture of the organisation. Box 10.4 gives a worked example.

BOX 10.4 Example

The problem
In one acute trust, swallow screening on admission of patients with stroke was a medical role with written medical referral required for full clinical assessment of swallowing by members of a speech and language dysphagia service. In practice, only around half of all patients admitted with acute stroke had their swallowing screened, screening was predominantly via non-valid methods and the referral process could be protracted (Perry & McLaren 2000). Good facilities were undermined by suboptimal processes, reflected in patient and carer complaints and staff dissatisfaction (see Table 10.1).

The proposed solution
Screening by nurses. This change had been originally identified via a broad consultation process involving all grades of relevant practitioners, patients and carers.

Planning the change
This entailed several steps (Table 10.2).

1. Identification of a valid and reliable method of screening swallowing function. This was undertaken by a consensus development panel chosen as the opinion leaders of their professions. Elements of the epidemiological approach were evident in choice of tool and manner of presentation, exemplifying a rigorous process expressed in clear and user-friendly documentation. Incorporation of the tool within the stroke pathway and proforma was intended to act as a visual prompt for medical and nursing staff during admission procedures. Costs of this component entailed time of project team members, photocopying and library costs accessing literature. The project manager's salary was an additional cost, funded through regional research funding streams. All other costs were subsumed within normal trust budgets.

2. Education and training of nursing and medical staff to use this screening tool. In addition to practical preparation interventions aimed to ensure professional acceptance of new role activities, e.g. nurses siting and checking placement of feeding tubes; doctors using new screening procedures. For nurses, training sessions were accommodated within the established Scope of Professional Practice programme, comprising educational input and skills training in aspects considered to be core role functions of the nursing grades. Ward leaders and influential senior staff were encouraged to attend first sessions. Preparation combined theory and practice away from the ward with a minimum of five practical sessions conducted on the wards screening real patients. In addition to teaching and assessing nurses' skills, this aimed to insert the behaviour into

its natural context, to associate it with daily nursing practice. Junior doctors' teaching occurred within their regular weekly programme. Costs of this component derived from extra study time required for nurses and time spent on teaching delivered by speech and language therapists and in-service trainers. Project time pressures enforced rapid implementation; this entailed use of some additional bank nurses to provide cover and locum speech and language therapy time.

3. Changes in role remit enabling nurses to contact the dysphagia service about patients with swallowing problems. Superficially an organisational change, recruiting support for this entailed multiple approaches. Audit and feedback of baseline practice highlighted aspects for change. Local consultants, nationally acknowledged for work in this area, addressed local clinicians and chaired discussion sessions. The intervention was widely promoted at ward and team meetings, in internal and neighbouring trust newsletters, the local newspaper, cable TV, and at local, national and international conferences. The trust board and internal professional groups circulated statements of support; influential figures role-modelled changed practice. Members of the stroke team and the project manager monitored and reported progress. The costs of this component were represented largely by project manager time, photocopying and two fees for external lecturers.

TABLE 10.2 STRATEGIES EMPLOYED TO IMPLEMENT SWALLOW SCREENING GUIDELINES

Requirements prior to implementation	Strategies employed to address this
Identification of a valid and reliable swallow screening tool	1. Consensus development panel composed of all relevant groups 2. Consensus development panel comprised opinion leaders of the professions 3. Choice of tool with demonstrated validity and reliability, including when tested with nurses 4. Presentation of the tool within guidelines developed by rigorous process 5. Clarity and user-friendliness of format 6. Incorporation within care pathway and proforma as visual prompts

(Continued)

TABLE 10.2 (CONTINUED)

Requirements prior to implementation	Strategies employed to address this
Education and training required to use the tool	1. Sessions incorporated within established uniprofessional education programmes. This facilitated access to staff and supported identification of screening as role 'norm' 2. Sessions function as discussion for a re role changes 3. Nurses' practical sessions take place on their wards; facilitates access to staff and associates screening with routine nursing practice 4. Ward sisters/charge nurses and senior staff encouraged to achieve competence and model changed practice
Changes in role remit to enable nurses to alert the dysphagia service of patients needing full clinical swallowing assessment	1. Support indicated via widespread consultation process, grassroots to management levels 2. Audit and feedback of baseline working of the referral system; identification of problems 3. Recruitment of support for changing referral system from all consultants; 1:1 discussions 4. Input and discussion session with nationally acknowledged opinion leader 5. Overt and widespread high-level support for changes expressed via public statements, memos and role modelling 6. 'Selling' the project through internal and local media, nationally and internationally 7. Implementation within evaluation framework allows assessment of merit of changes

Summary – how to implement the changes

A range of approaches to change management and a variety of strategies have been shown to be effective for guideline implementation.

- Approaches and strategies need to be planned to achieve their objectives within the context of the individual organisation.
- No one approach will be adequate alone; mix and match to meet individual requirements.
- Ensure that resourcing and management issues have been addressed, goals and time frames are realistic, interim and final review dates set.

Evaluating the progress and effects of the changes

It is important to maintain close contact with the progress of implementation interventions. Be prepared to make changes if things do not work as expected. For example, the practical swallow screening sessions were originally planned to take place whenever therapists were on the ward seeing patients. This proved unworkable; it was not possible to co-ordinate the activities of therapists with those of nursing staff and tie them in with patient needs on an opportunistic basis. This was changed to a programme of timed appointments; although it entailed administration time, this was successful.

Maintain the focus on sustainability. Project activities should shift from being seen as something different and special to everyday practice, 'business as usual'. Ways to address this will have been identified from the outset and include use of existing structures and processes, and involvement of clinical staff in all aspects. Members of the health-care team can be encouraged to assume responsibility for project activities within their areas of practice and as time progresses, the role of the project manager will need to change to reflect this. For changes in practice to be sustainable, there must be an effective transfer of activities and responsibilities from within a project framework to normal clinical practice. Whilst it is important that someone takes responsibility to drive dissemination and implementation of the guidelines, continued reliance upon a single individual weakens the long-term sustainability of guideline-supported practice. Withdrawal of the project leader should be planned, possibly around a staged progress of relinquishing responsibilities and adoption by practitioners.

Full incorporation of project activities within normal daily practice may be a lengthy process; it may be necessary to plan for an interim stage focused on continuing establishment of the changes as self-sustaining. It should not be assumed that this will occur naturally. For example, evaluation of a STEP project which initiated substantial changes in stroke management indicated need for a named individual to continue championing new practices and driving service development. A business plan was agreed for appointment of a stroke nurse co-ordinator; however, delayed funding resulted in a 1-year hiatus between departure of the project co-ordinator and appointment to the clinical post. During this time, erosion of nurse swallow screening practices (a key component of changed practice) was observed through falling numbers attending training programmes and reduced referrals for full clinical assessment of swallowing based on screening outcomes. The 9-month implementation stage of the project had not been adequate to

---

BOX 10.5 Changes effected by the STEP projects

- Significant gains in staff knowledge and positive attitude change towards family intervention for schizophrenia
- Significant reduction in work-related psychological distress
- Increased information delivered antenatally re infant feeding
- Increased skin-to-skin contact
- Increased continuance of breastfeeding to 12 weeks
- In stroke rehabilitation, significant improvements in multidisciplinary involvement and communication with carers
- Dramatic reductions in average costs of leg ulcer dressings per patient per week
- Improvements in numbers of patients with ulcers healed in 1–3 months and 3–6 months
- More complete assessment of continence problems in elderly patients
- Significant increases in nurses' knowledge of incontinence and its management
- Increased reportage of information given, involvement and satisfaction of older people with the discharge process
- Significant improvements in appropriate referrals for nutritional support; faster referral processes
- Significant reduction in time spent with nil orally prior to institution of nutrition support and throughout patient stay
- Fewer feeding tubes and X-rays required, feed quantities delivered closer to prescription
- Significant reduction in incidence of infective episodes – chest and urinary tract, sepsis of unidentified origin

---

achieve self-sustainability and an additional, clinically led phase of activities was required. This situation has been reported by a number of projects; for example, Goodman & Steckler (1988) described a health promotion programme which won a national award but terminated on the day that project funding ended.

Once formal evaluation of the changes has occurred, ensure that the information is disseminated to everyone involved and give public recognition for the time, energy and commitment of those who made things happen. Consider wider publication of both the processes experienced and results achieved. What has been learnt about the process of change may be as valuable to colleagues as the effects for patient care. Avenues to disseminate findings include local and national conferences, fora and interest group meetings, papers and publications ranging from major international journals to society newsletters. There are also implementation fora such as Impact, a section of *Bandolier*, accessible online at www.ebandolier.com and via the NeLH.

Conclusion

This chapter has sought to draw together information covered in preceding chapters and illustrate how this has been applied within real-life projects. Examples have been drawn from a wide range of implementation and evaluation projects to demonstrate things which worked and pitfalls to avoid. It would be misleading to suggest that following the processes detailed will guarantee success; changing practice is never easy and no two situations are identical. However, in the world of practice development there is a wealth of experience to draw on, and some of the outcomes of the STEP projects (Box 10.5) demonstrate that efforts to implement practice that is explicitly evidence based may be well rewarded.

References

Aboderin I, Venables G 1996 Stroke management in Europe. Pan European Consensus Meeting on Stroke Management. Journal of Internal Medicine 240(4):173–180

ACHCEW (Association for Community Health Councils for England and Wales) 1997 Hungry in hospital? ACHCEW, London

Adams H, Adams R, Del Zoppo G et al 2005 Guidelines for the early management of patients with ischemic stroke. 2005 Guidelines Update. A scientific statement from the Stroke Council of the American Heart Association/American Stroke Association. Stroke 36:916–921

Bignell V, Getliffe K, Forester L 2000 The South Thames Evidence-based Practice Project. The promotion of continence for elderly people in primary care: the role of community nurses. St George's Hospital Medical School and Kingston University, London

Bowers L, McCann E 2002 The promotion of rapid recovery from acute psychotic episodes: the application of recent research findings to the practice of psychiatric nursing on acute wards. Report to the Foundation of Nursing Studies and the Tompkins Trust. City University, London. Available online at: www.city.ac.uk/sonm/dps/research/research_reports/bowers_l/Rapid. pdf 10 September 2005

Bowling A 1997 Research methods in health. Open University Press, Buckingham

British Medical Association (BMA) 1999 Withholding and withdrawing life-prolonging medical treatment. Guidance for decision making. BMJ Publishing, London

Clarke H F, Bradley C, Whytock S et al 2005 Pressure ulcers: implementation of evidence-based nursing practice. Journal of Advanced Nursing 49(6):578–590

Clinical Standards Advisory Group 1998 Report on clinical effectiveness using stroke as an example. Stationery Office, London

Cluzeau F, Littlejohns P, Grimshaw J et al 1999 Development and application of a generic methodology to assess the quality of clinical guidelines. International Journal of Quality in Health Care 11(1):21–28. See also: www.sghms.ac.uk/depts/phs/hceu/clinguid.htm

Council of Europe 2003 Resolution ResAP(2003)3 on food and nutritional care in hospitals. Available online at: wcd.coe.int/ViewDoc.jsp?id=85747&BackColorInternet=9999CC&BackColorIntranet=FFBB55&BackColorLogged= FFAC75 10 Semember 2005

Deighan M, Boyd K 1996 Defining evidence-based health care. NT Research 1(5):332–339

Department of Health 2000a Research and development for a first class service. R & D funding in the new NHS. Department of Health, Leeds

Department of Health 2000b An organisation with a memory: report of an expert group on learning from adverse events in the NHS. Available online at: www.dh.gov.uk/assetRoot/04/08/89/48/04088948.pdf 10 September 2005

Department of Health 2001a The essence of care. Patient-focused benchmarking for health care practitioners. Available online at: www.modern.nhs.uk/home/key/docs/Essence%20of%20Care.pdf 10 September 2005

Department of Health 2001b The national service framework for older people. Available online at: www.dh.gov.uk/asset Root/04/07/12/83/04071283.pdf 10 September 2005

Department of Health 2005 The national service framework for long-term conditions. Available online at: www.dh.gov.uk/assetRoot/ 04/10/53/69/04105369.pdf 3 September 2005

Doherty D, Ross F, Yeo L et al 2000 The South Thames Evidence-based Practice Project. Leg ulcer management in an integrated service. St George's Hospital Medical School and Kingston University, London

Duncan P W, Zorowitz R, Bates B et al 2005 Management of adult stroke rehabilitation care: a clinical practice guideline. Stroke 36(9): e100–143

Dunn V, Crichton N, Roe B et al 1997 Using research for practice: a UK experience of the BARRIERS scale. Journal of Advanced Nursing 26(6):1203–1210

Funk S G, Tornquist E M, Champagne M T 1995 Barriers and facilitators of research utilisation. Nursing Clinics of North America 30(3):395–407

Gerrish K, Clayton J 2004 Promoting evidence-based practice: an organisational approach. Journal of Nursing Management 12:114–123

Goodman R M, Steckler A 1988 The life and death of a health promotion program – an institutionalization perspective. International Quarterly Journal of Community Health Education 8:5–19

Greenhalgh T, Robert G, Bate P et al 2004 How to spread good ideas. A systematic review of the literature on diffusion, dissemination and sustainability of innovations in health service delivery and organisation. Report for the National Co-ordinating Centre for NHS Service Delivery and Organisation R & D (NCCSDO). Available online at: www.sdo.lshtm.ac.uk/pdf/changemanagement_greenhalgh_report.pdf 10 September 2005

Grol R 1997 Beliefs and evidence in changing clinical practice. British Medical Journal 315:418–421

Intercollegiate Stroke Working Party 2004 National clinical guidelines for stroke, 2nd edn. Clinical Effectiveness and Evaluation Unit, Royal College of Physicians, London. Available online at: www.rcplondon.ac.uk/pubs/books/stroke/stroke_guidelines_2ed.pdf 10 September 2005

Kelson M, Ford C and the Intercollegiate Working Party for Stroke 1998 Stroke rehabilitation. Patient and carer views. Royal College of Physicians and College of Health, London

Kilbride C, Meyer J, Flatley M, Perry L 2005 Stroke units: the implementation of a complex intervention. Education Action Research 13(4):479

Lewin K 1951 Field theory in social science. Harper, New York

Love C, McLaren S, Smits M 2000 The South Thames Evidence-based Practice Project. Nutritional management for patients with acute stroke. St George's Hospital Medical School and Kingston University, London

Marshall J L, Mead P, Jones K et al 2001 The implementation of venous leg ulcer guidelines: process analysis of the intervention used in a multi-centre, pragmatic, randomised, controlled trial. Journal of Clinical Nursing 10(6):758–766

Miller C, Scholes J, Freeman P 1999 Evaluation of the 'assisting clinical effectiveness' programme. In: Humphris D, Littlejohns P (eds)

Implementing clinical guidelines. A practical guide. Radcliffe Press, Oxford

National Heart, Stroke and Vascular Health Strategies Group 2004 National strategy for heart, stroke and vascular health in Australia. Publication number 3402(JN8301). Available online at: www.health.gov.au/ May 2006

National Stroke Foundation 2003 National clinical guidelines for acute stroke management. Available online at: www.strokefoundation.com.au/ pages/image.aspx?assetId=RDM38248.6090587269 10 September 2005

Newman M, Papadopoulos I, Sigsworth J 1998 Barriers to evidence-based practice. Clinical Effectiveness in Nursing 2:11–20

NHS CRD (Centre for Reviews and Dissemination) 1999 Getting evidence in to practice. Effective Health Care 5:1

NHS Executive 1996 Clinical guidelines. Using clinical guidelines to improve patient care within the NHS. NHS Executive, Leeds

Nolan M, Grant G, Brown J et al 1998 Assessing nurses' work environment: old dilemmas, new solutions. Clinical Effectiveness in Nursing 2:145–156

O'Tuathail C, Ross F, Stubberfield D 2000 The South Thames Evidence-based Practice Project. Standardised multidisciplinary assessment of older people on discharge from hospital. St George's Hospital Medical School and Kingston University, London

Pantall J 2001 Benchmarking in health care. NT Research 6(2):568–580

Perry L 2003 Dilemmas and decisions in evaluation research: the project co-ordinator's tale. Royal College of Nursing Research Society Conference, Manchester

Perry L 2006 Promoting evidence-based practice in stroke care in Australia. Nursing Standard 20(34):35–42

Perry L, McLaren S 2000 An evaluation of implementation of evidence-based guidelines for dysphagia screening and assessment following acute stroke: phase 2 of an evidence-based practice project. Journal of Clinical Excellence 2:147–156

Perry L, McLaren S, Bennett M 2000 The South Thames Evidence-based Practice Project. Nutritional support for patients with acute stroke. St George's Hospital Medical School and Kingston University, London

Redfern S, Christian S, Murrells T et al 2000 Evaluation of change in practice: South Thames Evidence-based Practice Project (STEP). King's College, London

Ross F, McLaren S 2000 The South Thames Evidence-based Practice Project. An overview of aims, methods and cross-case analysis of nine implementation projects. St George's Hospital Medical School and Kingston University, London

Royal College of Physicians/British Geriatrics Society 1992 Standardized assessment scales for older people. Royal College of Physicians/British Geriatrics Society, London

Rycroft-Malone J 2000 Pressure ulcer risk assessment and prevention. Royal College of Nursing, London

Rycroft-Malone J, Harvey G, Seers K et al 2004 An exploration of the factors that influence the implementation of evidence into practice. Journal of Clinical Nursing 13(8):913–924

Sackett D L, Richardson W S, Rosenberg W et al 1996 Evidence-based medicine. How to practice and teach EBM. Churchill Livingstone, New York

Stegmayr B, Asplund K 1992 Measuring stroke in the population. Quality of routine statistics in comparison with a population-based stroke registry. Neuroepidemiology 11:204–213

Thompson C 2003 Clinical experience as evidence in evidence-based practice. Journal of Advanced Nursing 43(3):230–237

Thompson C, McCaughan D, Cullum N et al 2001 Issues and innovations in nursing practice. Journal of Advanced Nursing 36(3):376–388

Upton T, Brooks B 1995 Managing change in the NHS. Kogan Page, London

Wigfield A, Boon E 1996 Critical care pathway development: the way forward. British Journal of Nursing 5(12):732–735

Further reading

Easton N, Getliffe K, Mundy K 2000 The South Thames Evidence-based Practice Project. Rehabilitation care options for stroke patients. St George's Hospital Medical School and Kingston University, London

Grant J, Fletcher M, Warwick C 2000 The South Thames Evidence-based Practice Project. Supporting breastfeeding women. St George's Hospital Medical School and Kingston University, London

Lancashire S, Gournay K, Firn S et al 2000 The South Thames Evidence-based Practice Project. Disseminating family intervention for schizophrenia in routine clinical practice. St George's Hospital Medical School and Kingston University, London

Perry L 2001 Screening swallowing function of patients with acute stroke: part one: identification, implementation and initial evaluation of a screening tool for use by nurses. Journal of Clinical Nursing 10(4):463–473

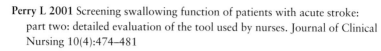

Perry L 2001 Screening swallowing function of patients with acute stroke: part two: detailed evaluation of the tool used by nurses. Journal of Clinical Nursing 10(4):474–481

Perry L, Love CP 2001 Screening for dysphagia and aspiration in acute stroke: a systematic review. Dysphagia 16(1):1–12

Tarpey A, Gould D, Rhodes V 2000 The South Thames Evidence-based Practice Project. Management of pressure areas in the acute setting. St George's Hospital Medical School and Kingston University, London

11

CHAPTER

How can we develop an evidence-based culture?

Carl Thompson

KEY POINTS

- The national policy imperative.
- What is meant by culture generally and an evidence-based culture specifically.
- Potential barriers to changing organisational culture.
- The need for diagnosis, planning and marketing.
- What works and what doesn't work in changing behaviours.
- What we can learn from case studies of evidence-based change.

Introduction

Culture shapes the beliefs and behaviours of those who deliver health care. Without an awareness of the impact of culture on the implementation and utilisation of research evidence, strategies for change will almost certainly fail. However, cultural change is hard to achieve in ways that are simple to predict (Davies et al 2000, Parker 2000, Scott et al 2003). Real-world, realistic strategies for evidence-based change in organisations require well-planned, targeted, informed strategies which incorporate what we know about both culture and the foreseeable effects of general and specific change interventions. Organisations such as the UK's NHS Service Delivery and Organisation Research and Development Programme (NHS SDO) and research teams such as the Performance and Culture group in the Centre for Health Economics at the University of York, UK, have extended our empirical and theoretical knowledge considerably since the first edition of this book. This chapter aims to steer a course through some of these developments.

National imperatives

A greater role for knowledge derived from scientific research in improving the quality of health services is a policy objective for many developed countries. Since the late 1990s, the UK government has pursued a systematic approach to quality improvement in the National Health Service (NHS). Clinical governance (Secretary of State for Health 1998) is the term intended to encapsulate this approach: 'A framework through which NHS organisations are accountable for continuously improving the quality of their services and safeguarding high standards of care by creating an environment in which excellence in clinical care will flourish' (p.33).

The boards of NHS organisations now have a formal duty to ensure that quality is improved and new bodies, such as the National Institute for Health and Clinical Excellence (NICE), National Service Frameworks (NSF), and the Health-care Commission, have been established in order to assist this process (Figure 11.1). Poor practice will be ever less acceptable. Chief executives will be subject to audit of the overall performance of their organisation (Secretary of State for Health 2000) and therefore they will increasingly be scrutinising the quality of health-care provision in individual clinical areas. In the United States, the Agency for Healthcare Research and Quality is a federal subagency of the Department of Health and Human Services. Since the late 1990s it has made an explicit commitment to fostering evidence-based provision of health care by supporting a range

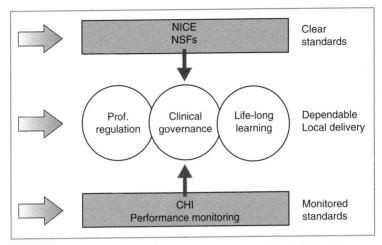

Figure 11.1 The NHS quality structure (from Department of Health 1998, with permission. Reproduced under the terms of the Click-Use Licence)

of evaluative initiatives in key areas such as using information technology to improve health and reducing disparities between communities.

Individual professional groups are similarly experiencing a policy 'push' towards evidence-based decision making. Indeed, the Department of Health (1999) is explicit in seeking a nursing profession that is made up of 'knowledgeable doers'. As the executive arm of government, individual employer organisations and the profession itself are firmly committed to addressing the difficult task of aligning quality, knowledge and the action of practitioners so the question 'How can we best develop an evidence-based practice culture?' looks more relevant than ever.

What does an evidence-based culture look like?

Organisational culture: what is it?

Culture is a contested concept. Despite the many ways of conceptualising it, two discernible strands emerge: culture as something that an organisation *is*, and something that an organisation *has* – in the form of attributes or variables that can be identified and shaped (Davies et al 2000). This distinction is important, for if organisations are the products of culture then there is considerably less scope for manipulating

> **BOX 11.1** Ten key features of organisational culture (adapted from Davies et al 2000)
>
> **Attitudes to innovation and risk taking:** the degree to which the organisation encourages and rewards new ways of doing things or, conversely, values tradition
>
> **Degree of central direction:** the extent of central setting of objectives and performance versus devolved decision making
>
> **Patterns of communication:** the degree to which instruction and reporting are channelled via formal hierarchies rather than informal networks
>
> **Outcome or process orientation:** whether the organisation values (focuses on) outcomes and results as opposed to tasks
>
> **Internal or external focus:** whether the organisation looks inward and restricts itself to organisational issues as opposed to looking at the needs of customers
>
> **Uniformity or diversity:** the organisational propensity towards consistency or diversity
>
> **People orientation:** valuation of the human resources available to an organisation
>
> **Team orientation:** does the organisation reward individualism or is it geared more towards teamwork?
>
> **Aggressiveness/competitiveness:** the extent to which the organisation seeks to dominate or co-operate with external competitors or players
>
> **Attitudes to change:** the extent to which the organisation demonstrates a predilection for stability in preference to dynamic change

and shaping progress towards organisational goals. On the other hand, if organisations possess attributes and values, then shaping and actively managing culture in order to reinforce strategic aims and goals becomes a possibility. Davies and colleagues (2000) suggest 10 key aspects of organisational culture (Box 11.1) that may be the focus of management efforts to align an organisation towards its goals and strategic aims (for example, the provision of increasingly evidence-based decisions as a route to better quality patient care).

An evidence-based practice culture

Muir Gray (1997) suggests that the basis for health-care provision is the decisions made within its structures and organisations. An evidence-based practice culture is one in which more good decisions are made than bad, and where research evidence, patient preferences, the available resources and

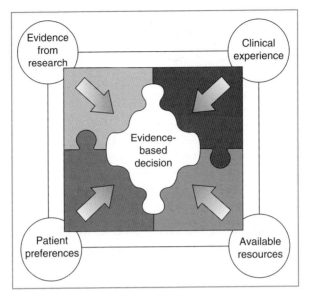

Figure 11.2 An evidence-based health-care decision

clinical expertise play an active part in decision-making processes (DiCenso et al 1998, Sackett et al 2000).

The key components of an evidence-based organisation, then, are: 'a built-in . . . capability to generate, and the flexibility to incorporate, evidence and individuals and teams who can find, appraise and use research evidence' (Muir Gray 1997, p.155). In order to achieve these characteristics, the organisation is dependent on the cultures, systems and structures contained within it. Moreover, all these elements share a degree of interdependence: systems that promote evidence-based decisions are no use unless accompanied by supportive structures and a facilitative cultural environment.

Evidence-based health care has five key processes:

1. converting health-care problems into focused health-care questions
2. searching for the best available research evidence
3. critically appraising the evidence retrieved
4. implementing the evidence
5. auditing the implementation.

Evidence-based organisational culture is one in which individuals and groups are totally committed to each of these stages and at all organisational levels. Brown (1999) notes that an organisational culture for evidence-based health care requires commitment at the level of:

- the individual
- clinical teams or practice groups
- health-care systems and organisations.

Before embarking on any attempt to change the culture of an organisation or group, key questions need addressing (Illes & Sutherland 2001), the most important of which is establishing why change is required and who and what can change. Only when this vital element of context has been mapped is it possible to plan for change.

Step one: diagnosing the challenges to changing practice – understanding complexity

Because changing cultures is complex, it is necessary to spend time trying to understand this complexity. In order to make sense of the context surrounding any planned change, a number of frameworks are available to help the manager or nurse. These include the 7s model, soft systems methodology, content context and process modelling and the '5 Whys' approaches (Illes & Sutherland 2001). These approaches vary in the effort and scope required to put them into practice. Accordingly, readers who require more detail of the methods are encouraged to look at the review by Illes & Sutherland (www.sdo.lshtm.ac.uk/pdf/changemanagement_review.pdf). However, some of the techniques are relatively simple to operationalise. For example, the '5 Whys' approach involves simply asking the question 'Why?' of a situation in which the focus is a single problem (see Box 11.2).

Any approach chosen as the basis for making sense of the complexity of a situation should:

- identify all the groups involved in, affected by or influencing the proposed change(s) in practice
- assess the characteristics of the proposed change that might influence its adoption
- assess the preparedness of health professionals to change and other potentially relevant internal factors within the target group
- identify the potential external barriers to change

BOX 11.2 The '5 whys' approach to understanding complexity

Problem: nurses are routinely ordering (unnecessary) urine tests on children who do not require them.

Why does this happen? It is seen as a necessary routine part of admission screening.

Why? Nurses do not understand the clinical value of looking at signs and symptoms and prevalence alongside the 'dipstick' urinalysis test they undertake.

Why? Nurses do not know about the positive predictive value of a test such as urinalysis.

Why? Nurses do not know what positive predictive value means and how to estimate it 'on the fly' in routine practice.

Why? Because they have not been introduced to the concept in practice and had its application reinforced.

- identify the likely enabling factors, including resources and skills (NHS CRD 1999).

Whilst these approaches are useful frameworks, they require gathering data as the means of providing answers to the questions generated. Techniques to consider as means of generating these data include:

- surveying key stakeholders (such as senior staff, managers and patient representatives) to identify the research appraisal and change management skills available. Similarly, some of the perceived barriers to research utilisation could be explored using survey approaches such as Funk's 'Barriers' Scale (Funk et al 1991). It is important to recognise, however, that reported barriers to utilisation may only capture those dimensions that individuals feel comfortable revealing. Moreover, in the field of research utilisation, what people say they do and what they actually do are often separate (Covell et al 1985, McCaughan et al 2005). The diagnostic value of this tool has not been established and so it is probably best considered as part of a broader suite of diagnostic activity

- adapting ward meetings or clinical supervision sessions so that potential problems can be identified, recorded and fed into the strategic planning process

- establishing focus groups of professionals, managers and, where appropriate, patient representatives, to identify pertinent barriers and drivers. Cameron & Wren (1999) used this approach by forming 'buzz' groups of 6–8 people who used 'reflection-on-action' (Schon 1983) to identify their values. These were typed and distributed to the group who then worked towards a collective understanding of the values identified.

Step two: how can evidence-based innovation and culture be encouraged?

Evidence-based innovation includes those new behaviours, routines and ways of working that are intended to improve health outcomes (Greenhalgh et al 2004). These innovations rarely happen by themselves; rather, they are planned and deliberate. Whilst there is no magic formula or bullet (Oxman et al 1995) for developing innovations, much is known about the ingredients required, even if the optimal 'mixes' remain hidden.

There are three major dimensions that must be addressed by anyone considering cultural change – to the point where it is manifest as changes in behaviour:

- the innovation itself
- the individuals and groups involved
- the system in which the innovation must operate.

Because none of the three elements operates in isolation from the others it is useful to add a fourth dimension to this list: the linkages between the innovation, its systemic context and the individuals involved.

The innovation

Those characteristics of the innovation itself associated with positive uptake in organisations are highlighted in Box 11.3.

The individual

Individuals within organisations work creatively with those organisations, and the individual differences that mark out team members also extend to the ways in which they interact with innovations. In order to maximise the chances of change adoption by a team and its members, it is important to understand some key characteristics and how they appear in the individual, team or work unit involved. Box 11.4 summarises the key dimensions to be charted.

BOX 11.3 Attributes of an innovation associated with adoption

Standard or universal attributes

Relative advantage: the degree to which a clear and unambiguous effectiveness or cost-effectiveness beyond 'where we are now' is present. Remembering that 'advantage' is often constructed by negotiations between stakeholders

Compatibility: fit with the values and norms of the workplace

Complexity: simple (or the ability to break down the innovation into a simple form) equates with higher chances

Trialability: can the innovation be tried out and experimented within the workplace?

Observability: observable benefits increase adoption

Reinvention: the ability to shape an innovation to suit one's own needs equates to a higher chance of adoption

Operational or context-specific attributes

Innovation: has to be seen as relevant for the adopter's work tasks

Performance improving: an innovation should be seen to improve performance in a given task

Perceived feasibility: in a given context

Divisibility: the ability to break it down into manageable components

Codified and transferable knowledge: the degree to which the knowledge needed to actually make use of the innovation can be separated from one context and transferred to another

---

The organisation as a knowledge-driven system

Using management to develop an organisation's structural and cultural components is a necessary step in encouraging assimilation of evidence-based innovations. The structural components of an organisation and their relationship to innovativeness (a key component of an evidence-based culture) are summarised in Table 11.1.

As can be seen from Table 11.1, a number of elements of culture can be manipulated in an organisation's drive to foster innovation. Not all the elements of an organisational system are within the direct control of a clinician or individual manager; they are, however, important elements of context to be borne in mind when developing change strategies.

BOX 11.4 Considerations at the level of the individual

Psychological precursors: cognitive and social psychology literature suggests that the degree to which someone is tolerant of ambiguity, their intellect and general values towards change will influence their propensity for trying new ideas. If the individual has identified a need and the innovation meets that need then change is more likely.

Meaning: the meaning that an innovation may have for an adopter needs to be established. If this meaning fits the meaning associated with management and other stakeholding groups then adopting an innovation is more likely.

Adoption decision nature: is the decision to opt into the innovation contingent (i.e. does it depend on someone else in the organisation?) or authoritative (a compulsory activity)? Whilst authoritative decisions may appear to increase chances of initial adoption, they also reduce the chances of long-term adoption.

Adoption decision stage concerns: it is important to remember that adoption is a process rather than a single event. Different concerns arise at different points in this process.

Before adoption – individuals need to be aware of the pending change and be given enough information to decide how it will affect them.

During the early stages – training and support to a level which will enable individuals to shape the change to their own working practices must be provided.

Once the change is established – feedback of the consequences enable individuals to continue to refine the innovation for their own environments.

Another important antecedent for developing an evidence-based culture at the level of systems is the organisation's capacity for absorbing new knowledge. Knowledge in service organisations underpins action; and the degree to which an organisation can codify what it does, capture new information, place it in the organisational context (so that it then becomes knowledge) and then design it into its work practices and decision-making machinery is an important determinant of the service that the public eventually receives (Ferlie et al 2001).

The knowledge that shapes social action, provides feedback on performance and 'feed-forward' (or task guidance) is socially constructed in health care. For example, a particular drug may objectively be 'effective' but the integration of patient values, its link to available resources and the expertise of the person delivering it all vary from context to context and, often, is negotiable. Once the contested nature of the knowledge

TABLE 11.1 ORGANISATIONAL SYSTEMIC CHARACTERISTICS AND RELATIONSHIP WITH INNOVATIVENESS IN ORGANISATIONS

Characteristic	Definition	Direction (positive or negative)
Administrative intensity	Administrative costs	+
Centralisation	Autonomy in decision making	−
Complexity	Degrees of professionalism and specialisation	+
External communication	Extent of workers' participation in professional activity outside the organisation	+
Formalisation	Degree of rule following and procedures	No significant relationship
Functional differentiation	Number of different work units	+
Internal communication	Communication between units	+
Managerial attitude to change		+
Managers' experience		No significant relationship
Professionalism	Degree of professional knowledge in the organisation	+
'Slackness'	The resources in an organisation that go beyond the minimum required to do the job	+
Specialisation	Number of specialties	+
Technical capacity	Amount of technical resource	+
Hierarchical levels	How many levels there are in the organisation	No significant relationship

required for managing decisions in health care, what Sackett and others (2000) term 'foreground' knowledge, is acknowledged, then the importance of the science of communication, knowledge management and transfer becomes apparent. As Greenhalgh and colleagues put it:

'... before it [knowledge] can contribute to organisational change initiatives, knowledge must be enacted and made social, entering into the stock of knowledge constructed and shared by other individuals. Knowledge depends for its circulation on interpersonal networks and will spread only when these social factors and barriers are overcome.' (Greenhalgh et al 2004, p.607)

Introducing new knowledge into an environment which is not receptive to change (or the possibility of it) is likely to lead to failure to innovate or change values, motivations and ultimately practice. Greenhalgh and colleagues (2004) suggest a number of indicators of receptive environments: strong leadership skills; clear strategic vision accompanied by managerial relations that help support that vision; key staff with a sense of shared vision; a risk-taking environment where trialling ideas is supported; and good systems of data capture. This last point is an essential component: data form the basis of information which, through the addition of context, then becomes knowledge.

Step three: how can change happen?

Thus far, I have concentrated on outlining some important components of what might be termed a framework for thinking about complexity and innovation in health-care settings. Considering these components is a necessary step for thinking about cultural change – not least in order to form a contextual backdrop for any planned action. Whilst all these elements are controllable to a greater or lesser degree, it is the level of specific change interventions (or, more accurately, combinations of specific change interventions) that provides the most fertile ground for most nurses to think about changing behaviour and impacting of values and goals relating to health-care provision.

The previous sections were aimed at diagnosing the change problem, mapping the antecedents of that problem most amenable to intervention, approaching the implementation of change in a planned and systematic way, and considering ways of evaluating its impact. A good start point for this generic approach to managing change generally is the *Clinical*

Effectiveness: What It's All About resource pack for nurses and health-care professionals produced by the NHS Executive (1999). Similarly the NHS Service Delivery and Organisation Programme produces a range of publications designed to aid change managers, details of which are presented at the end of the chapter.

Developing an evidence-based change toolkit

There is a surprising volume of material that summarises what we know about changing behaviour and managing the transition from abstract research knowledge into improved, and research-informed, professional decisions. Much of the high-quality material derived from randomised controlled trials has been summarised by the Cochrane Collaboration's Effective Practice and Organisation of Care Group (www.epoc.uottawa.ca/). Before considering specific elements of a change strategy, it is worth taking the time to think about the nature of the information used as the basis for day-to-day change and how this can be quality assured and the return for the time invested maximised.

Developing evidence-based ward literature: systems, synopses, syntheses and studies

The need to develop a store of good-quality information at ward or unit level arises out of a general recognition that nurses have limited time available for consulting written sources of information and that many resources are out of date and not evidence based. Moreover, obtaining a clinical bottom line for the patient in front of you is often difficult and involves the translation of hard-to-interpret research findings. Many sources are poorly organised, with few individuals being able to rapidly lay their hands on useful written information for every clinical problem. Moreover, nurses often invest time and considerable amounts of money in compiling these inadequate resources. Because of these human traits, wherever possible, change should be supported by a good-quality decision support system. Such systems are rare in nursing but they do exist (in anticoagulation clinics, for example) and in primary care in the (albeit limited) form of PRODIGY (www.prodigy.nhs.uk). Where such systems exist, they have the advantage of tailoring research-based clinical knowledge to the uncertainties associated with individual patients.

Where decision support systems do not exist, another efficient means of getting high-quality research messages, with the minimum of effort and maximum applicability, is in the form of synopses. The best forms of accessing synopses of information are the various evidence-based journals (such as *Evidence-based Nursing* and *Evidence-based Medicine*). An alternative that can be used for interventions other than simple pharmaceutical options is *Clinical Evidence* (www.clinicalevidence.com). These resources have the advantage that the critical appraisal and quality assurance are done for you (saving you time), with 'context' injected by virtue of the accompanying clinical commentary in the evidence-based journals.

Syntheses in the form of systematic reviews offer summarised information but have the relative disadvantage of requiring critical appraisal. Finally, searching for individual studies, even using computerised technology is labour intensive, relatively ineffective and uses up scarce time.

Other chapters in this book will deal with searching for resources, but what Brian Haynes calls the 4s approach to setting up an information strategy (Haynes 2001; Figure 11.3) should be the starting point for anyone seeking to use information to support clinical change.

As the NHS embraces electronic information technology (through, for example, NHSNet and the National Library for Health), it is crucial that

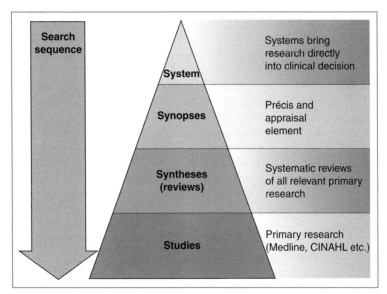

Figure 11.3 Derived from Haynes' 4s model of searching (and provision) of information sources

nurses acquire the skills to handle information effectively. There is no short-cut available to learning the computer and keyboard skills needed to use a personal referencing system or online database, but the investment will pay dividends. A first port of call for nurses employed by the NHS or by academic institutions within the UK is the National Library for Health (www.library.nhs.uk). This provides an invaluable source of quality-assured information including links to many of the resources listed below.

Table 11.2 gives some examples of evidence-based written and electronic sources of knowledge.

What works and what doesn't?

Empirical scrutiny of what works in terms of the behavioural element of getting evidence into practice has led to some tentative estimates of the 'effect size' of various strategies for changing practice and impacting on culture. These effect sizes are sobering. It is clear that the likely gains in performance based on what we know about changing practice may be far lower, and with greater variability, than is often assumed by those developing interventions. Moreover, it appears unlikely that simply combining interventions in the hope that more will be necessarily better exerts a greater or more predictable improvement in performance or its cultural component.

Continuing education: 'study days'

Study days, professional development courses, conference attendance and postregistration courses are all common features of many nurses' career trajectories and plans. However, as a stand-alone intervention, study days are not particularly effective. Five systematic reviews (Beaudry 1989, Bertram & Brooks-Bertram 1977, Davis et al 1995, Lloyd & Abrahamson 1979, Waddell 1991) all examine the impact of educational approaches to changing health-care professional behaviours. Waddell (1991) focuses specifically on nurses. The results are contradictory, with most reviews reporting at least some effect, but the validity of the reviews is hampered by the poor quality of many of the primary research reports. It is significant, however, that the high-quality systematic reviews (Davis et al 1995) conclude that continuing educational approaches are a relatively ineffective way of changing practice. Conversely, those reviews of lesser quality tend towards viewing study days as more effective (Waddell 1991). Grimshaw et al (2004) reported a 1% absolute improvement in performance attributable to educational meetings.

TABLE 11.2 SOURCES OF EVIDENCE-BASED HEALTH-CARE KNOWLEDGE FOR A WARD OR UNIT LIBRARY

Source	Description
Effective Healthcare Bulletins	Based around systematic reviews of effectiveness and cost-effectiveness studies. Produced by the NHS CRD at the University of York. Dealing with a range of clinical and management topics. Available through the National Library for Health (NLH): www.library.nhs.uk and www.york.ac.uk
Effectiveness Matters	Complements *Effective Healthcare*, provides updates on the effectiveness of important health interventions for practitioners and decision makers in the NHS. Covers topics in a shorter, more journalistic style, summarising the results of high-quality systematic reviews. Available through the NLH and www.york.ac.uk
Centre for Reviews and Dissemination (CRD) reports	Detailed reports of the systematic reviews carried out by CRD (in-depth, detailed and comprehensive). Available through the NLH and www.york.ac.uk
Evidence-based journals	Journals such as *Evidence-Based Nursing*, *Evidence-Based Medicine*, *Evidence-Based Mental Health*, *Evidence-Based Healthcare Management*, and *ACP Journal Club* offer concise summaries and clinical commentaries of the best quality research evidence. *Evidence-Based Nursing* available through www.evidencebasednursing.com
Epidemiologically based needs assessments	Published by the NHS Executive to support the commissioning process
Health Technology Assessments (HTA)	Some of the NHS HTA programme consists of systematic reviews. Available through the NLH and www.hta.nhsweb.nhs.uk
Clinical Evidence	*Clinical Evidence* is a 6-monthly, updated compendium of evidence on the effects of common clinical interventions, published by the BMJ Publishing Group. It provides a concise account of the current state of knowledge, ignorance and uncertainty about the prevention and treatment

(Continued)

TABLE 11.2 (CONTINUED)

Source	Description
	of a wide range of clinical conditions based on thorough searches of the literature. It is not a textbook of medicine or a book of guidelines. It summarises the best available evidence, and where there is no good evidence, it says so. Available through the NLH and www.clinicalevidence.com/
Cochrane Library	The Cochrane Library contains 4 databases which can be accessed via the internet (and NHSNet) and local CD ROM: 1. Cochrane Database of Systematic Reviews: a database of systematic reviews and planned reviews carried out for the Cochrane Collaboration 2. Database of Abstracts of Reviews of Effectiveness (DARE): critically appraised abstracts of systematic reviews. The abstracts are produced by reviewers from the NHS CRD at the University of York 3. Cochrane Review Methodology Update: articles, links and resources for those considering or undertaking a review 4. Cochrane Controlled Trials Register: a register of controlled trials identified by reviewers for the Cochrane Collaboration. Available through the NLH and www.cochranelibrary.com
National Clinical Guidelines	The RCN is beginning to produce guidelines (so far in the management of leg ulcers and pain in children). The NICE is set to produce clinical guidelines based on reviews of good-quality research evidence. At present organisations such as the Scottish Intercollegiate Guidelines Network and the North of England Guidelines Group also produce evidence-based clinical guidelines. Available through the NLH and www.rcn.org.uk
MEDLINE and CINAHL	Databases such as MEDLINE and CINAHL are invaluable, especially where the above sources fail to yield relevant information. An internet version of MEDLINE, PubMed, is available through the NLH and www.ncbi.nlm.nih.gov/entrez/query.fcgi

Clinical guidelines

Clinical guidelines have proved an influential and attractive mechanism for influencing behaviour in nursing, with the Royal College of Nursing in the UK committed to sponsoring, and co-operating in, their production. However, as in the case of continuing professional development, their success should not be assumed uncritically. Thomas et al (1999) have undertaken a systematic review of the role of clinical guidelines as a route to reducing inappropriate variations in practice and promoting the delivery of evidence-based health care (see Chapter 7 for details about the systematic review). They suggest that the best advice for a nurse wishing to use guidelines to change practice is to learn from the experiences of other groups – notably medicine – and to develop strategies that draw on evidence-based theoretical perspectives (Grol 1992). The NHS CRD (1999) found that properly developed guidelines can influence practice, but work best if adapted to local circumstance, used in conjunction with supportive educational strategies and use specific reminders to help professionals in their decision making.

Of course, some strategies such as integrated care pathways manage to combine at least some of these elements. Pathways are commonly based around local systems and processes, supported by clinical and managerial teams, based on a guideline format and have reminders built into documentation and monitoring technologies which are often part of larger scale clinical audit. However, we have only limited evidence of their success (Marrie et al 2000), as they have not been exposed to large-scale evaluation.

Other broad approaches

A number of systematic reviews examine the effectiveness of broad dissemination and implementation strategies (Oxman et al 1995, Wensing & Van Der Weijden 1998, Yano et al 1995), providing research information alone, management approaches and social influence approaches. Most of the reviews concur with Oxman et al's (1995) assertion that there are 'no magic bullets' when it comes to changing professional practice or attitudes. Based on the evidence, multifaceted approaches to change, whilst more expensive, have the most impact. However, this impact is unpredictable and doesn't always work across every situation.

Specific interventions

A number of systematic reviews examine whether or not specific approaches are useful for clinicians or managers seeking to introduce change. It should be stressed that, in examining these interventions, good-quality evaluative methodology has been weighted above nurse-specific content.

Educational outreach/detailing

Academic or educational detailing involves trained individuals going out to practice environments to help promote the utilisation of research findings in practice. We have used this approach at York in the area of compression bandaging for venous leg ulceration, but it has proved particularly successful in the prescribing arena. Until now, most of the work has been conducted in North American settings with doctors, but the approach may be useful in attempting to change practice amongst nurses. The effect of outreach approaches is maximised when they are conducted alongside a social marketing framework. The National Research Register (www.update-software.com/NRR/) gives contact details of researchers currently examining the value of educational outreach in the UK and some of these studies are specific to nursing, for example, 'An evaluation of the effectiveness and cost effectiveness of audit and feedback and educational outreach in improving nursing practice and outcomes' and 'Educational outreach in diabetes to encourage practice nurses to respond to guidelines to control hypertension and hyperlipidaemia in primary and shared care (EDEN): a randomised trial using a blocked reciprocal control design'. Generally, 'interactive' approaches to educating groups of professionals may yield positive results (Bero et al 1998). Grimshaw et al's (2004) analysis of educational outreach (both on its own and alongside other strategies) provides an estimate of a 6% improvement in absolute performance. Based on their analysis it is possible to suggest that:

- educational outreach alone may be relatively ineffective
- combinations of educational materials, educational meetings and educational outreach may have only modest to moderate effects
- there is no clear relationship between number of interventions and effect size.

Reminders

Reminders, whether manual or electronic, have been shown to be effective in improving preventive care (Shea et al 1996) and general management of patients. Grimshaw et al (2004) suggest that improvements in performance of up to 14% can be possible. However, as nurses increasingly diagnose and treat common conditions (such as asthma), their effect in relation to improving diagnostic behaviour is uncertain (Hunt et al 1998). Additionally, the evidence in favour of reminders as a component of a change strategy is strengthened as evaluations have been derived from a wide range of populations and clinical areas.

Audit and feedback

It is doubtful that clinical audit, on its own, is a sufficient mechanism for sustained change. Those studies looking at whether audit and feedback approaches to change result in improved behaviours (Balas et al 1996, Buntinx et al 1993, Thomson et al 1999) report at best only moderate effects and see it as less effective than less labour-intensive methods (such as reminders). Audit and feedback, as part of a wider strategy, has some merit but as a stand-alone approach to change, it should not be relied upon.

Local opinion leaders

Thomson et al (1999) report that local opinion leaders as conduits for change have mixed effects on professional practice. However, we don't always know what local opinion leaders do and descriptions of their characteristics are often lacking. Thomson et al (1999) suggest that further research is required to determine the identifying characteristics of leaders and the circumstances in which they are likely to influence the practice of their peers. Bero et al (1998) suggest that colleagues nominated by peers as 'educationally influential' might be a useful characteristic to focus on. Our own work, however, suggests that it is 'clinical credibility' (in the form of experience) rather than research competence or awareness that proves influential in getting nurses to engage with imparted information (Thompson et al 2000). In this multiple case site study, we found that nurses often perceived other nurses as a very influential block on them using research. Local opinion leaders (often those embodying the clinical nurse specialist role) were a powerful force for change.

Local consensus approaches

Mulhall & Le May (1999, p.200) recognise that 'ownership of the [change] project by nurses is important' and this statement is borne out by the evidence. Bero et al (1998) report that inclusion of stakeholder professionals in discussions to ensure their perception of the change problem as 'important' is developed and their response defined as 'appropriate' can exert some effect. However, the results of their scrutiny are mixed and consensus alone should not be relied upon.

Patient-mediated interventions

If a patient asked you to justify your choice of wound dressing or urinary catheter, would it change your approach? This kind of question lies at the core of patient-mediated interventions. Providing information to patients to use in a specific way in professional consultations can, in theory, exert an impact on the behaviour of clinicians. For example, many professionals are increasingly encountering the 'internet-informed' patient and anecdotally, I have encountered health-care professionals who claim that this 'makes them think twice' about the sorts of information and care provided. However, here too results are mixed and patient-mediated approaches are not a sufficient stand-alone mechanism for cultural shift.

Multifaceted interventions

In general, successful change interventions are multifaceted and targeted to combat specific local contextual factors or barriers to change. The theoretical basis for the combining of interventions is often unclear and results in something akin to a 'kitchen sink' (as in 'everything but the') approach to strategy. This may explain the empirical truth that 'more is not necessarily better' (Grimshaw et al 2004).

Making the most of what is on offer: why 'passive' approaches to change may not be as bad as we think

Those sources of research-based knowledge which many nurses rely on, such as didactic lecture-style study days, passively disseminated clinical practice guidelines, lecture notes, educational videos and protocols, seem to generate only marginal (at best) gains on performance. Freemantle et al (1999), in a review of printed educational materials, found no statistically significant improvements in practice. Similarly, Bero and colleagues (1998) report that didactic-style educational meetings are not useful for inducing change in practice. However, it is clear that whilst gains in performance may only be marginal, the gains in performance for expensive multifaceted interventions may – in absolute terms – not be that much higher, particularly where those interventions are not targeted or lack a strong theoretical foundation. Any strategy must take into account the costs involved. Comprehensive, multifaceted interventions which are ill thought out and expensive may be less useful than passive strategies that are cheaper.

Real-life examples of changing practice and culture

Case 1: A national approach

In the course of teaching nurses about evidence-based health care, the comment is often made that evidence-based health care is only for the 'technical' aspects of nursing or those roles that are seen as 'cutting edge' in nursing and health care (such as nurse practitioners or the emerging discipline of advanced practitioners). In the UK, however, policy makers and the professions are using a series of national benchmarks alongside audit, education and practice development to apply the principles of evidence-based health care to the basics of essential aspects of patient care in areas such as maintaining privacy and dignity, communication, continence and pressure area care. The policy initiative – called the 'essence of care' – focuses on a series of standards (benchmarks) that are derived from research evidence and adjusted in response to structured consultation with patients, carers and other stakeholders.

The benchmarks are designed to be tailored to local service delivery contexts via the PDSA framework (Plan, Do, Study, Act), a technique for testing 'change ideas'. Local operationalisation of the benchmarks has exposed the variations between services with respect to their location in the cycle of PDSA. Conversely, the local nature of the operationalisation has resulted in systems that are planned, implemented and evaluated with local context in mind. The national governmental, policy and professional 'steer' has many advantages, some of which are present in the review of the characteristics of innovation offered by Greenhalgh and colleagues (2004).

The standards themselves are evidence based, represent policy concerns and incorporate the values of users and the input of expert clinicians. The nature of the implementation process allows for trialling of the change ideas associated with progress towards the standards. The linkage to local and national audit processes allows for demonstration of progress (or, conversely, the possibility of a lack of it) – a powerful driver in an era of (limited) competition between providers for patients and interprovider comparisons of performance. The standards have high degrees of work relevance and are designed to produce improved and visible task performance. Through the link with audit activity, there is the potential for feedback of task performance and the standards' roles as frameworks for action offer a degree of feed-forward guidance for specific tasks associated with nursing roles. Despite having uniform standards to adhere to, different UK health-care providers are at different locations in the PDSA cycle. For an example of the variation in a single geographical area in the UK, look at www.berkshire. nhs.uk/tvsc/groups/Directory.htm.

Changes in the 'culture' of the national workforce are much harder to demonstrate than changes in the activities of individuals or teams charged with implementing this policy. Many of the UK reports on progress towards meeting these standards detail the 'activity' that surrounds the implementation – for example, the establishment of a forum, the appointment of 'champions' and the drafting of best practice. What is less common is the reporting of changes in patient outcome and workforce culture arising from the kind of multifaceted and targeted interventions that develop locally in response to national initiatives such as this. The link between changes in outcome and targeted multifaceted interventions is clearer in Case 2.

Case 2: A co-ordinated approach in the context of high-quality evaluation

Horbar and colleagues (2004) used a cluster randomised clinical trial as an opportunity to evaluate the success of a collaborative multifaceted change intervention to increase the uptake of surfactant (a substance that reduces the surface tension in fragile lungs) in neonatal infants in 57 neonatal intensive care units. The intervention was based around three key components:

- *audit* and *individualised confidential feedback* on peer comparison-related performance regarding administration and timing of surfactant, and delivery room practice for infants of 23–29 weeks' gestation
- a *workshop* made up of didactic sessions, facilitated site team exercises, and multi-institutional group exercises. The intervention was designed to promote four key cultural 'habits' (change, evidence-based practice, systems thinking, and collaborative learning). The sites were all supported via quarterly conference calls and an email discussion list. Control sites simply received centre-specific, confidential performance reports.

The effect of the intervention on routine administration in the delivery room was clinically and statistically significant. The relative benefit increase associated with the intervention was 200% (95% CI 176–228) with 55% of the intervention group (as opposed to 18% of the controls) routinely administering surfactant. The study failed to detect changes in mortality (it was not designed to do so) but does illustrate that theoretically informed multifaceted interventions can exert a powerful effect on the processes of health-care delivery – processes that are influenced (and maintained) by the culture of the organisation.

Change as a result of attempts at specifically influencing culture is often characterised by a series of decidedly non-linear periods of growth, plateaus, apparent demise and re-emergence: it is transformational (Illes & Sutherland 2001) (see Figure 11.4).

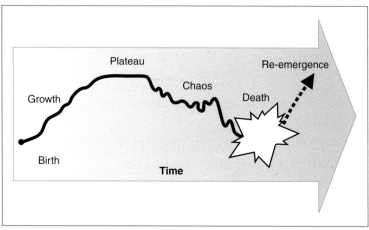

Figure 11.4 Transformational organisational change (derived from Illes & Sutherland 2001)

Case 3: The mediating effects of transformational change and local context

Newman et al (2000) developed a theoretically informed, locally tailored multifaceted intervention explicitly designed to change the prevailing culture of practice. The developers used a combination of specific change interventions ('link nurses', clinical supervision and educational outreach) nested within a broader action research framework. Perhaps crucially, they chose not to inject extra resources to support the change intervention, ostensibly to increase its 'realism'. They chose problems that were raised by the ward staff involved and used the generic evidence-based skills and techniques of question formulation, searching, appraisal, changing practice and evaluation to address them. Changes in culture and processes of health-care delivery were measured by using a combination of indicators such as staff sickness (believed to be linked to morale), patient complaints, the numbers of PICO questions generated (see Chapter 2) and searches undertaken, the nurses' perception of the impact of the project, and the quality of nursing documentation.

The strategic intervention met with only partial success. On the positive side, the project resulted in a number of improvements in work role and design (team and named nurses were introduced, better patient assessment, a standardised format for handing over patients – with accompanying clinical questions – team and self duty rostering and performance review). The strategy also reduced sickness by 10 days per month (95% CI 5.3–14.3) and was perceived as enhancing communication, confidence, leadership and teamwork.

On the less positive side, however, many of the organisational changes were not sustained, systems to link question formulation and searching failed to be fully operationalised, some nursing cultural subgroups actively resisted the project and the ward manager served as a negative role model for evidence-based practice. In the words of the researchers, 'changes were fragile and easily reversed'.

The evaluation took place over 10 months and what was observed may only have captured a small element of the transformational change sequence. The absence of extra resources – if only as a marker of organisational commitment and 'buy-in' – was possibly also a contributory factor to the intervention's relatively small long-term impact. Ultimately, the project leaders concluded that clinical units are unlikely to operationalise evidence-based practice without considering local professional and organisational contexts. As well as local contexts, they highlight particular structural issues such as the priority afforded to evidence-based practice by organisations; the matching of resources to workloads; preparing clinical leaders and nurses for using evidence-based practice skills and deploying new knowledge; and the need for ongoing development of 'generic' critical thinking and problem-solving skills (Newman et al 2000).

This last example represents a form of caveat for those considering trying to change organisational culture. Even with diagnosis, a theoretical framework and a multi-approach strategy using validated techniques, the results are often far from certain and nothing can be assumed.

Two examples from the King's Fund report *Getting Better with Evidence* (Wye & McClenahan 2000) suggest that sustainable change is possible with attention to the kinds of local, contextual and structural issues highlighted by Newman and colleagues.

Case 4: A nurse-led anticoagulation clinic

A group of secondary care trusts were targeted by the local health authority as suitable for the establishment of nurse-led anticoagulation clinics. Their strategy focused on using a combination of clinical guidelines, training and local opinion leaders to influence the approach. Guidelines were drawn up by consultant haematologists for nurses in conjunction with safety objectives and a short two-page protocol for the management of deep vein thrombosis and pulmonary embolism. To complement this, two nurses were given intensive (14 sessions in the first 3 months) and personalised training by two consultants. The two nurses also visited well-established nurse-led clinics in other areas. The overall leadership and 'steer' for the project was provided by the two respected and enthusiastic medical consultants. The project was audited every 3 months and the results fed back into the service planning and implementation loop. Data collected were a combination of clinical outcomes (such as mortality in stroke inpatients) and more qualitative end-user (patient and doctor) views on the service. The service also utilised a paper reminder in the form of a questionnaire on atrial fibrillation sent to local GPs that acted to reinforce the presence of the service.

The service is now well established in two main sites and being developed in a third. Numbers of patients on warfarin have increased and the general feeling is that nurses run the clinics well and that as a model of service delivery, the framework is successful and sustainable. However, the project did have to contend with funding and information technology problems. Despite the perceived success of the project, the outcomes audit reveals that admissions for strokes have not fallen from the 212 and 198 per year established at baseline in each site. The authors are at a loss as to how to explain this but the project does highlight the issue that perceived improvements in a service might not be accompanied by a change in patient outcomes. Change is often long term and measures of 'success' multidimensional and sensitive and because of this, it may be advantageous to examine 'softer' indicators of success such as the levels of satisfaction with the process of care delivery.

Case 5: Primary care leg ulcer clinics

In this example, a group of inner-city tissue viability specialist nurses (TVNs) wanted to develop, implement and audit their local guidelines on managing leg ulcers and then go on to set up two community-based leg ulcer clinics. The aim of this was to reduce variations in practice and outcomes across the trust and to reduce inappropriate referrals to an already busy complex wound clinic.

The nurses developed a fivefold strategy:

- *locally developed guidelines*: based on an inclusive, multidisciplinary development process that was actively 'marketed' in trust settings at lunch times
- *opinion leaders*: the two well-respected TVNs worked with nurses on a part-time basis and ensured that they also worked with consultants and local GPs
- *educational workshops*: these took place 'in-service' and were aimed at familiarising nurses with the guidelines and, crucially, learning to relate the guidelines to real patients and patient problems

- *targeted meetings and multidisciplinary training*: these focused on generating sufficient interest in practitioners so that they wanted to host clinics. Moreover, these involved targeting the most enthusiastic practitioner in a local team in order that they would persuade their more sceptical colleagues
- *training and feedback*: the TVNs visited each clinic once a month and offered real-time training, support and, crucially, the application of the guidelines during patient consultations.

This approach has led to the development of two clinics with a third in progress with broad cross-disciplinary support for the new ways of working. However, the team failed to collect patient data before or after the development of the clinics, which meant they had no baseline criteria for measuring their success. As well as this design fault, the team had to struggle against the very real constraints of underfunding, recruitment difficulties, competing priorities and variable morale and enthusiasm amongst staff. The qualitative comments of staff, in particular, reveal that relatively small changes such as changing the ways in which clinical nurse specialists work (giving them a trust-wide remit with responsibility for individual training and professional development) can yield good results, even in the context of a far from perfect strategy: 'Having (the clinical nurse specialist) there to discuss different things makes a difference. When you are seeing seven leg ulcers in a row, it leads to better practice. We are using the leg ulcer care programme lots . . . the professional development is the best part of it' (p.36).

So a relatively small change can have a significant impact on the development of others' expertise and professional development. Importantly, the team involved learned from their mistakes and were trying to factor in the solutions for the future: 'We would invest a proportion of the project's resources in a baseline audit because demonstrating improvement in healing rates provides the ultimate proof that an initiative to upgrade the care of patients with leg ulcers is working' (p.36).

Ultimately, the researchers conclude that the team's greatest (cultural) achievement was their contribution to the replacement of '. . . a severely fragmented, demoralised organisation with one where staff are enthusiastic and open to learning'.

Conclusion: culture, practice change and evidence-based health care

This chapter has shown how complex an entity organisational culture is and how difficult it is to try and mould something that is, by definition, malleable and contingent on so many other factors. Despite this complexity, I have outlined a number of strategies which, if used in conjunction with broad and specific interventions, could reasonably be expected to yield some results.

Most people would agree that evidence-based health care should be a reality but very often tips on how to deliver the necessary behavioural (and, by implication, cultural) changes are lacking. This chapter has argued that strategy and working with proven approaches can help add the local detail necessary to complement the national directives.

As Oxman et al (1995) point out, there are 'no magic bullets' when attempting organisational change. However, by strategically arming yourself with a number of different techniques for changing culture and behaviour, you can at least give yourself and your team a fighting chance of successfully introducing change.

To conclude, then, the clinician or manager considering change should employ a good diagnostic work-up of the factors likely to hinder or promote research use in decisions. This should focus on the levels of individuals, teams and the organisation and consider strategically targeting barriers and subgroups within each of these elements. Moreover, initial efforts should focus on those areas over which the team has a modicum of control (for example, the text-based ward resources amassed by the ward, unit or practice; the roles of key individuals such as the clinical nurse specialist or the link nurse; or the support and nature of skills training). Whilst being aware of the likely time scale involved and the non-linear progress of change, ensure that the process is seen as cyclical, with audit and feedback designed into the strategy.

Summary points

- Evidence-based change is a national policy imperative and unavoidable in practice.
- Evidence-based culture is one which is totally committed to balanced decisions which give due weight to research evidence, patient preference, available resources and clinical expertise. This commitment is manifest at the levels of the individual, clinical teams and health-care systems.
- Successful strategies for change are likely to be multifaceted, targeted at specific cultural groups in the organisation.
- Specific groups for targeted and planned change interventions are best identified through sensitive diagnostic strategies.

- Common barriers to change amongst nurses often relate to the information they have available, professional cultural resistance to some forms of evidence, environmental factors such as the availability of evidence, and individual psychology relating to change.
- Theoretical models such as social marketing may prove useful as a way of structuring change strategies, but evidence to date is lacking.
- Consistently effective interventions include educational outreach, electronic or paper-based reminders and multifaceted approaches.
- Audit and feedback alone has a mixed and unpredictable impact on changing professional behaviour and culture.
- Didactic study days, clinical guidelines and protocols that are passively disseminated have little or no effect on practice.

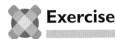 ## Exercise

Take a common clinical or managerial problem and try and answer the following questions.

- How can we understand the complexities and interdependence that surround the problem?
- Why does my organisation need to change?
- Who and what can change?
- How can this change happen?

Now read the publication *Developing change management skills. A resource for health care professionals and managers* (freely available at: www.sdo.lshtm. ac.uk/publications.htm). Then try and answer the questions above again, applying some of the tools and techniques introduced in the publication.

References

Balas E A, Austin S M, Mitchell J et al 1996 The clinical value of computerized information services: a review of 98 randomised clinical trials. Archives of Family Medicine 5:271–278

Beaudry J S 1989 The effectiveness of continuing medical education: a quantitative synthesis. Journal of Continuing Education for the Health Professions 9:285–307

Bero L A, Grilli R, Grimshaw J M et al 1998 Closing the gap between research and practice: an overview of systematic reviews of interventions to promote the implementation of research findings. British Medical Journal 317:465–468

Bertram D A, Brooks-Bertram P A 1977 The evaluation of continuing medical education: a literature review. Health Education Monographs 5:330–362

Brown S J 1999 Knowledge for health care practice: a guide to using research evidence. W B Saunders, London

Buntinx F, Winkens R, Grol R et al 1993 Influencing diagnostic and preventative performance in ambulatory care by feedback and reminders. A review. Family Practice 10:219–228

Cameron G, Wren A M 1999 Reconstructing organisational culture: a process using multiple perspectives. Public Health Nursing 16(2):96–101

Covell D G, Gwen C, Uman R N, Manning P R 1985 Information needs in office practice: are they being met? Annals of Internal Medicine 103: 596–599

Davies H T O, Nutley S M, Mannion R 2000 Organisational culture and quality of health care. Quality in Health Care 9:111–119

Davis D A, Thomson M A, Oxman A D et al 1995 Changing physician performance: a systematic review of the effect of continuing medical education strategies. Journal of the American Medical Association 274:700–705

Department of Health 1998 A first class service. Stationery Office, London

Department of Health 1999 Making a difference: strengthening the nursing, midwifery and health visiting contribution to health and health care. HMSO, London

DiCenso A, Cullum N, Ciliska D 1998 Implementation forum. Implementing evidence-based nursing: some misconceptions. Evidence-based Nursing 1(2):38–40

Ferlie E J, Gabbay L, Fitzgerald L E, Dopson S 2001 Evidence-based medicine and organisational change. In: Ashburner L (ed) Organisational behaviour and organisational studies in health care: reflections on the future. Palgrave, Basingstoke

Freemantle N, Harvey E L, Wolf F et al 1999 Printed educational materials to improve the behaviour of health care professionals and patient outcomes (Cochrane Review). Cochrane Library, Issue 1. Update Software, Oxford

Funk S, Champagne M T, Wiese R A, Tornquist E M 1991 Barriers: the Barriers to Research Utilization Scale. Applied Nursing Research 4(1):39–45

Greenhalgh T, Glenn R, Bate P et al 2004 Diffusion of innovations in service organisations: systematic review and recommendations. Millbank Quarterly 82(4):581–629

Grimshaw J M, Thomas R E, MacLennan G et al 2004 Effectiveness and efficiency of guideline dissemination and implementation strategies. Health Technology and Assessment 8(6):i–iv, 1–72

Grol R 1992 Implementing guidelines in general practice care. Quality in Health Care 1:184–191

Haynes R B 2001 Of studies, syntheses, synopses, and systems: the '4S' evolution of services for finding current best evidence. ACP Journal Club 134: A11–A13

Horbar J D, Carpenter J H, Buzas J et al 2004 Collaborative quality improvement to promote evidence-based surfactant for preterm infants: a cluster randomised trial. British Medical Journal 329:1004

Hunt D L, Haynes R B, Hanna S E et al 1998 Effects of computer based decision support on physician performance and patient outcomes. A systematic review. Journal of the American Medical Association 280:1339–1346

Illes V, Sutherland K 2001 Organisational change: a review for health care managers, professionals and researchers. NCC SDO, London

Lloyd J S, Abrahamson S 1979 Effectiveness of continuing medical education: a review of the evidence. Evaluation and the Health Professions 2:251–280

Marrie T J, Lau C Y, Wheeler S L, Wong C J, Vandervoort M K, Feagan B G 2000 A controlled trial of a critical pathway for treatment of community-acquired pneumonia. Journal of the American Medical Association 283(6):749–755

McCaughan D, Thompson C, Cullum N, Sheldon T A, Raynor P 2005 Nurse practitioner and practice nurses' use of research information in clinical decision making: findings from an exploratory study. Family Practice 22(5):490–497

Muir Gray J A 1997 Evidence-based health care: how to make health policy and management decisions. Churchill Livingstone, Edinburgh

Mulhall A, Le May A 1999 Nursing research: dissemination and implementation. Churchill Livingstone, London

Newman M, Papadopoulos I, Melifonwu R 2000 Developing organisational systems and culture to support evidence-based practice: the experience of the Evidence-based Ward Project. Evidence-based Nursing 3:103–105

NHS Centre for Reviews and Dissemination (CRD) 1999 Getting evidence into practice. Effective Health Care Bulletin 5(1):1–16

NHS Executive 1999 Clinical effectiveness:what it's all about. Available online at: www.doh.gov.uk/pub/docs/doh/aep.pdf

Oxman A, Thomson M A, Davis D A, Haynes R B 1995 No magic bullets: a systematic review of 102 trials of interventions to improve professional practice. Canadian Medical Association Journal 153(10):1423–1431

Parker M 2000 Organisational culture and identity: unity and division at work. Sage, London

Sackett D L, Strauss S E, Richardson W S, Rosenberg W, Haynes R B 2000 Evidence-based medicine: how to practise and teach EBM. Churchill Livingstone, London

Schon D 1983 The reflective practitioner: how professionals think in action. Basic Books, New York

Scott T, Mannion R, Davies H T O, Marshall M 2003 Implementing culture change in health care: theory and practice. International Journal for Quality in Health Care 15(2):111–118

Secretary of State for Health 1998 A first class service: quality in the new NHS. Department of Health, London

Secretary of State for Health 2000 The NHS plan. Department of Health, London

Shea S, DuMouchel W, Bahamonde L 1996 A meta-analysis of 16 randomised controlled trials to evaluate computer-based clinical reminder systems for preventative care in the ambulatory setting. Journal of the American Medical Informatics Association 3:399–409

Thomas L, Cullum N, McColl F, Rousseau N, Soutter J, Steen N 1999 Clinical guidelines in nursing, midwifery and other professions allied to medicine (Cochrane Review). Cochrane Library, Issue 1. Update Software, Oxford

Thompson C, McCaughan D, Cullum N, Sheldon T A, Thompson D R, Mulhall A 2000 Nurses' use of research information in clinical decision making: a descriptive and analytical study – final report. NHS R&D, NCC SDO, London

Thomson M A, Oxman A D, Davis D A, Haynes R B, Freemantle N, Harvey E L 1999 Outreach visits to improve health professional practice and health care outcomes (Cochrane Review). Cochrane Library, Issue 1. Update Software, Oxford

Waddell D L 1991 The effects of continuing education on nursing practice: a meta-analysis. Journal of Continuing Education in Nursing 22:113–118

Wensing M, Van Der Weijden T R G 1998 Implementing guidelines and innovations in general practice: which interventions are effective? British Journal of General Practice 48:991–997

Wye L, McClenahan J 2000 Getting better with evidence: experiences of putting evidence into practice. King's Fund, London

Yano E M, Fink A, Hirsch S H et al 1995 Helping practices reach primary care goals. Lessons from the literature. Archives of Internal Medicine 155:1146–1156

Glossary

Absolute risk reduction (ARR) & increase (ARI) This figure tells us the size of the difference between outcomes in the intervention (or exposure) group and outcomes in the control group. It is the absolute arithmetical difference between the experimental (or exposure) event rate (EER) and the control event rate (CER). To calculate: [EER − CER].

Allocation concealment Ensuring that the person who enrols individuals into a study is unaware of the group to which that individual will be allocated. Techniques include using sequentially numbered, sealed, opaque envelopes, with each envelope containing details of the group to which that individual is to be allocated (e.g. group A or group B). Central randomisation services are also used, where people not involved in the study hold the randomisation details. At the time of allocating the individual to a group, the investigator contacts the service to find out whether that individual is to go into group A or group B.

Bias Systematic error in the design, conduct or interpretation of a study that may distort the results of the study away from the 'truth'.

Blinding (masking) Concealing whether or not the participant is receiving (or has received) the experimental intervention. In an ideal study, the research participant, the people administering the intervention(s), the people assessing the outcomes and the data analysts will be blinded. The terms single-blind, double-blind or triple-blind are sometimes used to indicate the level of blinding. For example, where both the participants and the investigators assessing the outcomes are blinded, the trial may be classified as double-blind. However, it is important to note that these terms are not used consistently.

Boolean operators Used when searching electronic databases to combine search terms. They include AND, OR and NOT.

Case–control study An observational study where a group of individuals with the target disorder (cases) and a group of individuals without the target disorder (controls) are identified. Researchers look back in time to try and identify whether the exposure of interest was more prevalent in one group than the other.

Case series A study reporting on a series of patients who have all experienced an outcome of interest, and where there is no control group.

CATs & CATmaker software CAT is the abbreviated term for critically appraised topic. It is a summary of individual item(s) of evidence that you create yourself in response to an information need. The Centre for Evidence-Based Medicine produces CATmaker software which can be used to create CATs and which includes a facility to calculate figures such as the number needed to treat, etc.

Clinical effectiveness This term is used in two ways. First, as shorthand for the processes used to improve the quality of health care. Second, to refer to the extent to which a specific clinical intervention, when deployed in the field for a particular patient or population, delivers the intended outcomes such that the benefits outweigh the harms.

Clinical governance A framework through which health-care organisations are accountable for continuously improving the quality of health services and safeguarding high standards of care.

Cohort study An observational study where patients exposed to a drug or other agent are identified and followed forward in time to see whether they develop particular outcomes. People not exposed to the agent (i.e. a control group) may be included in the study.

Confidence interval (CI) Research studies use samples from the population. If the same study was carried out 100 times on different samples of the same population, 100 different results would be obtained. These results would spread around a true but unknown value. The confidence interval estimates this sampling variation. Thus we can think of the confidence interval as the range within which it is probable that the population value lies. It is possible to calculate this range from the data obtained in a single study. By convention, the 95% confidence interval is often used, i.e. the true population value will lie between the specified range in 95% of cases. For example, if a study reported a difference in mortality rates between two groups as 10% with an upper 95% CI limit of 13% and lower 95% confidence limit of 7%, we know that in 95% of cases the true mortality difference, for the population, is between 7% and 13%.

Confounder A factor that affects the observed relationship between the variables under investigation.

Constant comparative analysis Used in qualitative studies, the researcher constantly seeks out cases in the dataset during the collection of the data that support or 'shape' provisional hypotheses.

Control event rate (CER) This is the proportion of individuals in the control group in whom the outcome (event) is observed.

Control group The control group in a study is that group of individuals who do not receive the intervention or exposure, or who receive a placebo. Their outcomes are compared with those of the intervention group (the group receiving the intervention or exposure). They serve to 'control' for whether the patients in the intervention group would have improved or deteriorated regardless of the intervention or exposure.

Critical appraisal The process of systematically evaluating a piece of evidence to assess its validity (believability), importance and applicability.

Cross-sectional study Data are collected from a representative sample of individuals at the same point in time.

Experimental event rate (EER) This is the proportion of participants in the treatment (intervention) group in whom the outcome (event) is observed.

Incidence The number of new cases of a disease occurring in the population at risk, in a specified period of time.

Index term A controlled vocabulary term/keyword(s) used by indexers to ensure consistency in assigning terms to articles on the same topic. For example, a search using the index term 'kidney transplant' also retrieves papers where the author refers to the procedure as 'renal transplant'.

Intention-to-treat analysis This means that study participants are analysed in the groups to which they were randomised even if they did not receive the planned intervention or if they deviated from the study protocol. Intention-to-treat analysis mimics real-life situations because it investigates the outcomes following a management decision to use a particular treatment.

Inter-rater (or interobserver) reliability measures the extent to which an instrument or test gives consistent results when applied by different investigators under exactly the same circumstances and where the variable being measured remains unchanged.

Intraobserver reliability measures the extent to which an instrument or test gives consistent results when applied by the same investigator at two or more time points under exactly the same circumstances and where the variable being measured remains unchanged.

Kappa coefficient (κ) A statistical test used to indicate the extent of agreement between observers' measurements, adjusted for the amount of agreement that could be expected due to chance alone. The results are reported between 0 and 1. The nearer the result is to 1, the better the agreement between the observers' measurements.

Likelihood ratio *See* negative and positive likelihood ratios.

Median The midpoint on a scale. Half of the observations have a value less than or equal to the median and half have a value greater than or equal to the median.

Meta-analysis Used in systematic reviews, this is the process of statistically combining the results from a number of studies. Meta-analysis is not appropriate in all systematic reviews.

Naturalistic enquiry Relating to qualitative research, phenomena are studied within their natural setting rather than within a superficial or controlled one. The approach aims to minimise investigator manipulation of the study setting and places no prior constraint on what the outcomes will be.

Negative case analysis Used in qualitative research, the process of actively searching for cases that appear to be inconsistent with the emerging analysis.

Negative likelihood ratio The ratio of true-negative results to false-negative results. A negative likelihood ratio of 0.5 means that a negative test result is half as likely to occur in patients with the condition as in patients without the condition.

Negative predictive value The proportion of people with negative test results who do not have the target disorder (should be high).

Number needed to harm The number of patients to receive the intervention for one additional person to experience an episode of harm, over a specified period of time. To calculate: 1/ARR.

Number needed to treat The number of patients that need to be treated if a beneficial outcome is to occur in one additional person. To calculate: 1/ARR.

Odds The probability of an event happening, i.e. the ratio of the number of people having the outcome of interest to the number of people not having the outcome of interest.

Odds ratio The ratio of the odds of an event in the treatment (or exposure) group compared to the odds of the event in the control (or unexposed) group.

Placebo In the context of a placebo-controlled clinical trial, a biologically inert substance given to participants in the control arm of a trial. The placebo is similar in every other way to the biologically active intervention administered to participants in the treatment arm of the trial. It is used to conceal which arm of the trial the participants are in.

Positive likelihood ratio The ratio of true-positive results to false-positive results. A positive likelihood ratio of 8.5 means that a positive test result is 8.5 times as likely to occur in patients with the condition as in patients without the condition. (A positive likelihood ratio of 1 means that a positive test is equally as likely to occur in patients with the condition as in patients without the condition.)

Positive predictive value The proportion of people with positive test results who have the target disorder (should be high).

Prevalence This is the number of cases of the outcome of interest (e.g. a disease) in a defined population at a given point in time.

Quantitative research Seeks to describe phenomena through measuring and quantifying the relationship between the variables or characteristics being studied.

Qualitative research Seeks to describe phenomena through the meanings, experiences, practices and views of individuals within their natural settings. Qualitative research aims to understand real-world situations as they unfold, from the point of view of the people who live in these worlds.

Random allocation Individuals participating in the trial have a defined probability (usually 50%, i.e. an equal chance) of being allocated to either the intervention or the control group. Computer packages or printed random number tables are usually used to generate a list of random numbers (i.e. numbers with no discernable sequence or order) which indicate the group to which each individual is to be randomised. So, for example, even numbers might indicate allocation to the intervention group and odd numbers to the control group. The group to which each individual is to be allocated is not predictable.

Randomised controlled trial (RCT) A study in which individuals are assigned to the experimental intervention group or to the comparison group(s) by random allocation.

Reflexivity A technique used in qualitative research, especially in the analysis of data, where the author reflects on how she or he may have shaped or influenced the research findings.

Relative benefit increase (RBI) The proportional increase in rates of beneficial events between the experimental and control group. To calculate: [EER − CER]/CER.

Relative risk (RR) The ratio of the risk in one group compared to the other.

Relative risk increase (RRI) The proportional increase in rates of harmful or undesirable events between the experimental and control group. To calculate: [EER − CER]/CER.

Relative risk reduction (RRR) The proportional reduction in rates of harmful or undesirable events between the experimental and control group. To calculate: [EER − CER]/CER.

Reliability *See* inter-rater and intraobserver reliability.

Respondent (member) checking Used in qualitative research, the process of feeding back the researcher's interpretations of the data to informants to determine whether they recognise and agree with them.

Sample Research is carried out on a subgroup of the population. This subgroup is often referred to as the study sample. A variety of sampling methods can be employed to select the sample depending on the purpose of the research.

Sensitivity When applied to diagnostic tests, sensitivity refers to the proportion of people with a target disorder who have a positive test result.

Specificity When applied to diagnostic tests, specificity refers to the proportion of people who do not have a target disorder who have a negative test result.

Statistical significance The likelihood of a result occurring by chance. By convention, the level at which a result is said to be statistically significant is set at 5%, i.e. when there is less than a 5% probability that the result happened by chance, it is said to be statistically significant. This is usually written in the form of $p < 0.05$. The p-value does not, however, tell us how clinically important the result is.

Systematic review A summary of research evidence pertinent to a specified question in which systematic and explicit methods are used to identify, select, critically appraise and synthesise the available research evidence. Systematic reviews are research studies in their own right and are sometimes called 'secondary research'.

Thick description A term used in qualitative research. A very detailed account of the methodological and interpretive strategy in the form of fieldnotes.

Triangulation A strategy for strengthening the credibility of qualitative research. Multiple sources, methods, investigators or theories are used in combination to assess whether the findings are similar.

Truncation Used in searching electronic databases, truncation ensures that all terms that have the same text stem are found. For example, a truncation mark at the end of 'child' will retrieve articles containing the terms child, childhood, childless, children, etc. The truncation mark may be an asterisk (child*), a dollar sign (child$) or a % sign (child%) but varies according to the database provider.

Wildcard Used in searching electronic databases, a wildcard is a character (in some databases it is a ?) that can be used to replace one or more characters within a word so that articles will be retrieved regardless of the way in which the word is spelt. For example, if the term 'p?ediatric' is searched, articles using the American spelling (pediatric) and articles using the British spelling (paediatric) will be retrieved.

Index